Clinical Dilemmas in

# Non-Alcoholic Fatty Liver Disease

# Clinical Dilemmas in

# Non-Alcoholic Fatty Liver Disease

EDITED BY

**Roger Williams**, CBE
The Institute of Hepatology
Foundation for Liver Research
London, UK

**Simon D. Taylor-Robinson**
Digestive Diseases Division
Imperial College London
London, UK

WILEY Blackwell

This edition first published 2016 © 2016 by John Wiley & Sons, Ltd

*Registered Office*
John Wiley & Sons, Ltd, The Atrium, Southern Gate, Chichester, West Sussex, PO19 8SQ, UK

*Editorial Offices*
9600 Garsington Road, Oxford, OX4 2DQ, UK
The Atrium, Southern Gate, Chichester, West Sussex, PO19 8SQ, UK
111 River Street, Hoboken, NJ 07030-5774, USA

For details of our global editorial offices, for customer services and for information about
how to apply for permission to reuse the copyright material in this book please see our website
at www.wiley.com/wiley-blackwell

*Library of Congress Cataloging-in-Publication Data*

Names: Williams, Roger, 1931–, editor. | Taylor-Robinson, Simon D., author.
Title: Clinical dilemmas in non-alcoholic fatty liver disease /
   [edited by] Roger Williams, Simon Taylor-Robinson.
Description: Chichester, West Sussex ; Hoboken, NJ : John Wiley & Sons Inc., 2016. |
   Includes bibliographical references and index.
Identifiers: LCCN 2015040510 | ISBN 9781118912034 (pbk.)
Subjects: | MESH: Non-alcoholic Fatty Liver Disease.
Classification: LCC RC848.F3 | NLM WI 700 | DDC 616.3/62–dc23
LC record available at http://lccn.loc.gov/2015040510

A catalogue record for this book is available from the British Library.

Wiley also publishes its books in a variety of electronic formats. Some content that appears in
print may not be available in electronic books.

Set in 8.75/12pt Minion by SPi Global, Pondicherry, India

Printed in Singapore by C.O.S. Printers Pte Ltd

1   2016

# Contents

**Part V: What Does the Future Hold?**

# List of contributors

**Dr Quentin M. Anstee**
Institute of Cellular Medicine
Newcastle University
Newcastle upon Tyne, UK;
Liver Unit, Freeman Hospital
Newcastle upon Tyne, UK

**Professor Curtis K. Argo**
Division of Gastroenterology and Hepatology
University of Virginia
Charlottesville, VA, USA

**Professor Elizabeth M. Brunt**
Department of Pathology and Immunology
Washington University School of Medicine
St. Louis, MO, USA

**Professor Stephen H. Caldwell**
Division of Gastroenterology and Hepatology
University of Virginia
Charlottesville, VA, USA

**Dr Jeremy F. L. Cobbold**
Oxford University Hospitals NHS Trust
Oxford, UK

**Dr Paul Cordero**
Institute for Liver and Digestive Health
University College London
London, UK

**Professor Christopher P. Day**
Institute of Cellular Medicine, Newcastle University
Newcastle upon Tyne, UK;
Liver Unit, Freeman Hospital
Newcastle upon Tyne, UK

**Professor Anil Dhawan**
Paediatric Liver Centre, King's College London School of Medicine
King's College Hospital
London, UK

**Professor Anna Mae Diehl**
Division of Gastroenterology
Department of Medicine
Duke University, Durham, NC, USA

**Dr Joanna K. Dowman**
Department of Gastroenterology and Hepatology
Queen Alexandra Hospital, Portsmouth, UK

**Professor Jean-François Dufour**
University Clinic for Visceral Surgery and Medicine
Inselspital University of Berne
Bern, Switzerland

**Dr Jonathan Fallowfield**
MRC/University of Edinburgh Centre for Inflammation Research
Queen's Medical Research Institute
University of Edinburgh
Edinburgh, UK

**Professor Geoffrey C. Farrell**
The Canberra Hospital
Australian Capital Territory, Australia;
Department of Hepatic Medicine
Australian National University
Canberra, Australia

**Professor Nicholas Finer**
Centre for Weight Loss, Metabolic and Endocrine Surgery
University College London Hospitals,
London, UK

National Centre for Cardiovascular Prevention and Outcomes
UCL Institute of Cardiovascular Science
London, UK

**Dr Emer Fitzpatrick**
Paediatric Liver Centre, King's College London School of Medicine
King's College Hospital
London, UK

**Dr Shareen Forbes**
Endocrinology Unit, University/BHF Centre for Cardiovascular Science
Queen's Medical Research Institute
University of Edinburgh
Edinburgh, UK

**Dr Ian F. Godsland**
Division of Diabetes Endocrinology and Metabolism
Department of Medicine
Faculty of Medicine
Imperial College London
London, UK

**Dr Stephen A. Harrison**
Division of Gastroenterology
Department of Medicine
San Antonio Military Medical Center
Fort Sam Houston
San Antonio, TX, USA

**Dr Jonathan M. Hazlehurst**
Centre for Diabetes, Endocrinology and Metabolism
School of Clinical and Experimental Medicine
University of Birmingham
Birmingham, UK

**Professor Hero K. Hussain**
Department of Radiology and MRI
University of Michigan Health System
Ann Arbor, MI, USA

**Mr Andrew Jenkinson**
Clinical Lead Department of Metabolic
and Bariatric Surgery, University College
London Hospital, London, UK

**Professor Desmond
G. Johnston**
Department of Medicine, Faculty of Medicine
Imperial College London, London, UK

**Dr David E. Kleiner**
Laboratory of Pathology
National Cancer Institute
National Institutes of Health
Bethesda, MD, USA

**Professor Jay H. Lefkowitch**
Department of Pathology and Cell Biology
College of Physicians and Surgeons
Columbia University, New York, NY, USA

**Dr Nader Lessan**
Imperial College London Diabetes Centre
Abu Dhabi, United Arab Emirates,
Imperial College London, United Kingdom

**Ms Jiawei Li**
Institute for Liver and Digestive Health
University College London, London, UK

**Dr Soo Lim**
Department of Internal Medicine,
Seoul National University College of Medicine
Seoul National University Bundang Hospital
Seoul, Korea

**Dr Yang-Lin Liu**
Institute of Cellular Medicine
Newcastle University
Newcastle upon Tyne, UK

**Dr Haripriya Maddur**
Division of Gastroenterology and Hepatology
Saint Louis University, St. Louis, MO, USA

**Dr Cristina Margini**
Hepatology, Department of Clinical Research
University of Bern, Bern, Switzerland

**Dr Natasha McDonald**
MRC/University of Edinburgh Centre for
Inflammation Research
Queen's Medical Research Institute
University of Edinburgh, Edinburgh, UK

**Dr Sanjeev Mehta**
London North West Healthcare NHS Trust
and Department of Diabetes and
Endocrinology
Imperial College London, Ealing Hospital
London, UK

**Dr Fabian Meienberg**
Department of Diabetology
Endocrinology and Metabolism
University Hospital Basel
Basel, Switzerland

**Dr Brent
A. Neuschwander-Tetri**
Division of Gastroenterology and Hepatology
Saint Louis University
St. Louis, MO, USA

**Professor Philip Newsome**
Institute of Biomedical Research
The Medical School
University of Birmingham
Birmingham, UK

**Dr Jude A. Oben**
Institute for Liver and Digestive Health,
University College London
London, UK;
Department of Gastroenterology and
Hepatology, Guy's and St Thomas' Hospital
NHS Foundation Trust
London, UK

**Professor Massimo Pinzani**
Institute for Liver and Digestive Health
University College London
Royal Free Hospital
London, UK

**Professor Vlad Ratziu**
Service d'hépatogastroentérologie
Hôpital Pitié salpêtrière
Institute for Cardiometabolism and Nutrition
Université Pierre et Marie Curie
Paris, France

**Dr Arun J. Sanyal**
Virginia Commonwealth University
Richmond, VA, USA

**Dr Mohammad Bilal Siddiqui**
Department of Internal Medicine
University of Texas Medical School
Houston, Texas, USA

**Mohammad Shadab
Siddiqui**
Virginia Commonwealth University
Richmond, VA, USA

**Dr Wing-Kin Syn**
Foundation for Liver Research
Institute of Hepatology
London, UK

**Professor
Simon D. Taylor-Robinson**
Digestive Diseases Division
Imperial College London
London, UK

**Professor
Jeremy W. Tomlinson**
Oxford Centre for Diabetes,
Endocrinology and Metabolism
University of Oxford
Churchill Hospital
Headington, UK

**Dr Dawn M. Torres**
Division of Gastroenterology
Department of Medicine
Walter Reed National Military Medical
Center
Bethesda, MD, USA

**Dr Emmanuel A. Tsochatzis**
Institute for Liver and Digestive Health
University College London
Royal Free Hospital
London, UK

**Professor
Roger Williams, CBE**
The Institute of Hepatology
Foundation for Liver Research
London, UK

**Dr Michael Yee**
Metabolic Medicine Unit
St Mary's Hospital
London, UK

**Professor Yusuf Yilmaz**
Department of Gastroenterology
School of Medicine, Marmara University
Istanbul, Turkey

**Professor
Hannele Yki-Järvinen**
Department of Medicine
University of Helsinki
Helsinki, Finland

# Preface

In this further volume in the Clinical Dilemmas series, we have attempted to provide for nonalcoholic fatty liver disease the latest and most critical information regarding the nature of the condition and the factors that lead to disease progression. How best to assess severity and value of currently available different treatment measures, including the role of bariatric surgery and its quite remarkable effects on diabetes, have separate sections. The final chapter is a look ahead—what does the future hold—and includes coverage of the new molecular targeted agents that are currently in preclinical and phase I clinical trial development.

With obesity constituting a worldwide epidemic with prevalent figures for NAFLD in some Western countries as high as 30–40% of the population, there are yet few signs of it being controlled by public health measures. Understanding the cross talk that underlies the involvement of a number of other organs and systems leading to cardiac and respiratory events and cancers of various organs is of critical importance. We hope that this volume will encourage the necessary investment in preventative, diagnostic, and treatment facilities needed if the effect of this lifestyle related and preventable condition on the health of many nations is to be reduced.

As editors we are grateful to the contributors worldwide who have made it possible with their expertise and commitment to produce what we believe is an outstanding volume. A personal thanks to Jasmine Chang, Project Editor; Jon Peacock, Senior Project Editor; Oliver Walter, Publisher at Wiley-Blackwell; and also to Enda O'Sullivan, Editorial Assistant in the Institute of Hepatology, London.

**Professor Roger Williams, CBE**
**Professor Simon D. Taylor-Robinson**

# PART I
# Nature of the Condition

# 1 Non-alcoholic fatty liver disease: Hype or harm?

**Stephen H. Caldwell and Curtis K. Argo**

Division of Gastroenterology and Hepatology, University of Virginia, Charlottesville, VA, USA

Few potentially fatal diseases have ever been referred to as "trash" in a serious and critical treatise on the topic [1] or have been specifically the subject of an unsuccessful legal action aimed at shutting down a particular form of animal-derived food production (Caldwell S, personal experience) or have at one time been, rather accurately, referred to as "big" and "little" varieties to indicate early recognized variability in severity from mild and essentially inconsequential to potentially fatal (McCullough AJ, personal communication). However, all of these attributes are true of non-alcoholic fatty liver disease (NAFLD) and its potentially more severe subset non-alcoholic steatohepatitis (NASH).

In many ways, NASH remains a very challenging disorder over 30 years after pathologist Jurgen Ludwig first coined the term "NASH" for a "hitherto unnamed" form of steatohepatitis [2], and in doing so, he and his colleagues ushered in the modern era of clinical and basic research into the various forms of nonalcohol-related fatty liver—a field that has grown from a few published papers per year to many publications per week or month. On a practical level, much of the persistent challenge hinges on questions about the natural history and prognosis of fatty liver when it is encountered in a given individual—currently an almost daily occurrence in many clinics whether on its own or in combination with other liver disorders. The patient usually presents with asymptomatic, mild to moderate range of abnormal liver enzymes, negative additional diagnostic testing, and fatty changes noted on diagnostic ultrasound. This raises a frequent clinical question: is fatty liver a benign physiological finding (possibly an ancient adaptation to feast or famine, where nowadays feast exceeds famine), is it a disease warranting liver biopsy (with inherent risk) and directed intervention, or is it an epiphenomenon of a metabolic disorder encompassing diabetes mellitus, vascular disease, and cancer risks with clinical consequences that supersede the significance of the fatty liver [3]? All of these posits have some truth in NAFLD/NASH

*Clinical Dilemmas in Non-Alcoholic Fatty Liver Disease*, First Edition. Edited by Roger Williams and Simon D. Taylor-Robinson.
© 2016 John Wiley & Sons, Ltd. Published 2016 by John Wiley & Sons, Ltd.

and constitute the pressing clinical challenge to discern hype and harm.

"Big" NASH and "little" NASH are now somewhat forgotten terms used casually in the discussion of early natural history studies, which indicated a dichotomy in the clinical course: long-term stability of the liver in many patients and progression to cirrhosis and liver-related mortality in a smaller but substantial fraction [4]. Since those early days, the nomenclature has obviously evolved with recognition of potentially progressive "big" NASH, characterized by cellular injury and fibrosis, as a subset of the more global term, NAFLD, which indicates liver fat exceeding 5–10% triglyceride by weight. Subsequently, long-term natural history studies of NAFLD have consistently demonstrated this dichotomous natural history: non-NASH fatty liver tends to be stable over years with low liver-related mortality, while NASH carries a significant, tangible risk of progression to cirrhosis and associated liver-related mortality [5–8]. Most of these studies have focused on mortality rather than morbidity, and overall mortality is clearly dominated by cardiovascular disease and nonliver malignancy. These findings suggest that the emphasis on the liver disease itself may be somewhat misplaced. However, this overlooks the fact that a substantial number of patients, especially those with histological NASH will progress to cirrhosis and suffer many of the typical cirrhosis-related complications. Moreover, the development of cirrhosis and coexisting vascular disease or neoplasm significantly complicates the management of either condition. Thus, directing specific therapy at the liver is appropriate in some patients, but careful patient selection is essential, and unless a therapy is very safe and inexpensive (such as diet and exercise), many NAFLD patients warrant only conservative management. Riskier interventions should be directed at those with histological NASH especially with more advanced fibrosis stages.

Is steatosis ever physiologically adaptive? To some extent it can be viewed as such under certain circumstances [9]. This is most evident in certain species of migratory *Palmipedes* spp. (geese and ducks) where the development of steatosis is a normal premigratory process and presumably provides a source of energy during the long flight with little calorie intake. This process was recognized long ago, and for thousands of years, "foie gras" production has hinged on it. However, our own work in cooperation with several individuals in France demonstrated that the *Palmipedes* develop only non-NASH fatty liver. Hence, the

effort by People for the Ethical Treatment of Animals (PETA) to block foie gras production in the United States—on the grounds that the meat represented a disease state—failed due to the absence of NASH. No doubt, the grounds for the attempted legal action were the result of some of the media publicity that has surrounded NAFLD.

On the other hand, humans with histological NASH are at risk for progression of fibrosis through stages to cirrhosis. Serial biopsy studies suggest that this is a slow, steady march when it occurs [10]. However, it remains unclear whether or not the progression is uniform over time, and it is conceivable that NASH progression may occur in subclinical "fits and starts" with peaks and troughs of disease activity rather than by a slow, steady process. It has also been shown that some patients with non-NASH fatty liver may transition to histological NASH [11]. Presumably, changes in activity, diet, or weight with resultant worsening insulin resistance may trigger such a transition. Once cirrhosis develops in patients with NASH, complications of portal hypertension develop at a steady rate but somewhat slower than that seen with cirrhosis due to hepatitis C [12]. Patients are also at significantly increased risk of hepatocellular cancer usually, but perhaps not always, in the setting of coexisting cirrhosis [13].

Adding to the clinical diagnostic challenge, when cirrhosis develops in NASH, steatosis, a hallmark of NASH, tends to diminish significantly, sometimes leaving a picture of "cryptogenic cirrhosis," especially in patients without a confirmed antecedent diagnosis of NASH [14–16]. Such patients often present with minor findings, such as asymptomatic and previously unexplained thrombocytopenia, often labeled in prior encounters as idiopathic thrombocytopenia purpura ("ITP") or with cirrhosis, incidentally discovered at the time of elective surgery, especially for suspected or confirmed gallbladder disease. The mechanisms underlying diminished liver fat remain uncertain but may involve altered insulin exposure through changes in blood flow or repopulation of the liver from stem cells with altered physiology and fat metabolic capacity. Clearly, there are also other causes of cryptogenic cirrhosis, including silent autoimmune hepatitis, occult ethanol abuse, or as yet unrecognized viral infection, but NASH appears to be the leading etiology in many areas of the world [17].

Although it is well established that NAFLD has a largely dichotomous natural history, based on initial histology (NASH vs. non-NASH fatty liver), it is perplexing that certain aspects of NASH histology remain challenging.

While there are a number of characteristic histological findings, the key features that usually are used to define NASH are steatosis, inflammation, cellular ballooning, and fibrosis; the first three of these parameters define the commonly utilized NAFLD activity score (NAS) [18, 19]. Perhaps not surprisingly, histological fibrosis appears to be a reliable finding with low interobserver variation rates and a reliable indicator of prognosis. However, agreement between scoring systems and individual parameters remains a potentially significant problem that can muddy clinical trials and natural history studies [20–22]. Defining criteria for cellular ballooning has been especially problematic although emergence of keratin staining as a means of characterizing pathological processes within these cells may lead to beneficial refinements of histological criteria [23–26].

ASH, NASH, BASH (indicating both alcohol exposure and risks for metabolic fatty liver), chemical-associated steatohepatitis (CASH), and drug-associated steatohepatitis (DASH): the nomenclature for the recognized varieties of steatohepatitis has continued to evolve over the years [27]. While by no means uniformly accepted, the term "BASH" ("B" for both alcohol and metabolic fatty liver) denotes possibly the most significant of these, as it indicates the presence of metabolic risks for NASH such as obesity, diabetes, and inactivity together with ethanol use above safe levels but below levels at which the risk of ASH rises steeply [28]. This represents a potentially important gray area, and it highlights the fact that the diagnosis of "NASH" is truly both a clinical- and pathology-based exercises that is not always clear cut [29, 30].

What about the individual patient who is seen in the clinic and presents with the "chief complaint" of abnormal liver enzymes, negative additional testing, and fatty changes on diagnostic ultrasound? Is it a benign finding, a marker for comorbid vascular disease and cancer risk, or a disease warranting liver biopsy and more aggressive therapeutic management recommendations than diet and exercise? Recent advances in genetic risks promise to further help sort hype from harm in NAFLD. PNPLA3 and TM6SF2 polymorphisms code for gene products that appear to be intimately involved with small fat droplet and lipoprotein metabolism and impart significant risk for steatosis and related organ injury [31–34]. Although far from being available as clinical tools, this work points out the continued clinical importance of the family history in NASH/NAFLD [35]. Indeed, we recommend earlier consideration

of biopsy when, as often is the case, a family member is significantly affected even if the relative was reported to have had alcohol-related liver disease. Moreover, preliminary work from our group suggests that PNPLA3 polymorphism may predict response to such mild agents as omega-3 fatty acid supplements.

Clearly, NASH progresses to advanced stages of fibrosis, cirrhosis, and hepatocellular cancer reasonably often, and it may shed some its histological hallmarks in the process, which can complicate the diagnosis. Recognition of this phenomenon has allowed clinicians to avoid Dr. Ludwig's "embarrassment" in diligently attempting to ferret out the occult alcoholic when actually confronted with frank NASH. Without doubt, the emergence of this field coexists with a degree of hype, which has likely been magnified due to the parallel obesity epidemic. It is all the more important to sort out, within the limitations of existing literature, the hype from the harm in order to best tailor emerging pharmacological treatment strategies and match risks and benefits.

## References

1. Cassiman D, Jaeken J. NASH may be trash. Gut 2008;57:141–4.
2. Ludwig J, Viggiano TR, McGill DB, Ott BJ. Nonalcoholic steatohepatitis: Mayo Clinic experiences with a hitherto unnamed disease. Mayo Clin Proc 1980;55:434–8.
3. Anstee QM, Targher G, Day CP. Progression of NAFLD to diabetes mellitus, cardiovascular disease or cirrhosis. Nat Rev Gastroenterol Hepatol 2013;10:330–44.
4. Matteoni CA, Younossi ZM, Gramlich T, Boparai N, Liu YC, McCullough AJ. Nonalcoholic fatty liver disease: a spectrum of clinical and pathological severity. Gastroenterology 1999;116:1413–9.
5. Adams LA, Lymp JF, St Sauver J, Sanderson SO, Lindor KD, Feldstein A, Angulo P. The natural history of nonalcoholic fatty liver disease: a population-based cohort study. Gastroenterology 2005;129:113–21.
6. Ekstedt M, Franzen LE, Mathiesen UL, Thorelius L, Holmqvist M, Bodemar G, Kechagias S. Long-term follow-up of patients with NAFLD and elevated liver enzymes. Hepatology 2006;44:865–73.
7. Ong JP, Pitts A, Younossi ZM. Increased overall mortality and liver-related mortality in non-alcoholic fatty liver disease. J Hepatol 2008;49:608–12.
8. Rafiq N, Bai C, Fang Y, Srishord M, McCullough A, Gramlich T, Younossi ZM. Long-term follow-up of patients with nonalcoholic fatty liver. Clin Gastroenterol Hepatol 2009;7:234–8.

9. Caldwell SH, Ikura Y, Iezzoni JC, Liu Z. Has natural selection in human populations produced two types of metabolic syndrome (with and without fatty liver)? J Gastroenterol Hepatol 2007;22 Suppl 1:S11–9.

10. Argo CK, Northup PG, Al-Osaimi AM, Caldwell SH. Systematic review of risk factors for fibrosis progression in non-alcoholic steatohepatitis. J Hepatol 2009;51:371–9.

11. Pais R, Charlotte F, Fedchuk L, Bedossa P, Lebray P, Poynard T, Ratziu V; LIDO Study Group. A systematic review of follow-up biopsies reveals disease progression in patients with non-alcoholic fatty liver. J Hepatol 2013;59:550–6.

12. Sanyal AJ, Banas C, Sargeant C, Luketic VA, Sterling RK, Stravitz RT, Shiffman ML, Heuman D, Coterrell A, Fisher RA, Contos MJ, Mills AS. Similarities and differences in outcomes of cirrhosis due to nonalcoholic steatohepatitis and hepatitis C. Hepatology 2006;43:682–9.

13. Baffy G, Brunt EM, Caldwell SH. Hepatocellular carcinoma in non-alcoholic fatty liver disease: an emerging menace. J Hepatol 2012;56:1384–91.

14. Powell EE, Cooksley WG, Hanson R, Searll J, Halliday JW, Powell LW. The natural history of nonalcoholic steatohepatitis: a follow-up study of forty-two patients for up to 21 years. Hepatology 1990;11:74–80.

15. Caldwell SH, Oelsner DH, Iezzoni JC, Hespenheide EE, Battle EH, Driscoll CJ. Cryptogenic cirrhosis: Clinical characterization and risk factors for underlying disease. Hepatology 1999;29:664–9.

16. Caldwell SH, Lee VD, Kleiner DE, Al-Osaimi AM, Argo CK, Northup PG, Berg CL. NASH and cryptogenic cirrhosis: a histological analysis. Ann Hepatol 2009;8:346–52.

17. Ayata G, Gordon FD, Lewis WD, Pomfret E, Pomposelli JJ, Jenkins RL, Khettry U. Cryptogenic cirrhosis: clinicopathologic findings at and after liver transplantation. Hum Pathol 2002;33:1098–104.

18. Kleiner DE, Brunt EM, Van Natta ML, Behling C, Contos MJ, Cummings OW, Ferrell LD, Liu YC, Torbenson MS, Unalp-Arida A, Yeh M, McCullough AJ, Sanyal AJ. Nonalcoholic Steatohepatitis Clinical Research Network. Design and validation of a histologic scoring system for NAFLD. Hepatology 2005;41:1313–21.

19. Brunt EM, Kleiner DE, Wilson LA, Belt P, Neuschwander-Tetri BA. NASH Clinical Research Network (CRN). Nonalcoholic fatty liver disease (NAFLD) activity score and the histopathologic diagnosis in NAFLD: distinct clinicopathologic meanings. Hepatology 2011;53:810–20.

20. Younossi ZM, Stepanova M, Rafiq N,Makhlouf H, Younoszai Z, Agrawal R, Goodman Z. Pathologic criteria for nonalcoholic steatohepatitis: interprotocol agreement and ability to predict liver-related mortality. Hepatology 2011;53:1874–82.

21. Juluri R, Vuppalanchi R, Olson J, Unalp A, Van Natta ML, Cummings OW, Tonascia J, Chalasani N. Generalizability of the NASH-CRN histologic scoring system for nonalcoholic fatty liver disease. J Clin Gastroenterol 2011;45:55–8.

22. Gawrieh S, Knoedler DM, Saeian K, Wallace JR, Komorowski RA. Effects of interventions on intra- and interobserver agreement on interpretation of nonalcoholic fatty liver disease histology. Ann. Diagn. Pathol. 2011;15:19–24.

23. Lackner C, Gogg-Kamerer M, Zatloukal K, Stumptner C, Brunt EM, Denk H. Ballooned hepatocytes in steatohepatitis: the value of keratin immunohistochemistry for diagnosis. J Hepatol 2008;48:821–8.

24. Guy CD1, Suzuki A, Burchette JL, Brunt EM, Abdelmalek MF, Cardona D, McCall SJ, Ünalp A, Belt P, Ferrell LD, Diehl AM. Nonalcoholic Steatohepatitis Clinical Research Network. Costaining for keratins 8/18 plus ubiquitin improves detection of hepatocyte injury in nonalcoholic fatty liver disease. Hum Pathol 2012;43:790–800.

25. Caldwell S, Ikura Y, Dias D, Isomoto K, Yabu A, Moskaluk C, Pramoonjago P, Simmons W, Scruggs H, Rosenbaum N, Wilkinson T, Toms P, Argo CK, Al-Osaimi AM, Redick JA. Hepatocellular ballooning in NASH. J Hepatol 2010; 53:719–23.

26. Kakisaka K1, Cazanave SC, Werneburg NW, Razumilava N, Mertens JC, Bronk SF, Gores GJ. A hedgehog survival pathway in 'undead' lipotoxic hepatocytes. J Hepatol 2012;57: 844–51.

27. Brunt EM. What's in a NAme? Hepatology 2009;50:663–7.

28. Becker U, Deis A, Sørensen TI, Grønbaek M, Borch-Johnsen K, Müller CF, Schnohr P, Jensen G. Prediction of risk of liver disease by alcohol intake, sex, and age: a prospective population study. Hepatology 1996;23:1025–9.

29. Tiniakos DG. Liver biopsy in alcoholic and non-alcoholic steatohepatitis patients. Gastroenterol Clin Biol 2009;33:930–9.

30. Tannapfel A1, Denk H, Dienes HP, Langner C, Schirmacher P, Trauner M, Flott-Rahmel B. Histopathological diagnosis of non-alcoholic and alcoholic fatty liver disease. Virchows Arch 2011;458:511–23.

31. Valenti L, Al-Serri A, Daly AK, Galmozzi E, Rametta R, Dongiovanni P, Nobili V, Mozzi E, Roviaro G, Vanni E, Bugianesi E, Maggioni M, Fracanzani AL, Fargion S, Day CP. Homozygosity for the patatin-like phospholipase-3/adiponutrin I148M polymorphism influences liver fibrosis in patients with nonalcoholic fatty liver disease. Hepatology 2010;51:1209–17.

32. Kozlitina J, Smagris E, Stender S, Nordestgaard BG, Zhou HH, Tybjærg-Hansen A, Vogt TF, Hobbs HH, Cohen JC. Exome-wide association study identifies a TM6SF2 variant that confers susceptibility to nonalcoholic fatty liver disease. Nat Genet 2014;46:352–6.

33. Mahdessian H, Taxiarchis A, Popov S, Silveira A, Franco-Cereceda A, Hamsten A, Eriksson P, van't Hooft F. TM6SF2 is a regulator of liver fat metabolism influencing triglyceride secretion and hepatic lipid droplet content. Proc Natl Acad Sci U S A 2014;111:8913–8.

34. Liu YL, Reeves HL, Burt AD, Tiniakos D, McPherson S, Leathart JB, Allison ME, Alexander GJ, Piguet AC, Anty R, Donaldson P, Aithal GP, Francque S, Van Gaal L, Clement K, Ratziu V, Dufour JF, Day CP, Daly AK, Anstee QM. TM6SF2 rs58542926 influences hepatic fibrosis progression in patients with non-alcoholic fatty liver disease. Nat Commun 2014;5:4309.

35. Struben VMD, Hespenheide EE, Caldwell SH. Nonalcoholic steatohepatitis and cryptogenic cirrhosis within kindreds. Am J Med 2000;108:9–13.

## 2 NAFLD: A worldwide problem

**Joanna K. Dowman[1], Geoffrey C. Farrell[2,3], and Philip Newsome[4]**

[1] Department of Gastroenterology and Hepatology, Queen Alexandra Hospital, Portsmouth, UK
[2] The Canberra Hospital, Australian Capital Territory, Australia
[3] Department of Hepatic Medicine, Australian National University, Canberra, Australia
[4] Institute of Biomedical Research, The Medical School, University of Birmingham, Birmingham, UK

### LEARNING POINTS

- The prevalence of worldwide obesity has nearly doubled since 1980, now exceeding 50% in some regions. Obesity prevalence has also increased in children, with ~23% of children in developed countries and 13% of children in developing countries now either overweight or obese.

- The close association between obesity and non-alcoholic fatty liver disease (NAFLD) has resulted in this now representing the most common cause of liver disease in Western countries, where it affects 20–30% of the adult population.

- Prevalence of NAFLD in countries such as Asia, Latin America and the Caribbean has risen as a result of increasingly urban and westernised lifestyles.

- The lowest estimates of NAFLD prevalence in Asia are from rural areas inhabited by more physically active, less affluent and lean populations.

- Estimates from biopsy series indicate an overall prevalence of the more advanced form of NASH of 3–5% in the United States, rising to 12% in some populations.

- In Europe and the United States, NAFLD is usually associated with obesity and insulin resistance. However in Asian countries the disease can manifest at a lower BMI; therefore application of ethnic-specific BMI thresholds is important to ensure accurate identification of higher-risk individuals.

- The incidence of NASH-related HCC is rapidly increasing, with NASH now the second leading aetiology of HCC-related liver transplantation in the United States and an increasingly frequent cause of HCC in Asia.

- Significant ethnic variations in propensity to NAFLD exist, which are largely accounted for by genetic factors. The extensively validated genetic modifier of NAFLD is the PNPLA3 polymorphism, which increases propensity to NAFLD, severity of disease and risk of HCC.

- NAFLD frequently acts as a cofactor with viral hepatitis, alcohol and other liver diseases to increase severity of liver injury.

## Introduction

NAFLD is a complication of over-nutrition, being closely associated with obesity, diabetes and insulin resistance (IR), dyslipidaemia and hypertension. It is therefore recognised to represent the hepatic manifestation of the metabolic syndrome. The increasing global levels of obesity, IR and metabolic syndrome, driven by the trend of post-industrialised countries towards urban and inactive lifestyles, with easy access to cheap processed foods, have led to an estimated 20-fold increase in the prevalence of NAFLD since 1983 [1]. NAFLD now represents the most common cause of abnormal liver tests and chronic liver disease in the Western world [2–4] and is projected to become the leading cause of cirrhosis and most common indication for liver transplantation in the United States by 2030 [5]. More recent data demonstrate that the trend towards more urban and Westernised lifestyles occurring in many countries, which until the last few decades have been less well-developed, has resulted in NAFLD

*Clinical Dilemmas in Non-Alcoholic Fatty Liver Disease*, First Edition. Edited by Roger Williams and Simon D. Taylor-Robinson.
© 2016 John Wiley & Sons, Ltd. Published 2016 by John Wiley & Sons, Ltd.

now playing an equally important role in Asia, Latin America and the Caribbean, establishing it as a truly global disease.

Although NAFLD is highly prevalent worldwide, the epidemiology and demographic characteristics vary in different populations. In Europe and the United States, NAFLD is associated with obesity and IR in the great majority of cases; however in Asian countries the disease can manifest at a lower BMI, albeit most often after a period of weight gain and with central adiposity. NAFLD also frequently acts as a cofactor with other liver diseases, and its impact is therefore influenced by the prevalence of other injurious factors such as viral hepatitis and alcohol consumption in different populations.

## Prevalence of NAFLD worldwide

A variety of methodologies have been used to study the prevalence of NAFLD in different populations (Table 2.1). Although histology provides the most definitive data, liver biopsy is invasive and not amenable to population studies. The most commonly used diagnostic modalities for such studies have been ultrasonography and/or elevations in liver transaminase levels, although data has also been obtained from autopsy studies and MRI imaging.

### Europe

Two large ultrasound-based studies in Italian and Spanish populations indicate a prevalence of NAFLD of between 20 and 30% in Europe. The Dionysos nutrition and liver study demonstrated the prevalence of NAFLD in a general Italian population to be 25 and 20% in subjects with and without suspected liver disease, respectively [6]. A Spanish multicentre population study demonstrated a prevalence of NAFLD of 33% in men and 20% in women [7].

**TABLE 2.1** Estimated prevalence of NAFLD in different geographical regions

| Region | Estimated prevalence (%) |
| --- | --- |
| United States | 20–46 |
| Europe | 20–30 |
| South/South East Asia | 5–32 |
| East Asia | 11–45 |
| Australasia | 20–30 |

### United States

A large multi-ethnic, population-based study of 2287 individuals using proton magnetic resonance spectroscopy (MRS) to measure intrahepatic triglyceride content demonstrated NAFLD to be present in approximately one third of American adults [8]. A higher ultrasonographic NAFLD prevalence of 46% was demonstrated in a study of over 300 middle-aged patients performed at the Brooke Army Medical Center. In this study, 30% of those with NAFLD were confirmed by liver biopsy to have NASH [9]. Importantly, these figures mask significant ethnic variations in disease prevalence, with significantly higher rates in Hispanics > white populations > African Americans [8, 9]. The lower frequency of hepatic steatosis in blacks is not explained by ethnic differences in BMI or IR [8] and is fully accounted for by genetic factors (see later). Such studies, and the >30% obesity prevalence in the adult population, suggest an estimated NAFLD prevalence in the United States of at least 30%.

Although there are limited data from Latin America, the prevalence of NAFLD in this area has been reported to range between 17 and 35% [10]. A 2007 study reported an ultrasonographic NAFLD prevalence of 35% in community-dwelling middle-aged and older adults in Brazil, a high proportion of whom had metabolic syndrome [11]. The population prevalence of NAFLD in Mexico is estimated at 20–30%, based on an approximate 30% prevalence of obesity [12], with steatosis demonstrated in 83% of a cohort of 198 Mexican subjects with metabolic syndrome [13].

### Asia

NAFLD was originally regarded as a disease of highly industrialised Western nations, occurring as a consequence of increasingly sedentary behaviour with abundant availability of energy-dense foods. However, the major lifestyle and dietary changes observed in many Asian countries in recent decades, resulting from increased urbanisation and industrialisation, have led to a marked increase in the prevalence of NAFLD, with recent studies reporting levels similar to those in Europe and the United States [1, 14]. Further, genetic predisposition to type 2 diabetes is higher in many Asian populations, and such predisposition is very relevant to both the prevalence and severity of NAFLD [15–17]. Prevalence of NAFLD in Japan increased from 13% in 1989 to 30% by 1998 and ~32% in men and 17% in women by 2008 [18]. This rise was associated with a significant increase in fat intake and number of registered motor vehicles, increasing urbanisation and GDP, increased import of soft drinks and processed foods from outside Asia, and increasing availability and consumption of fast food [1, 18]. A similarly high NAFLD prevalence of 11–45% has been reported in Korea, China and Taiwan [1, 19–21].

The prevalence of NAFLD in South and South East Asian countries has been reported to range from 5 to 32% [1, 22–25]. A population-based study in a rural south Indian community demonstrated a NAFLD prevalence of 32%, based on ultrasound and measurement of metabolic risk factors [24].

The lowest estimates of NAFLD prevalence in Asia are from rural areas inhabited by more physically active, less affluent and lean populations. A large study of >11 000 residents of Indian railway colonies demonstrated an overall prevalence of ultrasonographic NAFLD of 17%, and 19% in individuals over 20 years [26], with a prevalence of only 8.7% in a large study in a rural community in West Bengal [22].

## Australasia and Pacific Islands

The prevalence of NAFLD in Australia and New Zealand is reported to be similar to Northern Europe at between 20 and 30% [27]. Although there are few data from the Pacific Islands, the strikingly high prevalence of obesity and diabetes, which exceeds 50% in several populations including Tonga, Nauru, Federated States of Micronesia, Tonga and Samoa [28], predicts a high burden of NAFLD in these areas.

## Africa

A paucity of data exists on the prevalence of NAFLD in Africa, and further research is required in this area. One study reported a NAFLD prevalence of ~9% in Nigeria [29], but it is likely that similar differences between rural and urban areas to those observed in Asia will exist here. Given the high prevalence of fatty liver and diabetes associated with hepatitis C in Egypt (see later), it may be that NAFLD is also common in Egypt, but this requires further study.

## Disease severity

NAFLD encompasses a pathological spectrum of disease ranging from simple steatosis through steatohepatitis (NASH), characterised by lobular inflammation and hepatocyte ballooning, with increasing fibrosis to eventual cirrhosis with risk of hepatocellular carcinoma (HCC). Studies with up to 20 years follow-up have demonstrated that simple steatosis is usually associated with a relatively benign prognosis, whereas the diagnosis of NASH, particularly with the presence of fibrosis, is associated with increased liver- and cardiovascular-related morbidity and mortality [30, 31].

Despite many advances in the non-invasive assessment of NAFLD, liver biopsy is still required to make a definitive diagnosis of NASH. This precludes large population assessments of NASH prevalence, but recent smaller studies have shown a high prevalence of NASH among NAFLD cases ranging from 10 to 25%. Estimates from biopsy series indicate an overall prevalence of NASH of 3–5% in the United States, although in some populations this may be as high as 12% [9]. In European and US studies, histological NASH was present in up to 30% of patients with ultrasound-detected steatosis [9], in 20–33% of patients with elevated aminotransferases [32, 33], in 32–37% in morbidly obese patients [34, 35] and in 3–16% in apparently healthy, living liver donors [36, 37]. Data on the prevalence of NASH in Asian and African patients with NAFLD are lacking and represent an area requiring further study.

NAFLD-related cirrhosis is now the third most common indication for liver transplantation in the United States and is projected to overtake alcoholic liver disease and HCV as the leading indication in future decades. As cirrhosis usually takes several decades to develop, the prevalence of advanced disease is currently less common in Asian countries where the rise in NAFLD prevalence has been more recent. However, this is expected to increase in future decades as the current cohort ages, and as a result of the increasing prevalence of NAFLD in children and young people [1]. The incidence of HCC secondary to NASH is also increasing, with NASH now the second leading aetiology of HCC-related liver transplantation in the United States [5]. A notable increase in NAFLD-associated HCC has also been observed in Asia. A study of 329 patients in South Korea reported an increase in the proportion of cases of HCC associated with NAFLD from 3.8% in 2001–2005 to 12.2% in 2006–2010, at the same time as a decrease in HBV-attributable HCC [38], and NAFLD now accounts for 2% of HCC in Japan [1, 18, 39]. Although the estimated 2–3%/year risk of incident HCC in NASH is lower than in cirrhosis associated with HBV or HCV, the much greater number of patients with NASH renders the absolute burden of NASH-related HCC higher. While HCC most commonly occurs in the presence of cirrhosis, it is also increasingly observed in non-cirrhotic NASH [40, 41]. If confirmed by prospective studies with careful histological assessment, this finding has considerable implications for both screening and future disease burdens.

## Obesity and metabolic syndrome

### Obesity

Obesity is closely associated with NAFLD, and increased BMI is a risk factor for liver disease progression. The prevalence of worldwide obesity has nearly doubled since 1980, with more than 1.4 billion adults overweight and over 200 million men and nearly 300 million women obese worldwide by 2008 [42]. A recent systematic analysis of the worldwide changes in the prevalence of overweight and obesity reported that the global proportion of adults with a body mass index (BMI) of $25\,kg/m^2$ or greater increased from 28.8 to 36.9% in men and from 29.8 to 38.0% in women between 1980 and 2013 [28]. Estimated prevalence of obesity exceeded 50% in some regions, including several Pacific Islands, Kuwait, Libya and Qatar. Prevalence has also increased markedly in children and adolescents, with approximately 23% of children in developed countries and 13% of children in developing countries overweight or obese in 2013. Concerningly, despite the major global health challenge posed by obesity, no national success stories in addressing the issue have been reported in the past 33 years [28]. Unless unprecedented progress is made in reversing this trend, it is therefore expected that the prevalence of NAFLD and its complications will continue to proliferate worldwide.

### Metabolic syndrome

South and East Asians appear to be at increased risk of NAFLD, IR, type 2 diabetes and metabolic syndrome, and tend to develop these features at a lower BMI than in other ethnic groups. For a given BMI, both the percentage of fat and its distribution between the subcutaneous and visceral depots differ between European and South and East Asian people [1]. This ethnic difference in susceptibility to IR and metabolic syndrome accounts for the oft-cited observation that NAFLD is more common in 'lean' South and East Asians than individuals from other ethnic groups, and the term 'metabolically obese' has been given to such lean, but insulin resistant, individuals. The finding that IR, diabetes and NAFLD occur at a lower BMI in South and East Asians

has led to revision of the BMI thresholds for obesity in Asian people [43], and in fact only ~15% of Asians with NAFLD would be classified as lean using ethnic-specific anthropometric indices [1, 22, 44, 45]. Greater awareness and application of ethnic-specific BMI thresholds are essential to ensure accurate identification of higher-risk individuals.

## Genetic predisposition

Genetic studies, including several large genome-wide association studies (GWAS), have identified an increasing number of genetic single nucleotide polymorphisms (SNPs), which may be associated with increased risk of NAFLD and/or disease severity in different populations. To date, the most extensively investigated and validated genetic modifier of NAFLD is polymorphism in the adiponutrin or *PNPLA3* gene. In multiple studies, PNPLA3 variants have been shown to increase both prevalence and severity of NASH and, more recently, risk of HCC (in both NASH and alcoholic liver diseases) [46]. In one large GWAS study, this polymorphism was shown to fully account for the ethnic differences in prevalence of NAFLD between Hispanics, white populations and African Americans living in the United States [47].

Several other genetic polymorphisms have been identified, which may also contribute to ethnic differences in susceptibility to NAFLD. A GWAS study in a US population reported a strong association between NAFLD and the farnesyl-diphosphate farnesyltransferase 1 (FDFT1) genotype in non-Hispanic women [48]. Other SNPs associated with NAFLD include Kruppel-like factor 6 (KLF6) [49], PPARα [50], PPARγ [51] and APOC3 (the findings here are not consistent) [52], all of which play important roles in the regulation of insulin sensitivity and/or lipid metabolism. Ongoing research will undoubtedly identify more genetic modifiers and add to our understanding of individual and population differences in susceptibility to NAFLD, possibly facilitating identification of individuals at higher risk and potentially informing the development of novel therapies.

## NAFLD as a cofactor

NAFLD and the metabolic syndrome can also act as a cofactor with other liver diseases to enhance disease progression. This is of particular importance in many Asian countries with a high prevalence of viral hepatitis. Areas of highest hepatitis B prevalence include South East Asia, China, sub-Saharan Africa and the Amazon basin, where at least 8% of individuals are HBV carriers [53]. Although steatosis is less common in Asian patients with HBV than the general population, when present it is usually associated with the same metabolic factors as NAFLD [54–56], and the risk of cirrhosis is significantly higher in individuals with both hepatitis B and metabolic syndrome than in lean subjects with hepatitis B [57]. Further, HBV-infected patients with metabolic syndrome are more likely to have cirrhosis than those without [58], indicating interactions between fatty liver and hepatitis B can worsen disease progression.

Prevalence of hepatitis C is highest (>3.5%) in Central and East Asia and North Africa/Middle East, with moderate prevalence (1.5–3.5%) in South and South East Asia, sub-Saharan Africa, Latin America, Caribbean, Australasia and Europe [59]. The effects of fatty liver, obesity and diabetes on liver disease with chronic HCV infection include more rapid progression to cirrhosis, higher incidence of HCC and suboptimal response to interferon-based therapy. Further, chronic HCV infection increases incidence of type 2 diabetes several fold, and is associated with increased all-cause mortality largely attributable to cardiovascular and liver disease [60]. It is therefore predicted that coincidence of NAFLD with HCV will significantly increase the burden of chronic liver disease and HCC in future.

NAFLD can also exacerbate damage caused by other liver diseases, including haemochromatosis and alcoholic liver disease [55], whose prevalence also varies in different geographical regions.

## Conclusions

The incidence and prevalence of NAFLD is increasing worldwide as a consequence of the rising levels of obesity and metabolic syndrome. Recognition of the global importance of NAFLD and its complications of portal hypertension, liver failure and HCC, is reflected in the development of practice guidelines by Medical Societies encompassing all continents, including both the American [4] and European [61] Associations for the Study of Liver Disease, the Asia-Pacific Working Party for NAFLD [62], World Gastroenterological Association [63] and the Chinese Liver Disease Association [19]. NAFLD is more prevalent in certain ethnic groups, and identification of several genetic polymorphisms has helped to increase our understanding of these differences in susceptibility. The precise pathogenetic mechanisms underpinning the development and progression of

NAFLD are not yet fully understood and likely vary in different populations due to complex interactions between genetics, diet, hepatic lipid handling, microbiome and environmental influences [64].

Effective treatments for NAFLD are currently lacking, with existing treatment strategies primarily directed towards lifestyle modification and control of metabolic risk factors. Ongoing research into ethnic and genetic differences in susceptibility could help to further our knowledge of the pathogenesis of NAFLD and should inform the development of novel therapeutic strategies. There is a need for further longitudinal studies to delineate the natural history of the condition in different ethnic groups and to more accurately chart the changing prevalence in developing countries. The advances in non-invasive methods to diagnose and stage NAFLD without recourse to liver biopsy should facilitate such studies in the future. However, the most urgent priority remains reversal of the inexorable global trend of rising obesity levels, sedentariness and unhealthy eating behaviours, which underpin the burgeoning NAFLD epidemic. This will require education and public health interventions at both the individual and population levels.

## References

1. Farrell GC, Wong VW, Chitturi S. NAFLD in Asia – as common and important as in the West. Nat Rev Gastroenterol Hepatol 2013;10(5):307–318.
2. Vernon G, Baranova A, Younossi ZM. Systematic review: the epidemiology and natural history of non-alcoholic fatty liver disease and non-alcoholic steatohepatitis in adults. Aliment Pharmacol Ther 2011;34(3):274–285.
3. Younossi ZM, Stepanova M, Afendy M et al. Changes in the prevalence of the most common causes of chronic liver diseases in the United States from 1988 to 2008. Clin Gastroenterol Hepatol 2011;9(6):524–530.
4. Chalasani N, Younossi Z, Lavine JE et al. The diagnosis and management of non-alcoholic fatty liver disease: practice guideline by the American Gastroenterological Association, American Association for the Study of Liver Diseases, and American College of Gastroenterology. Gastroenterology 2012;142(7):1592–1609.
5. Wong RJ, Cheung R, Ahmed A. Nonalcoholic steatohepatitis is the most rapidly growing indication for liver transplantation in patients with hepatocellular carcinoma in the U.S. Hepatology 2014;59(6):2188–2195.
6. Bedogni G, Miglioli L, Masutti F et al. Prevalence of and risk factors for nonalcoholic fatty liver disease: the Dionysos nutrition and liver study. Hepatology 2005;42(1):44–52.

7. Caballeria L, Pera G, Auladell MA et al. Prevalence and factors associated with the presence of nonalcoholic fatty liver disease in an adult population in Spain. Eur J Gastroenterol Hepatol 2010;22(1):24–32.

8. Browning JD, Szczepaniak LS, Dobbins R et al. Prevalence of hepatic steatosis in an urban population in the United States: impact of ethnicity. Hepatology 2004;40(6):1387–1395.

9. Williams CD, Stengel J, Asike MI et al. Prevalence of nonalcoholic fatty liver disease and nonalcoholic steatohepatitis among a largely middle-aged population utilizing ultrasound and liver biopsy: a prospective study. Gastroenterology 2011;140(1):124–131.

10. Mendez-Sanchez N. Non alcoholic fatty liver disease. Ann Hepatol 2009;8(Suppl 1):S3.

11. Karnikowski M, Cordova C, Oliveira RJ et al. Non-alcoholic fatty liver disease and metabolic syndrome in Brazilian middle-aged and older adults. Sao Paulo Med J 2007;125(6):333–337.

12. Almeda-Valdes P, Cuevas-Ramos D, Aguilar-Salinas CA. Metabolic syndrome and non-alcoholic fatty liver disease. Ann Hepatol 2009;8(Suppl 1):S18–S24.

13. Castro-Martinez MG, Banderas-Lares DZ, Ramirez-Martinez JC, Escobedo-de la Pena J. Prevalence of nonalcoholic fatty liver disease in subjects with metabolic syndrome. Cir Cir 2012;80(2):128–133.

14. Eguchi Y, Hyogo H, Ono M et al. Prevalence and associated metabolic factors of nonalcoholic fatty liver disease in the general population from 2009 to 2010 in Japan: a multicenter large retrospective study. J Gastroenterol 2012; 47(5):586–595.

15. Chitturi S, Abeygunasekera S, Farrell GC et al. NASH and insulin resistance: insulin hypersecretion and specific association with the insulin resistance syndrome. Hepatology 2002;35(2):373–379.

16. Anjana RM, Lakshminarayanan S, Deepa M et al. Parental history of type 2 diabetes mellitus, metabolic syndrome, and cardiometabolic risk factors in Asian Indian adolescents. Metabolism 2009;58(3):344–350.

17. Loomba R, Abraham M, Unalp A et al. Association between diabetes, family history of diabetes, and risk of nonalcoholic steatohepatitis and fibrosis. Hepatology 2012;56(3): 943–951.

18. Okanoue T, Umemura A, Yasui K et al. Nonalcoholic fatty liver disease and nonalcoholic steatohepatitis in Japan. J Gastroenterol Hepatol 2011;26(Suppl 1):153–162.

19. Gao X, Fan JG. Diagnosis and management of non-alcoholic fatty liver disease and related metabolic disorders: consensus statement from the Study Group of Liver and Metabolism, Chinese Society of Endocrinology. J Diabetes 2013;5(4):406–415.

20. Park SH, Jeon WK, Kim SH et al. Prevalence and risk factors of non-alcoholic fatty liver disease among Korean adults. J Gastroenterol Hepatol 2006;21(1 Pt 1):138–143.

21. Tsai CH, Li TC, Lin CC. Metabolic syndrome as a risk factor for nonalcoholic fatty liver disease. South Med J 2008;101(9): 900–905.

22. Das K, Das K, Mukherjee PS et al. Nonobese population in a developing country has a high prevalence of nonalcoholic fatty liver and significant liver disease. Hepatology 2010;51(5): 1593–1602.

23. Dassanayake AS, Kasturiratne A, Rajindrajith S et al. Prevalence and risk factors for non-alcoholic fatty liver disease among adults in an urban Sri Lankan population. J Gastroenterol Hepatol 2009;24(7):1284–1288.

24. Mohan V, Farooq S, Deepa M et al. Prevalence of non-alcoholic fatty liver disease in urban south Indians in relation to different grades of glucose intolerance and metabolic syndrome. Diabetes Res Clin Pract 2009;84(1):84–91.

25. Amarapurkar DN, Hashimoto E, Lesmana LA et al. How common is non-alcoholic fatty liver disease in the Asia-Pacific region and are there local differences? J Gastroenterol Hepatol 2007;22(6):788–793.

26. Amarapurkar D, Kamani P, Patel N et al. Prevalence of non-alcoholic fatty liver disease: population based study. Ann Hepatol 2007;6(3):161–163.

27. Chitturi S, Farrell GC, Hashimoto E et al. Non-alcoholic fatty liver disease in the Asia-Pacific region: definitions and overview of proposed guidelines. J Gastroenterol Hepatol 2007;22(6):778–787.

28. Ng M, Fleming T, Robinson M et al. Global, regional, and national prevalence of overweight and obesity in children and adults during 1980–2013: a systematic analysis for the Global Burden of Disease Study 2013. Lancet 2014;384:766–781.

29. Onyekwere CA, Ogbera AO, Balogun BO. Non-alcoholic fatty liver disease and the metabolic syndrome in an urban hospital serving an African community. Ann Hepatol 2011;10(2):119–124.

30. Younossi ZM, Stepanova M, Rafiq N et al. Pathologic criteria for nonalcoholic steatohepatitis: interprotocol agreement and ability to predict liver-related mortality. Hepatology 2011;53(6):1874–1882.

31. Ekstedt M, Franzen LE, Mathiesen UL et al. Long-term follow-up of patients with NAFLD and elevated liver enzymes. Hepatology 2006;44(4):865–873.

32. Lédinghen V de, Ratziu V, Causse X et al. Diagnostic and predictive factors of significant liver fibrosis and minimal lesions in patients with persistent unexplained elevated transaminases. A prospective multicenter study. J Hepatol 2006;45(4):592–599.

33. Soderberg C, Stal P, Askling J et al. Decreased survival of subjects with elevated liver function tests during a 28-year follow-up. Hepatology 2010;51(2):595–602.

34. Machado M, Marques-Vidal P, Cortez-Pinto H. Hepatic histology in obese patients undergoing bariatric surgery. J Hepatol 2006;45(4):600–606.

35. Campos GM, Bambha K, Vittinghoff E et al. A clinical scoring system for predicting nonalcoholic steatohepatitis in morbidly obese patients. Hepatology 2008;47(6):1916–1923.

36. Minervini MI, Ruppert K, Fontes P et al. Liver biopsy findings from healthy potential living liver donors: reasons for disqualification, silent diseases and correlation with liver injury tests. J Hepatol 2009;50(3):501–510.

37. Nadalin S, Malago M, Valentin-Gamazo C et al. Preoperative donor liver biopsy for adult living donor liver transplantation: risks and benefits. Liver Transpl 2005;11(8):980–986.

38. Cho EJ, Kwack MS, Jang ES et al. Relative etiological role of prior hepatitis B virus infection and nonalcoholic fatty liver disease in the development of non-B non-C hepatocellular carcinoma in a hepatitis B-endemic area. Digestion 2011;84(Suppl 1):17–22.

39. Tokushige K, Hashimoto E, Horie Y et al. Hepatocellular carcinoma in Japanese patients with nonalcoholic fatty liver disease, alcoholic liver disease, and chronic liver disease of unknown etiology: report of the nationwide survey. J Gastroenterol 2011;46(10):1230–1237.

40. Dyson J, Jaques B, Chattopadyhay D et al. Hepatocellular cancer: the impact of obesity, type 2 diabetes and a multidisciplinary team. J Hepatol 2014;60(1):110–117.

41. Torres DM, Harrison SA. Nonalcoholic steatohepatitis and noncirrhotic hepatocellular carcinoma: fertile soil. Semin Liver Dis 2012;32(1):30–38.

42. WHO. Obesity and Overweight: World Health Organisation Fact sheet N°311. 2014.

43. WHO Expert Consultation. Appropriate body-mass index for Asian populations and its implications for policy and intervention strategies. Lancet 2004;363(9403):157–163.

44. Liu CJ. Prevalence and risk factors for non-alcoholic fatty liver disease in Asian people who are not obese. J Gastroenterol Hepatol 2012;27(10):1555–1560.

45. Park SH, Kim BI, Yun JW et al. Insulin resistance and C-reactive protein as independent risk factors for non-alcoholic fatty liver disease in non-obese Asian men. J Gastroenterol Hepatol 2004;19(6):694–698.

46. Liu YL, Patman GL, Leathart JB et al. Carriage of the PNPLA3 rs738409 C >G polymorphism confers an increased risk of non-alcoholic fatty liver disease associated hepatocellular carcinoma. J Hepatol 2014;61(1):75–81.

47. Romeo S, Kozlitina J, Xing C et al. Genetic variation in PNPLA3 confers susceptibility to nonalcoholic fatty liver disease. Nat Genet 2008;40(12):1461–1465.

48. Chalasani N, Guo X, Loomba R et al. Genome-wide association study identifies variants associated with histologic features of nonalcoholic Fatty liver disease. Gastroenterology 2010;139(5):1567–1576.

49. Miele L, Beale G, Patman G et al. The Kruppel-like factor 6 genotype is associated with fibrosis in nonalcoholic fatty liver disease. Gastroenterology 2008;135(1):282–291.

50. Chen S, Li Y, Li S et al. A Val227Ala substitution in the peroxisome proliferator activated receptor alpha (PPAR alpha) gene associated with non-alcoholic fatty liver disease and decreased waist circumference and waist-to-hip ratio. J Gastroenterol Hepatol 2008;23(9):1415–1418.

51. Hui Y, Yu-Yuan L, Yu-Qiang N et al. Effect of peroxisome proliferator-activated receptors-gamma and co-activator-1alpha genetic polymorphisms on plasma adiponectin levels and susceptibility of non-alcoholic fatty liver disease in Chinese people. Liver Int 2008;28(3):385–392.

52. Petersen KF, Dufour S, Hariri A et al. Apolipoprotein C3 gene variants in nonalcoholic fatty liver disease. N Engl J Med 2010;362(12):1082–1089.

53. Hou J, Liu Z, Gu F. Epidemiology and Prevention of Hepatitis B Virus Infection. Int J Med Sci 2005;2(1):50–57.

54. Wong VW, Wong GL, Chu WC et al. Hepatitis B virus infection and fatty liver in the general population. J Hepatol 2012;56(3):533–540.

55. Powell EE, Jonsson JR, Clouston AD. Steatosis: co-factor in other liver diseases. Hepatology 2005;42(1):5–13.

56. Shi JP, Fan JG, Wu R et al. Prevalence and risk factors of hepatic steatosis and its impact on liver injury in Chinese patients with chronic hepatitis B infection. J Gastroenterol Hepatol 2008;23(9):1419–1425.

57. Wong GL, Wong VW, Choi PC et al. Metabolic syndrome increases the risk of liver cirrhosis in chronic hepatitis B. Gut 2009;58(1):111–117.

58. Wong GL, Chan HL, Yu Z et al. Coincidental metabolic syndrome increases the risk of liver fibrosis progression in patients with chronic hepatitis B – a prospective cohort study with paired transient elastography examinations. Aliment Pharmacol Ther 2014;39(8):883–893.

59. Mohd HK, Groeger J, Flaxman AD et al. Global epidemiology of hepatitis C virus infection: new estimates of age-specific antibody to HCV seroprevalence. Hepatology 2013;57(4):1333–1342.

60. Negro F. Facts and fictions of HCV and comorbidities: steatosis, diabetes mellitus, and cardiovascular disease. J Hepatol 2014;61(S1):S69–S78.

61. Ratziu V, Bellentani S, Cortez-Pinto H et al. A position statement on NAFLD/NASH based on the EASL 2009 special conference. J Hepatol 2010;53(2):372–384.

62. Farrell GC, Chitturi S, Lau GK et al. Guidelines for the assessment and management of non-alcoholic fatty liver disease in the Asia-Pacific region: executive summary. J Gastroenterol Hepatol 2007;22(6):775–777.

63. LaBrecque DR, Abbas Z, Anania F et al. World Gastroenterology organisation global guidelines: non-alcoholic fatty liver disease and nonalcoholic steatohepatitis. J Clin Gastroenterol 2014;48(6):467–473.

64. Loomba R, Sanyal AJ. The global NAFLD epidemic. Nat Rev Gastroenterol Hepatol 2013;10(11):686–690.

# 3 Is insulin resistance the principal cause of NAFLD?

**Ian F. Godsland[1], Sanjeev Mehta[2], Shareen Forbes[3], Fabian Meienberg[4], Michael Yee[5], Simon D. Taylor-Robinson[6], and Desmond G. Johnston[7]**

[1] Division of Diabetes Endocrinology and Metabolism, Department of Medicine, Faculty of Medicine, Imperial College London, London, UK

[2] London North West Healthcare NHS Trust, and Department of Diabetes and Endocrinology, Imperial College London, Ealing Hospital, London, UK

[3] Endocrinology Unit, University/BHF Centre for Cardiovascular Science, Queen's Medical Research Institute, University of Edinburgh, Edinburgh, UK

[4] Department of Diabetology, Endocrinology and Metabolism, University Hospital Basel, Basel, Switzerland

[5] Metabolic Medicine Unit, St Mary's Hospital, London, UK

[6] Digestive Diseases Division, Imperial College London, London, UK

[7] Department of Medicine, Faculty of Medicine, Imperial College London, London, UK

## LEARNING POINTS

- Conditions where insulin resistance is a feature (e.g. obesity) are associated with a high prevalence of NAFLD.

- Insulin resistance is conventionally measured in terms of glucoregulatory insulin resistance, but antilipolytic insulin resistance may be more important with regard to fatty liver.

- Antilipolytic insulin resistance has mostly been evaluated in terms of the ability of plasma insulin to lower plasma non-esterified fatty acid (NEFA) or glycerol levels, although an agreed reference method has yet to be established.

- *De novo* lipogenesis in the liver is stimulated by the hyperinsulinaemia of insulin resistance, but most hepatic triglyceride derives from circulating NEFA of adipose tissue origin.

- Insulin stimulates fatty acid uptake into the liver, *de novo* lipogenesis and hepatic triglyceride synthesis, and it inhibits fatty acid oxidation and hepatic VLDL secretion. Accordingly, the hyperinsulinaemia of insulin resistance promotes hepatic fatty accumulation.

- Although hepatic steatosis may occur in the absence of insulin resistance, insulin resistance does appear to be an important pathogenetic factor. However, the importance of hepatic insulin resistance may have been exaggerated since hepatic steatosis appears to be largely a consequence of adipose tissue NEFA release.

## Introduction

A relationship between insulin resistance and non-alcoholic fatty liver disease (NAFLD) has been recognised for many years, but whether insulin resistance is an aetiological factor in NAFLD or simply an accompanying feature continues to be debated. In this chapter, we review some of the evidence. We begin with a brief examination of the mechanisms of insulin resistance and how insulin sensitivity is measured with particular emphasis on insulin resistance as it relates to lipid metabolism. Some of the clinical situations where insulin resistance and NAFLD coexist are reviewed. Potential aetiological mechanisms for NAFLD are discussed and potential causative links between insulin resistance and NAFLD are examined.

*Clinical Dilemmas in Non-Alcoholic Fatty Liver Disease*, First Edition. Edited by Roger Williams and Simon D. Taylor-Robinson.
© 2016 John Wiley & Sons, Ltd. Published 2016 by John Wiley & Sons, Ltd.

## What is meant by insulin resistance?

Insulin is a key factor in many physiological processes, ranging from its classically recognised effects on glucose metabolism to its influences on cell division and survival. In the context of NAFLD, the influence of insulin on lipid and glucose metabolism may be central. These influences include suppression of adipose tissue lipolysis; stimulation of *de novo* lipogenesis in the liver, adipose tissue and elsewhere; stimulation of fatty acid uptake by the liver; increased hepatic triglyceride synthesis; inhibition of release of very-low-density lipoprotein (VLDL) by the liver; stimulation of glucose uptake by peripheral tissues (skeletal muscle and adipose tissue) and provision of glycerol-3-phosphate for triglyceride synthesis; and suppression of hepatic gluconeogenesis and promotion of glycogen synthesis in the liver and other tissues.

Insulin resistance is conventionally measured in terms of the extent to which a unit change in plasma insulin concentration can lower plasma glucose levels, but it can equally be considered in terms of any of the other metabolic processes that insulin influences. In some circumstances, assessing these other actions is important, especially as they differ in their sensitivities to a given insulin concentration. For example, half-maximal velocity for stimulation of peripheral glucose uptake into peripheral tissues is achieved at a plasma insulin concentration of ~60 mU/L. By contrast, half-maximal velocity for suppression of hepatic gluconeogenesis and adipose tissue lipolysis by insulin occurs at ~15 mU/L.

Insulin-induced suppression of hepatic VLDL release occurs at lower levels still. Insulin resistance is obviously not a simple concept and should be considered in relation to the insulin-sensitive process being quantified. It is also important to recognise that knowledge of insulin action is far from complete. In a study of the mouse liver phospho-proteome, insulin stimulation led to phosphorylation of hundreds of proteins that were not previously known to be insulin sensitive [1]. Each of these phosphorylations may be differently affected by a given concentration of insulin, further emphasising the need to define what net physiological effect or discrete biochemical step is being measured with reference to the effects insulin is having.

It should be noted that, conventionally, the terms 'insulin sensitivity' and 'insulin resistance' are used interchangeably, a measure of insulin resistance being the inverse of a measure of insulin sensitivity. However, strictly speaking, 'insulin sensitivity' is the measurement, with 'insulin resistance' then being a state of abnormally low insulin sensitivity.

## How is insulin resistance measured *in vivo* in man?

In principle, insulin sensitivity could be measured with reference to any one of the many physiological or biochemical effects that insulin has in the body. As mentioned, insulin sensitivity is conventionally measured in terms of the effect of plasma insulin concentrations on plasma glucose concentrations, and there are a variety of techniques available for measuring so-called 'glucoregulatory' insulin sensitivity. Importantly for a discussion of insulin resistance in NAFLD, there are also available several approaches to measuring insulin sensitivity as it relates to lipid metabolism, and these concern primarily the influence of insulin on suppression of adipose tissue lipolysis, so-called 'antilipolytic' insulin sensitivity. Both approaches to the measurement of insulin sensitivity have been used in the study of insulin resistance in NAFLD [2–5].

### Measuring glucoregulatory insulin sensitivity: The euglycaemic hyperinsulinaemic clamp

The reference method for measuring the insulin sensitivity of an individual is the euglycaemic hyperinsulinaemic clamp [6]. This technique is designed to quantify the ability of insulin to lower blood glucose concentrations and aims to determine a steady-state rate of glucose infusion needed to maintain euglycaemia in the presence of a sustained elevation in plasma insulin concentrations. At steady state, this glucose infusion rate reflects the rate at which blood glucose levels would otherwise be falling, and with measurement of the accompanying steady-state plasma insulin concentration, this rate of fall can be expressed per unit insulin concentration. The rate of fall in plasma glucose concentrations comprises two components: uptake of glucose by peripheral tissues and suppression of hepatic glucose production. In principle, hepatic glucose production should be completely suppressed by the hyperinsulinaemia of the clamp procedure so that clamp insulin sensitivity measurements primarily reflect peripheral glucose disposal. In its simplest implementation, in which the rate of glucose infusion at steady state (the so-called '*M*' value) is taken as the measure of insulin sensitivity (the higher the *M* value, the greater the sensitivity to insulin), the reference clamp procedure primarily quantifies the influence of insulin on peripheral glucose uptake.

However, if there is insulin resistance at the liver, there may be incomplete suppression of hepatic glucose production during the clamp, and by incorporating an infusion of isotopically labelled glucose into the procedure, hepatic glucose production can be distinguished from peripheral glucose uptake [7]. Calculation of isotope dilution provides a measure of the net rate of entry of unlabelled glucose into the body, and since this is the sum of the steady-state exogenous glucose infusion rate, which is known, and the rate of hepatic glucose production, which is not known, the rate of hepatic glucose production can be calculated as the difference between the net rate of entry and the steady-state glucose infusion rate. The clamp may be modified to enable sensitive discrimination and quantification of both the sensitivity of suppression of hepatic glucose production to insulin and the sensitivity of peripheral glucose elimination to insulin by performance of the clamp at low followed by high rates of insulin infusion. The former elevates plasma insulin concentrations to the relatively low levels at which suppression of hepatic glucose production is most sensitive, whereas the latter elevates insulin concentrations to the relatively high levels at which stimulation of peripheral glucose elimination is most sensitive. Glucose and insulin concentrations during such a 'two-step' clamp are illustrated in Figure 3.1 (panels A–C). The clamp can therefore be adapted for differentiating peripheral glucose disposal from hepatic glucose production and, by carrying out clamps at different steady-state insulin concentrations, can provide full dose–response curves [9].

## The minimal model of intravenous glucose tolerance test glucose and insulin concentrations

The clamp provides a true measure of insulin sensitivity in terms of reduction in plasma glucose concentration relative to the accompanying insulin concentration. One other procedure can provide this, namely, analysis of the dynamic relationship between the fall in glucose concentrations and the accompanying changes in insulin concentrations following an intravenous glucose injection (the intravenous glucose tolerance test (IVGTT)), using the minimal model of glucose disappearance [10]. Typical IVGTT glucose and insulin concentration profiles are shown in Figure 3.2 (panels A and B), and the minimal model quantitatively relates the rate of fall in glucose concentrations at any given

moment during the IVGTT to the accompanying insulin concentration. Like the clamp, the minimal model approach returns a measure of insulin sensitivity that primarily reflects peripheral glucose disposal. However, while minimal modelling has been adapted to differentiate hepatic glucose production from peripheral glucose disposal [11], its particular strength lies in the fact that the IVGTT procedure can provide a widely used measure of beta cell function, the acute insulin response to glucose [12], and with measurement of plasma C-peptide concentrations and further modelling analyses, it can provide measures of insulin secretion into the hepatic portal vein and uptake of this newly secreted insulin by the liver [13, 14]. The minimal model method is also simpler to perform than clamp techniques.

## Surrogate measures of insulin sensitivity

The clamp involves a complex procedure but a relatively straightforward calculation, whereas the IVGTT with minimal model analysis involves a relatively straightforward procedure but with a complex calculation. The necessary complexity of these direct measurement approaches has motivated introduction of a range of more simple, surrogate indices of insulin sensitivity [15, 16]. These mainly depend for their validity on there being proportionality between the degree of insulin resistance and the degree of compensatory hyperinsulinaemia that accompanies it. However, this proportionality only holds if beta cell function can compensate adequately. Any beta cell deficiency will be accompanied by a rise in plasma glucose levels as well as a rise in insulin concentrations, and calculations for deriving surrogate indices of insulin sensitivity generally take this into account. Whether peripheral or hepatic insulin sensitivity is reflected in the index will depend on the extent to which fasting or post-glucose load insulin and glucose measurements are entered in the equations. In the fasting state, glucose and insulin concentrations are largely determined by hepatic glucose production (reflecting mainly gluconeogenesis), so these provide indices of hepatic insulin sensitivity. By contrast, changes in glucose and insulin concentrations following a glucose load (e.g. during an oral glucose tolerance test (OGTT)) are more determined by peripheral glucose elimination and therefore reflect peripheral insulin sensitivity.

Of various indices that have been proposed based on fasting measurements, the original and still most widely used is the homeostasis model assessment (HOMA) index

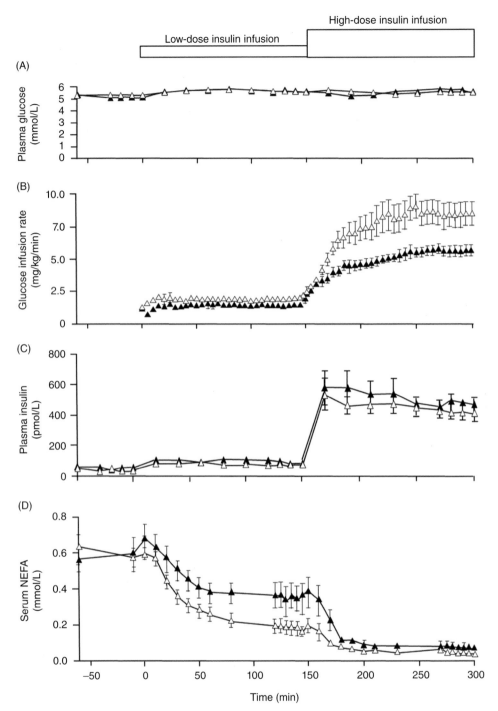

**FIG 3.1** The two-step, low- and high-insulin infusion rate, euglycaemic hyperinsulinaemic clamp. Eight volunteers with familial combined hyperlipidaemia (FCHL: closed triangles) were compared with eight healthy controls (open triangles). Plasma glucose concentrations (panel A) were kept constant by a variable rate glucose infusion (panel B) in the presence of small and large increases in plasma insulin concentrations (panel C). The sensitivity to insulin of glucose elimination from plasma (conventional insulin sensitivity) was quantified by the rate of glucose infusion needed to maintain euglycaemia in the presence of constantly elevated insulin concentrations. As shown in panel B, differences between the two groups in insulin sensitivity were most clearly discriminated at high insulin concentrations between 150 and 300 min. The sensitivity of suppression of lipolysis to insulin was quantified by the magnitude of the fall in plasma NEFA concentrations (panel D), which was most clearly discriminated between the two groups in the presence of the small increase in insulin concentrations between 0 and 150 min. The FCHL group showed appreciably less of a reduction in NEFA concentrations in response to a low insulin infusion rate compared with the controls, indicating resistance to the antilipolytic effects of insulin (*Source:* Aitman et al. [8]).

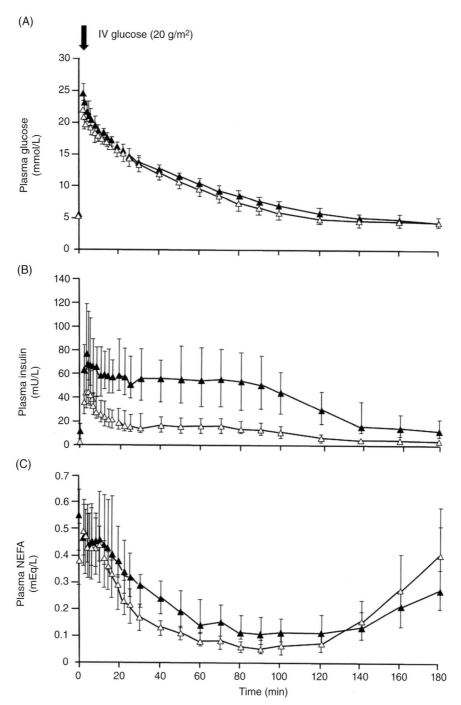

**FIG 3.2** Suppression of lipolysis during an intravenous glucose tolerance test. A group of eight volunteers with non-alcoholic fatty liver disease (NAFLD: closed triangles) was compared with eight healthy controls (open triangles). A rapid, bolus, intravenous injection of glucose stimulates insulin secretion from the pancreas. Panel A shows that the rate at which glucose concentrations returned to normal differed little between the two groups. However, as shown in panel B, this was achieved with a marked difference in insulin concentrations. To restore normoglycaemia, significantly higher insulin concentrations were necessary in the NAFLD group, indicating appreciable insulin resistance. The sensitivity to insulin of glucose elimination from plasma (insulin sensitivity) was quantified by relating the rate of fall in glucose concentrations to the accompanying insulin concentrations in a mathematical modelling analysis. Accompanying changes in NEFA concentrations are shown in panel C. The sensitivity of suppression of lipolysis to insulin was quantified as the ratio of the rate of fall in plasma NEFA concentrations between 16 and 40 min divided by the incremental area under the insulin concentration profile between 16 and 40 min. The NAFLD group showed an appreciably slower rate of reduction in NEFA concentrations despite higher accompanying insulin concentrations compared with the controls, indicating resistance to the anti-lipolytic effects of insulin (*Source*: From data reported in Mehta et al. [5]).

of insulin resistance [17]. The equation used to derive the HOMA index is simple ((fasting glucose in mmol/L × fasting insulin in mU/L)/22.5) but derives from a rigorous modelling analysis of the relationships between fasting insulin and glucose concentrations. Another approach based on fasting glucose and insulin concentrations, but developed *ad hoc* by comparison with reference clamp measures, is the quantitative insulin sensitivity check index (QUICKI = 1/ (log fasting glucose + log fasting insulin)) [18].

Surrogate indices of insulin sensitivity that derive from glucose and insulin concentrations during an OGTT have mainly been generated by *ad hoc* comparisons with clamp measures and, like the fasting indices, generally involve relatively simple calculations. Indices include the Matsuda [19], Stumvoll [20], Gutt [21], Belfiore [22] and Cederholm [23] insulin sensitivity indices. There is also a model-based index, the oral glucose insulin sensitivity (OGIS) index [24], and an approach to discriminating hepatic and peripheral insulin sensitivity using OGTT-derived data has been proposed [25].

Beyond clamp, minimal model and surrogate approaches to quantifying glucoregulatory insulin sensitivity or resistance, several other approaches have been adopted or proposed. The insulin tolerance test, measuring the rate of glucose decline following a bolus injection of insulin, offers a relatively simple and conceptually straightforward way of assessing insulin sensitivity [26]. Specifically relating to hepatic insulin resistance, DeFronzo's hepatic insulin resistance index is derived by multiplying overnight fasting glucose production measured isotopically by the fasting insulin concentration [27]. Furthermore, attempts have been made to assess the sensitivity to insulin of hepatic glucose uptake, measured either using glucose tracer (2H or 13C) methodology [28] or positron emission tomography with [18F]-labelled 2-fluoro-2-deoxyglucose [29].

## Measuring antilipolytic insulin sensitivity

Techniques for measurement of glucoregulatory insulin sensitivity have been extensively explored, primarily because of the importance of evaluating the role of insulin resistance in the pathogenesis of type 2 diabetes mellitus. Evaluation of antilipolytic insulin sensitivity has received less attention, probably because antilipolytic insulin resistance is not perceived as having the same importance as glucoregulatory insulin resistance in disease pathogenesis and possibly because it has been assumed by many that antilipolytic insulin resistance is quantitatively similar to glucoregulatory insulin resistance. However, there has been little rigorous investigation of this possibility, and such an equivalence cannot be assumed.

The perceived lesser importance of antilipolytic insulin sensitivity has meant that there has been appreciably less methodological development in this respect and there is no accepted reference method for measuring antilipolytic insulin sensitivity. Rather than dedicated methodological studies, techniques for quantifying antilipolytic insulin sensitivity have generally been adopted in the context of clinical investigations of lipid metabolism, with the approach taken generally depending on the type, size and depth of investigation intended. Nevertheless, if a reference approach were to be adopted, there would be a strong argument for basing it on evaluation of the suppression of plasma non-esterified fatty acid (NEFA) concentrations during a euglycaemic hyperinsulinaemic clamp. As mentioned previously, suppression of adipose tissue lipolysis has the same dose–response characteristics with respect to insulin as does suppression of hepatic gluconeogenesis. Evaluation of the extent of the reduction in plasma NEFA concentrations at steady state during a low insulin infusion rate clamp then provides a sensitive measure of antilipolytic insulin sensitivity. Use of this approach in the investigation of a clinical condition (familial combined hyperlipidaemia) that may have antilipolytic insulin resistance as an aetiological factor is illustrated in Figure 3.1 (panel D); the reduction in NEFA concentrations during the low-dose phase of a two-step clamp is seen to be appreciably less in the affected compared with the unaffected group. This approach has been used to evaluate both glucoregulatory and antilipolytic insulin resistance in association with a range of metabolic conditions [4] including hepatic fat deposition [2]. A particular advantage of the clamp is that the investigative procedure can be extended to incorporate quantification of the effects of insulin on a range of metabolic measurements, as seen in the use of isotopically labelled glucose to distinguish hepatic and peripheral insulin sensitivity. Accordingly, and in the context of studies of liver fat deposition, evaluation of the effects of insulin on lipid metabolism has been extended using the clamp to include measurement of rates of glycerol production and therefore rates of adipose tissue lipolysis, fatty acid appearance and lipid oxidation [3, 30].

The rapid rise in insulin concentrations at the outset of an IVGTT offers another context in which both glucoregulatory and antilipolytic insulin sensitivities can be quantified.

NEFA concentrations generally fall exponentially during the first hour following intravenous glucose injection, and the rate constant for this fall relative to the accompanying increment in insulin concentrations has been used to quantify antilipolytic insulin sensitivity [31]. Moreover, modelling approaches analogous to minimal model analysis have been proposed for quantifying antilipolytic insulin sensitivity using the IVGTT [32]. As with the clamp, both glucoregulatory and antilipolytic insulin resistance have been evaluated in the context of liver fat deposition using the IVGTT [5].

In principle, antilipolytic insulin sensitivity could be quantified in any situation that involves an excursion in insulin concentrations. For example, glycerol levels and appearance rates measured isotopically have enabled quantification of antilipolytic insulin sensitivity during a low-dose insulin infusion [33]. More straightforwardly, the extent of the decline in NEFA concentrations during an OGTT has been used [34], and a simple measure of adipose tissue insulin sensitivity (adipo-IR = fasting plasma insulin × fasting plasma NEFA concentration) has been proposed [35] and applied in studies of NAFLD [36].

While various approaches to measurement of antilipolytic insulin resistance have been adopted in clinical investigations, evaluations of the sensitivity to insulin of other insulin-dependent aspects of lipid and lipoprotein metabolism have generally been in the context of dedicated experimental studies in metabolic mechanisms. The effects of insulin on hepatic [37] and lipoprotein lipase activity [38], apolipoprotein CIII transcription [39] and hepatic assembly [40] and secretion of very-low-density lipoprotein [41, 42] have individually been the subject of dedicated investigations, but the few that have been in the context of clinical studies have generally been concerned with differences in the effects of insulin between defined groups rather than with quantifying a dose–response sensitivity.

None of the approaches to quantifying antilipolytic insulin sensitivity – or any other lipid metabolism-related insulin sensitivity – mentioned previously has been rigorously evaluated from the general methodological point of view, though all have provided biologically plausible information. Even less well explored, at least from the point of view of providing an index of insulin sensitivity, has been the possibility of combining a range of different metabolic measures to provide a working index, based on the net effects of variation in insulin sensitivity. This possibility is implicit in the Belfiore insulin sensitivity index, which derives from not only fasting and OGTT glucose and insulin concentrations but also NEFA concentrations [22], thus providing an index that could reflect aspects of both antilipolytic and glucoregulatory insulin sensitivity. However, the wider context for this possibility is provided by the concept of the metabolic syndrome, which acknowledges the broad intercorrelations that exist between a range of metabolic measures including fasting and glucose-stimulated insulin and glucose concentrations, triglycerides, high-density lipoprotein cholesterol, uric acid, blood pressure and total and central adiposity. The continuing widespread interest in this concept stems to a large extent from its origins in the possibility that combining these various measures might in some way provide a highly sensitive index of cardiovascular or diabetes risk. This possibility remains controversial [43], but to the extent that insulin resistance can be proposed as a unifying underlying mechanism for disturbances in this entire range of measures, these measures could, suitably combined, provide a guide to the global effects of insulin resistance on a broad range of insulin-dependent physiological and biochemical processes. This possibility has been explored and it was noted that while a measure of glucoregulatory insulin resistance did not predict cardiovascular mortality, a rigorously derived index of co-associated, insulin resistance-related disturbances did [44]. Methods for evaluating insulin resistance are summarised in Table 3.1.

## Insulin resistance and NAFLD

### Insulin actions and the consequences of insulin resistance for liver fat content

In classical insulin-sensitive tissues such as muscle, insulin binds to its membrane receptor, activating insulin receptor tyrosine kinase (reviewed in Ref [45]). This phosphorylates insulin receptor substrate 1 (IRS1), which in turn activates phosphatidylinositol 3-kinase. Glucose transporter 4 (Glut4) is translocated to the cell membrane following activation of a number of signalling molecules, resulting in increased muscle glucose uptake. In the liver also, insulin increases its receptor substrate phosphorylation. Suppression of hepatic gluconeogenesis occurs via downstream effectors, resulting in phosphorylation of the key metabolic regulator, FoxO1. An alternative downstream pathway is via SREBP-1c, another important metabolic regulator, in this case resulting in increased hepatic lipogenesis.

**TABLE 3.1**  Some methods of assessing insulin resistance

| Method | What is being assessed | References |
| --- | --- | --- |
| *Glucoregulatory insulin sensitivity* | | |
| Hyperinsulinaemic euglycaemic clamp reference method | Sensitivity of combined effects of insulin on suppression of gluconeogenesis and stimulation of peripheral glucose elimination | [6] |
| Hyperinsulinaemic euglycaemic clamp with isotopically labelled glucose and low and high insulin infusion rates | Hepatic (low insulin infusion rate) and peripheral (high insulin infusion rate) insulin sensitivity | [2, 4, 7] |
| Intravenous glucose tolerance test with minimal model analysis | Combined effects of insulin on suppression of gluconeogenesis and stimulation of peripheral glucose elimination | [10] |
| Fasting plasma insulin and glucose-derived indices (HOMA-IR and QUICKI) | Surrogate index of hepatic insulin sensitivity predominantly | [17, 18] |
| OGTT plasma insulin and glucose-derived indices (Matsuda, Stumvoll, Gutt, Belfiore, Cederholm) | Surrogate index of peripheral insulin sensitivity predominantly | [19–23] |
| OGTT plasma insulin and glucose identification (OGIS) or regression model-based measures | Indices of peripheral insulin sensitivity predominantly | [24, 25] |
| Insulin tolerance test | Combined effects of insulin on suppression of gluconeogenesis and stimulation of peripheral glucose elimination | [26] |
| Positron emission tomography with fluorodeoxyglucose and exogenous insulin infusion | Hepatic glucose uptake | [29] |
| Hepatic insulin resistance index (basal endogenous glucose rate of appearance × fasting plasma insulin) | Hepatic insulin sensitivity predominantly | [27] |
| *Antilipolytic insulin sensitivity* | | |
| Low insulin infusion rate hyperinsulinaemic euglycaemic clamp assessing plasma NEFA or glycerol concentration suppression | Sensitivity of suppression of the concentrations of products of lipolysis to insulin | [2, 4] |
| Low insulin infusion rate hyperinsulinaemic euglycaemic clamp with isotopic infusion to assess glycerol rate of appearance | Sensitivity of suppression of rate of lipolysis to insulin | [3, 30] |
| Low-dose insulin infusion with infusion of isotopically labelled glycerol | Sensitivity of suppression of rate of lipolysis to insulin | [33] |
| Intravenous glucose tolerance test with measurement of plasma NEFA and insulin concentrations | Sensitivity of suppression of the concentrations of products of lipolysis to insulin | [5, 31, 32] |
| Fasting measurements of NEFA and insulin concentrations (adipo-IR = fasting plasma insulin × fasting plasma NEFA concentration) | Sensitivity of suppression of the concentrations of products of lipolysis to insulin | [35, 36] |
| OGTT measurements of NEFA and insulin concentrations | Sensitivity of suppression of the concentrations of products of lipolysis to insulin | [34] |
| *Net effect indices of insulin sensitivity* | | |
| Fasting and OGTT glucose, insulin and NEFA concentrations – Belfiore's index | Glucoregulatory and antilipolytic insulin sensitivity | [22] |
| Insulin resistance syndrome index | Effects of variation in insulin sensitivity expressed in terms of co-associated variation in a range of metabolic measures affected by insulin sensitivity | [44] |

As insulin resistance develops, IRS1 phosphorylation in muscle is impaired, as are the subsequent downstream processes, and in consequence insulin-stimulated muscle glucose uptake diminishes. Circulating glucose levels rise.

In the liver, FoxO1 phosphorylation is reduced and gluconeogenesis increases. There is evidence that the sensitivity of the SREBP-1c pathway is preserved [46], even when insulin resistance is otherwise severe, such that despite

**TABLE 3.2** Portal venous insulin delivery before and during an intravenous glucose tolerance test in insulin-resistant men with NAFLD compared with controls

| Portal insulin delivery (pmol/min/mL) | Controls (*n* = 19) | NAFLD patients (*n* = 21) |
|---|---|---|
| Basal | 130 (63–216) | 247 (213–942) |
| Increment during IV glucose tolerance test | 168 (79–214) | 449 (197–902) |

*Source*: Derived from Mehta et al. [5].

diminished glucose-lowering effects, the hepatic lipogenic actions of insulin are preserved or even enhanced – the phenomenon of selective insulin resistance [47–49].

Hyperglycaemia results in increased insulin secretion, and the hyperinsulinaemia enhances the stimulatory effect on SREBP-1c. The resultant stimulation of *de novo* lipogenesis is further enhanced by the anatomical position of the liver, with insulin delivery directly into the hepatic portal vein. Portal venous insulin levels are much higher than in the peripheral circulation. In consequence, portal insulin delivery in insulin-resistant subjects with NAFLD has been observed to be 1.9-fold higher than in controls in the fasting state and 2.7 higher following glucose stimulation [5] (Table 3.2).

Although *de novo* lipogenesis is not the major source of hepatic lipid in NAFLD, it is relatively high when compared with people without NAFLD (23% vs. 10%; [50]). Most hepatic triglyceride derives from circulating NEFA of adipose tissue origin. There is a substrate cycle between triglycerides and fatty acids in adipose tissue, and insulin both suppresses lipolysis and increases fatty acid esterification. The metabolic fate of the fatty acids released after lipolysis in adipose tissue is to be re-esterified locally in the substrate cycle or released into the circulation as NEFA. Circulating NEFA are bound to albumin and subsequently oxidised as fuel by many tissues such as skeletal and heart muscle. Alternatively, NEFA may be taken up by the liver. There they cross the liver cell membrane facilitated by fatty acid transport proteins, of which FATP2 and FATP5 are the most important [51]. In the liver, the fatty acids may be oxidised completely to carbon dioxide and water or partially to generate ketone bodies for export and metabolism in many tissues. Alternatively, they may be esterified once more in the liver to triglycerides either for storage in hepatocytes or release into the circulation as VLDL triglyceride. Insulin

stimulates fatty acid uptake into the liver, *de novo* lipogenesis and hepatic triglyceride synthesis, and it inhibits fatty acid oxidation. It also reduces hepatic VLDL secretion, at least in part through promoting degradation of its major apolipoprotein B (apoB). This is the situation that pertains after an overnight fast. In the postprandial state with high insulin levels, *de novo* lipogenesis increases. Although most chylomicron triglyceride is hydrolysed and assimilated peripherally, 20% is taken up directly by the liver (reviewed in Ref [52]), and if food intake is high, more fatty acid is taken up by the liver through this mechanism.

There is evidence, poorly understood, that insulin-resistant states may actually be preceded by a phase of reduced fatty acid mobilisation. In non-diabetic women with previous gestational diabetes (who are at high risk of developing type 2 diabetes in later life), the rates of appearance of glycerol and palmitic acid measured isotopically are reduced after an overnight fast, indicating reduced lipolysis in comparison with matched controls [53, 54]. At this time, the rate of appearance of glucose is not elevated, but unlike normal controls, it fails to fall with more prolonged fasting. Thus, it appears that the early abnormalities are a subtle defect in glucose production and a phase of reduced lipolysis and fatty acid mobilisation. In prospective studies in Pima Indians, who as an ethnic group are at very high risk indeed of developing type 2 diabetes, high insulin sensitivity early in life is predictive of weight gain and insulin resistance later [55]. Clues to the evolution of insulin resistance may derive from prospective studies in subjects who are insulin resistant and at high risk of progression to diabetes. Current indications are that abnormalities compatible with disordered adipocyte function and impaired mitochondrial fatty acid oxidation are present at a very early stage [56]. The biological basis for such observations is unclear, but insulin resistance becomes the dominant feature for the rest of life.

Established insulin resistance, by definition, causes reduced biological effect, and the compensatory hyperinsulinaemia has consequences for lipid metabolism reflecting the balance between diminished insulin action and the effects of the hyperinsulinaemia. The sequelae vary in different tissues. In adipose tissue, lipolysis and fatty acid mobilisation during fasting, assessed as circulating NEFA or glycerol concentrations (or in kinetic studies), are elevated. In the liver, the major effects on lipid metabolism are predominantly those due to the secondary hyperinsulinaemia, with stimulated fatty acid uptake, reduced oxidation

**TABLE 3.3** Classical insulin-resistant states and NAFLD

| Condition | Insulin insensitivity | NAFLD | Reference |
|---|---|---|---|
| Previous GDM | HOMA | Increased 2.2-fold | [57] |
| Previous GDM | QUICKI | Increased 2.5-fold | |
| Previous GDM | OGIS | Hepatocellular lipid in PGDM $p < 0.05$ | [58] |
| Obesity (BMI > 30) | HOMA | Increased 2.0-fold | [59] |
| Obesity | HOMA | Odds ratio 0.11, $p < 0.01$ | [60] |
| Metabolic syndrome | HOMA | Increased 3.8-fold | [59] |
| Metabolic syndrome | HOMA | Increased 2.3-fold | [61] |
| Polycystic ovary syndrome | HOMA | 55% NAFLD (no controls) | [62] |
| Polycystic ovary syndrome | Various (meta-analysis) | Odds ratio (95% CI) 3.93 (2.17, 7.11) | [63] |

and increased triglyceride synthesis, an effect compounded by the relatively higher hepatic insulin exposure.

## Is insulin resistance always associated with NAFLD?

The common and classical clinical conditions where insulin resistance is a feature are associated with a high prevalence of NAFLD. This applies, for example, to obesity, the 'metabolic syndrome', polycystic ovary syndrome and prediabetic insulin-resistant states such as exists in women with a previous history of gestational diabetes. In obesity, NAFLD may be present in 60–70% and NAFLD rates are generally two- to fourfold elevated in insulin-resistant conditions compared with matched controls (Table 3.3).

The association is however not universal. Adult patients with conventionally treated hypopituitarism, who are deficient in growth hormone, are insulin resistant and have central adiposity, hypertension, hypertriglyceridaemia and low HDL cholesterol levels – metabolic syndrome features. Nonetheless, their rates of NAFD are no greater than those observed in weight-matched normal controls whose pituitary function is intact, at least in subjects of European origin. Growth hormone replacement, although it leads to reduced abdominal subcutaneous and visceral fat, does not reduce liver fat content [64]. The metabolic basis for this dissociation is unknown.

There are other clinical situations where there is a dissociation between insulin resistance and steatosis. One such is in the presence of a genetic insulin receptor mutation. These people have severe insulin resistance with normal liver fat content [65]. In a mouse model with a specific deletion of the *hepatic* insulin receptor, the animals are markedly insulin resistant without hepatic steatosis [66].

Despite the exceptions, insulin resistance and NAFD are generally very closely associated. Emphasis has been placed on the importance of resistance to insulin at the liver, so-called *hepatic* insulin resistance. The rationale for this emphasis is unclear as hepatic steatosis is largely driven by the excessive supply of fatty acids, most of which derive from peripheral or visceral adipose tissue (and visceral adipose tissue may be especially important in that it is more responsive than subcutaneous adipose tissue to catecholamine-mediated lipolysis [67]). Insulin resistance in muscle leads to diminished glucose uptake and hyperglycaemia, and the resultant increase in secretion of insulin favours triglyceride storage in the liver.

The importance of hepatic fatty acid uptake is illustrated in another mouse model with an adenovirus-induced knockdown of FATP2 or FATP5 (which normally induce transfer of fatty acids from the circulation into the liver). These animals have reduced hepatic triglyceride accumulation when fed a high-fat, insulin resistance-inducing diet [68]. Humans with a polymorphism of FATP5 readily develop hepatic steatosis and other components of the metabolic syndrome [51].

The possibility that hepatic steatosis is primary and that insulin resistance is the secondary phenomenon has also been considered (discussed in a thoughtful review by Farese et al. [69]). Hepatic steatosis can occur in the absence of insulin resistance, as has been observed in numerous animal models where there are abnormalities of fatty acid synthesis, oxidation, mobilisation or storage. In man also, mutations or variation in genes affecting triglyceride metabolism can result in liver fat accumulation without accompanying insulin resistance.

The roles of the specific fatty acid moieties in hepatic triglyceride, diglyceride, cholesterol ester and ceramides have been reviewed with accumulating evidence that some of these molecules, especially some diglycerides and ceramides, play a role in reducing insulin's actions [70]. Specific diglycerides, ceramides and fatty acyl CoAs have been associated with hepatic insulin resistance [71]. Plausible mechanisms have been described for this including diglyceride activation of protein kinase Cs and ceramide-induced activation of atypical protein kinase Cs and c-Jun N-terminal kinases. There are few data in man, but when circulating cholesterol ester and phospholipid fatty acid compositions are used as surrogates for what is present in the liver, relationships between individual fatty acid moieties and insulin sensitivity have been observed (as have ethnic differences). This is an area that warrants further study.

### Insulin resistance and steatohepatitis

The mechanisms underlying the development of inflammatory change and later fibrosis in relation to hepatic steatosis are uncertain, but insulin resistance probably plays a role. Insulin-resistant conditions are pro-inflammatory, with effects observed in adipose tissue, the liver and elsewhere. There is a low-grade chronic inflammatory state with increased levels of some cytokines and acute phase proteins, and activation of inflammatory signalling pathways. Cytokines, particularly IL-6, TNF-α and IL-1β, have been implicated and may lead to elevated circulating C-reactive protein (reviewed in Refs [48, 72]). Once excess fat is deposited in the liver, this may enhance inflammation locally as fatty acids in high quantities have pro-inflammatory effects in their own right.

Ketogenesis is extremely insulin sensitive and low levels of circulating 3-hydroxybutyrate and acetoacetate have been observed in obese people with steatohepatitis relative to those with steatosis alone [73]. Levels of liver RNA for some of the important genes regulating ketogenesis are also reduced. It is uncertain if the low ketone body and ketogenic enzyme levels are related to insulin sensitivity but levels did correlate significantly and positively with circulating NEFA and the adipose tissue insulin resistance index suggesting that this may be the case.

### Conclusions

Insulin resistance and liver triglyceride accumulation are highly associated and in most situations where one exists, so does the other. Although there are exceptions, the close association suggests at the least that there are common underlying mechanisms, perhaps even a causative relationship in most circumstances. The most plausible mechanism is that insulin resistance leads to increased adipose tissue lipolysis and enhanced fatty acid delivery to the liver. The liver itself is primed for fatty acid uptake and triglyceride accumulation by a combination of insulin resistance and hyperinsulinaemia, even if export in VLDL is elevated.

### References

1. Monetti M, Nagaraj N, Sharma K, Mann M. Large-scale phosphosite quantification in tissues by a spike-in SILAC method. Nat Methods. 2011;8:655–58.
2. Seppälä-Lindroos A, Vehkavaara S, Häkkinen AM, Goto T, Westerbacka J, Sovijärvi A, et al. Fat accumulation in the liver is associated with defects in insulin suppression of glucose production and serum free fatty acids independent of obesity in normal men. J Clin Endocrinol Metab. 2002;87:3023–8.
3. Bugianesi E, Gastaldelli A, Vanni E, Gambino R, Cassader M, Baldi S, et al. Insulin resistance in non-diabetic patients with non-alcoholic fatty liver disease: sites and mechanisms. Diabetologia. 2005;48:634–42.
4. Kotronen A, Juurinen L, Tiikkainen M, Vehkavaara S, Yki-Järvinen H. Increased liver fat, impaired insulin clearance, and hepatic and adipose tissue insulin resistance in type 2 diabetes. Gastroenterology. 2008;135:122–30.
5. Mehta SR, Godsland IF, Thomas EL, Pavitt DV, Morin SX, Bell JD, et al. Intrahepatic insulin exposure, intrahepatocellular lipid and regional body fat in nonalcoholic fatty liver disease. J Clin Endocrinol Metab. 2012;97:2151–9.
6. DeFronzo RA, Tobin JD, Andres R. Glucose clamp technique: a method for quantifying insulin secretion and resistance. Am J Physiol. 1979;237:E214–33.
7. Kolterman OG, Gray RS, Griffin J, Burstein P, Insel J, Scarlett JA, et al. Receptor and postreceptor defects contribute to the insulin resistance in noninsulin-dependent diabetes mellitus. J Clin Invest. 1981;68:957–69.
8. Aitman TJ, Godsland IF, Farren B, Crook D, Wong J, Scott J. Defects of insulin action on fatty acid and carbohydrate metabolism in familial combined hyperlipidaemia. Arterioscler Thromb Vasc Biol. 1997;17:748–54.
9. Kolterman OG, Insel J, Saekow M, Olefsky JM. Mechanisms of insulin resistance in human obesity: evidence for receptor and postreceptor defects. J Clin Invest. 1980;65:1272–84.
10. Bergman RN, Ider YZ, Bowden CR, Cobelli C. Quantitative estimation of insulin sensitivity. Am J Physiol. 1979;236:E667–77.
11. Caumo AC, Cobelli C. Hepatic glucose production during the labelled IVGTT: estimation by deconvolution with a new minimal model. Am J Physiol. 1993;264:E829–41.

12. Kahn SE, Prigeon RL, McCulloch DK, Boyko EJ, Bergman RN, Schwartz MW, et al. Quantification of the relationship between insulin sensitivity and beta-cell function in human subjects. Evidence for a hyperbolic function. Diabetes. 1993;42:1663–72.

13. Cobelli C, Pacini G. Insulin secretion and hepatic extraction in humans by minimal modelling of C-peptide and insulin kinetics. Diabetes. 1988;37:223–31.

14. Watanabe RM, Vølund A, Roy S, Bergman RN. Prehepatic beta-cell secretion during the intravenous glucose tolerance test in humans: application of a combined model of insulin and C-peptide kinetics. J Clin Endocrinol Metab. 1989;69:790–7.

15. Otten J, Ahrén B, Olsson T. Surrogate measures of insulin sensitivity vs the hyperinsulinaemic-euglycaemic clamp: a meta-analysis. Diabetologia. 2014;57:1781–8.

16. Simonson DC. Surrogate measures of insulin resistance: does one size fit all? Diabetologia. 2015;58:207–10.

17. Matthews DR, Hosker JP, Rudenski AS, Naylor BA, Treacher DF, Turner RC. Homeostasis model assessment: insulin resistance and ß-cell function from fasting plasma glucose and insulin concentrations in man. Diabetologia. 1985;28:412–19.

18. Katz A, Nambi SS, Mather K, Baron AD, Follmann DA, Sullivan G, et al. Quantitative insulin sensitivity check index: a simple, accurate method for assessing insulin sensitivity in humans. J Clin Endocrinol Metab. 2000;85:2402–10.

19. Matsuda M, DeFronzo RA. Insulin sensitivity indices obtained from oral glucose tolerance testing. Diabetes Care. 1999;22:1462–70.

20. Stumvoll M, Mitrakou A, Pimenta W, Jenssen T, Yki-Järvinen H, Van Haeften T, et al. Use of the oral glucose tolerance test to assess insulin release and insulin sensitivity. Diabetes Care. 2000;23:295–301.

21. Gutt M, Davis CL, Spitzer SB, Llabre MM, Kumar M, Czarnecki EM, et al. Validation of the insulin sensitivity index (ISI(0,120)): comparison with other measures. Diabetes Res Clin Pract. 2000;47:177–84.

22. Belfiore F, Iannello S, Volpicelli G. Insulin sensitivity indices calculated from basal and OGTT-induced insulin, glucose, and FFA levels. Mol Genet Metab. 1998;63:134–41.

23. Cederholm J, Wibell L. Insulin release and peripheral sensitivity at the oral glucose tolerance test. Diabetes Res Clin Pract. 1990;10:167–75.

24. Mari A, Pacini G, Murphy E, Ludvik B, Nolan JJ. A model based method for assessing insulin sensitivity from the oral glucose tolerance test. Diabetes Care. 2001;24:539–48.

25. Abdul-Ghani MA, Matsuda M, Balas B, DeFronzo RA. Muscle and liver insulin resistance indexes derived from the oral glucose tolerance test. Diabetes Care. 2007;30:89–94.

26. Gelding SV, Robinson S, Lowe S, Niththyananthan R, Johnston DG. Validation of the low dose short insulin tolerance test for evaluation of insulin sensitivity. Clin Endocrinol. 1994;40:611–5.

27. DeFronzo RA, Ferrannini E, Simonson DC. Fasting hyperglycemia in non-insulin-dependent diabetes mellitus: contributions of excessive hepatic glucose production and impaired tissue glucose uptake. Metabolism. 1989;38:387–9.

28. Radziuk J, Norwich KH, Vranic M. Experimental validation of measurements of glucose turnover in nonsteady state. Am J Physiol. 1978;234:E84–93.

29. Borra R, Lautamäki R, Parkkola R, Komu M, Sijens PE, Hällsten K, et al. Inverse association between liver fat content and hepatic glucose uptake in patients with type 2 diabetes mellitus. Metab Clin Exp. 2008;57:1445–51.

30. Sanyal AJ, Campbell-Sargent C, Mirshahi F, Rizzo WB, Contos MJ, Sterling RK, et al. Nonalcoholic steatohepatitis: association of insulin resistance and mitochondrial abnormalities. Gastroenterology. 2001;120:1183–92.

31. Zoratti R, Godsland IF, Chaturvedi N, Crook D, Stevenson JC, McKeigue PM. Relation of plasma lipids to insulin resistance, non-esterified fatty acid levels and body fat in men from three ethnic groups: relevance to variation in risk of diabetes and coronary disease. Metabolism. 2000;49:245–52.

32. Periwal V, Chow CC, Bergman RN, Ricks M, Vega GL, Sumner AE. Evaluation of quantitative models of the effect of insulin on lipolysis and glucose disposal. Am J Physiol Regul Integr Comp Physiol. 2008;295:R1089–96.

33. Gelding SV, Coldham N, Niththyananthan R, Anyaoku V, Johnston DG. Insulin resistance with respect to lipolysis in non-diabetic relatives of European patients with type 2 diabetes. Diabet Med. 1995;12:66–73.

34. Kooner JS, Baliga RR, Wilding J, Crook D, Packard CJ, Banks LM, et al. Abdominal obesity, impaired nonesterified fatty acid suppression, and insulin-mediated glucose disposal are early metabolic abnormalities in families with premature myocardial infarction. Arterioscler Thromb Vasc Biol. 1998;18:1021–6.

35. Gastaldelli A, Harrison SA, Belfort-Aguilar R, Hardies LJ, Balas B, Schenker S, et al. Importance of changes in adipose tissue insulin resistance to histological response during thiazolidinedione treatment of patients with nonalcoholic steatohepatitis. Hepatology. 2009;50:1087–93.

36. Lomonaco R, Ortiz-Lopez C, Orsak B, Webb A, Hardies J, Darland C, et al. Effect of adipose tissue insulin resistance on metabolic parameters and liver histology in obese patients with nonalcoholic fatty liver disease. Hepatology. 2012;55:1389–97.

37. Baynes C, Henderson AD, Richmond W, Johnston DG, Elkeles RS. The response of hepatic lipase and serum lipoproteins to acute hyperinsulinaemia in type 2 diabetes. Eur J Clin Investig. 1992;22:341–46.

38. Sadur C, Eckel R. Insulin stimulation of adipose tissue lipoprotein lipase. J Clin Invest. 1982;69:1119–25.

39. Patsch W, Franz S, Schonfeld G. Role of insulin in lipoprotein secretion by cultured rat hepatocytes. J Clin Invest. 1983;71:1161–74.

40. Lin MCM, Gordon D, Wetterau JR. Microsomal triglyceride transfer protein (MTP) in HepG2 cells: insulin negatively regulates MTP gene expression. J Lipid Res. 1995; 36:1073–81.

41. Lewis GF, Uffelman KD, Szeto LW, Weller B, Steiner G. Interaction between free fatty acids and insulin in the acute control of very low density lipoprotein production in humans. J Clin Invest. 1995;95:158–66.

42. Malmström R, Packard CJ, Caslake M, Bedford D, Stewart P, Yki-Järvinen H, et al. Defective regulation of triglyceride metabolism by insulin in the liver in NIDDM. Diabetologia. 1997;40:454–62.

43. Simmons RK, Alberti KG, Gale EA, Colagiuri S, Tuomilehto J, Qiao Q, et al. The metabolic syndrome: useful concept or clinical tool? Report of a WHO Expert Consultation. Diabetologia. 2010;53:600–5.

44. Godsland IF, Johnston DG. Co-associations between insulin sensitivity and measures of liver function, subclinical inflammation and hematology. Metabolism. 2008;57: 1190–7.

45. Shulman GI. Ectopic fat in insulin resistance, dyslipidemia, and cardiometabolic disease. N Engl J Med. 2014;371: 1131–41.

46. Raghow R, Yellaturu C, Deng X, Park EA, Elam MB. SREBPs: the crossroads of physiological and pathological lipid homeostasis. Trends Endocrinol Metab. 2008;19:65–73.

47. Brown MS, Goldstein JL. Selective versus total insulin resistance: a pathogenic paradox. Cell Metabolism. 2008;7: 95–6.

48. Sparks JD, Sparks CE, Adeli K. Selective hepatic insulin resistance, VLDL overproduction, and hypertriglyceridemia. Arterioscler Thromb Vasc Biol. 2012;32:2104–12.

49. Wu X, Chen K, Williams KJ. The role of pathway-selective insulin resistance and responsiveness in diabetic dyslipoproteinemia. Curr Opin Lipidol. 2012;23:334–44.

50. Donnelly KL, Smith CI, Schwarzenberg SJ, Jessurun J, Boldt MD, Parks EJ. Sources of fatty acids stored in liver and secreted via lipoproteins in patients with nonalcoholic fatty liver disease. J Clin Invest. 2005;115:1343–51.

51. Auinger A, Valenti L, Pfeuffer M, Helwig U, Herrmann J, Fracanzani AL, et al. A promoter polymorphism in the liver-specific fatty acid transport protein 5 is associated with features of the metabolic syndrome and steatosis. Horm Metab Res. 2010;42:854–9.

52. Berlanga A, Guiu-Jurado E, Porras JA, Auguet T. Molecular pathways in non-alcoholic fatty liver disease. Clin Exp Gastroenterol. 2014;7:221–39.

53. Forbes S, Robinson S, Dungu J, Anyaoku V, Bannister P, Forster D, et al. Sustained endogenous glucose production, diminished lipolysis and non-esterified fatty acid appearance and oxidation in non-obese women at high risk of type 2 diabetes. Eur J Endocrinol. 2006;155:469–76.

54. Forbes S, Godsland IF, Taylor-Robinson SD, Bell JD, Thomas EL, Patel N, et al. A history of previous gestational diabetes mellitus is associated with adverse changes in insulin secretion and VLDL metabolism independently of increased intrahepatocellular lipid. Diabetologia. 2013;56:2021–33.

55. Swinburn BA, Nyomba BL, Saad MF, Zurlo F, Raz I, Knowler WC, et al. Insulin resistance associated with lower rates of weight gain in Pima Indians. J Clin Invest. 1991;88:168–73.

56. Anderson SG, Dunn WB, Banerjee M, Brown M, Broadhurst DI, Goodacre R, et al. Evidence that multiple defects in lipid regulation occur before hyperglycemia during the prodrome of type-2 diabetes. PLoS ONE. 2014;9:e103217.

57. Forbes S, Taylor-Robinson SD, Patel N, Allan P, Walker BR, Johnston DG. Increased prevalence of non-alcoholic fatty liver disease in European women with a history of gestational diabetes. Diabetologia. 2011;54:641–7.

58. Prikoszovich T, Winzer C, Schmid AI, Szendroedi J, Chmelik M, Pacini G, et al. Body and liver fat mass rather than muscle mitochondrial function determine glucose metabolism in women with a history of gestational diabetes mellitus. Diabetes Care. 2011;34:430–6.

59. Browning JD, Szczepaniak LS, Dobbins R, Nuremberg P, Horton JD, Cohen JC, et al. Prevalence of hepatic steatosis in an urban population in the United States: impact of ethnicity. Hepatology. 2004;40:1387–95.

60. Bedogni G, Miglioli L, Masutti F, Tiribelli C, Marchesini G, Bellentani S. Prevalence of and risk factors for nonalcoholic fatty liver disease: the Dionysos nutrition and liver study. Hepatology. 2005;42:44–52.

61. Smits MM, Ioannou GN, Boyko EJ, Utzschneider KM. Non-alcoholic fatty liver disease as an independent manifestation of the metabolic syndrome: results of a US national survey in three ethnic groups. J Gastroenterol Hepatol. 2013;28:664–70.

62. Gambarin-Gelwan M, Kinkhabwala SV, Schiano TD, Bodian C, Yeh HC, Futterweit W. Prevalence of nonalcoholic fatty liver disease in women with polycystic ovary syndrome. Clin Gastroenterol Hepatol. 2007;5:496–501.

63. Ramezani-Binabaj M, Motalebi M, Karimi-Sari H, Rezaee-Zavareh MS, Alavian SM. Are women with polycystic ovarian syndrome at a high risk of non-alcoholic Fatty liver disease; a meta-analysis. Hepat Mon. 2014;14:e23235.

64. Gardner CJ, Irwin AJ, Daousi C, McFarlane IA, Joseph F, Bell JD, et al. Hepatic steatosis, GH deficiency and the effects of GH replacement: a Liverpool magnetic resonance spectroscopy study. Eur J Endocrinol. 2012;166:993–1002.

65. Semple RK, Sleigh A, Murgatroyd PR, Adams CA, Bluck L, Jackson S, et al. Postreceptor insulin resistance contributes to human dyslipidemia and hepatic steatosis. J Clin Invest. 2009;119:315–22.

66. Biddinger SB, Hernandez-Ono A, Rask-Madsen C, Haas JT, Alemán JO, Suzuki R, et al. Hepatic insulin resistance is sufficient to produce dyslipidemia and susceptibility to atherosclerosis. Cell Metab. 2008;7:125–3.

67. Wahrenberg H, Lönnqvist F, Arner P. Mechanisms underlying regional differences in lipolysis in human adipose tissue. J Clin Invest. 1989;84:458–67.

68. Doege H, Baillie RA, Ortegon AM, Tsang B, Wu Q, Punreddy S, et al. Targeted deletion of FATP5 reveals multiple functions in liver metabolism: alterations in hepatic lipid homeostasis. Gastroenterology. 2006;130:1245–58.

69. Farese RVJ, Zechner R, Newgard CB, Walther TC. The problem of establishing relationships between hepatic steatosis and hepatic insulin resistance. Cell Metab. 2012;15:570–3.

70. Galbo T, Perry RJ, Jurczak MJ, Camporez JP, Alves TC, Kahn M, et al. Saturated and unsaturated fat induce hepatic insulin resistance independently of TLR-4 signaling and ceramide synthesis in vivo. Proc Natl Acad Sci U S A. 2013; 30:12780–5.

71. Konstantynowicz-Nowicka K, Harasim E, Baranowski M, Chabowski A. New evidence for the role of ceramide in the development of hepatic insulin resistance. PLoS One. 2015; 10(1):e0116858.

72. Meshkani R, Adeli K. Hepatic insulin resistance, metabolic syndrome and cardiovascular disease. Clin Biochem. 2009; 42:1331–46.

73. Männistö VT, Simonen M, Hyysalo J, Soininen P, Kangas AJ, Kaminska D, et al. Ketone body production is differentially altered in steatosis and non-alcoholic steatohepatitis in obese humans. Liver Int. 2015; 35:1853–61.

# Paediatric NAFLD: A distinct disease with the propensity for progressive fibrosis

**4**

**Emer Fitzpatrick and Anil Dhawan**

Paediatric Liver Centre, King's College London School of Medicine, King's College Hospital, London, UK

## LEARNING POINTS

- To understand the burden of NAFLD in children, its presentation and difficulties in diagnosis and appreciate the differences between paediatric and adult NAFLD.

- To examine the developmental origins of paediatric NAFLD and understand how this may influence presentation and outcome.

- To explore how the histological pattern of paediatric NAFLD may have an association with more aggressive fibrotic disease and hence the outcome.

## Introduction

The global epidemic of obesity/overweight has been central to the appearance of fatty liver disease, both in adults and children in the last two decades. Several genetic and epigenetic factors have been attributed to explain the variability and severity of the disease in patients with comparable body mass indices. Body growth is unique to paediatric population, necessitating higher body weight to calorie requirements, compared to adults and could partly explain the historic practice of feeding children high-fat and high-sugar foods. Liver in childhood has lower probability of exposure to toxins like alcohol and other environmental toxins. However, the complex interaction between nutritional toxins (saturated fats and sugar) with the liver cells of the maturing liver is less well studied but with suggestions that fibrosis as end result of hepatocyte injury is somehow more exaggerated in the paediatric population than adults and could theoretically cause accelerated cirrhosis. Additional factors to consider are the effects of under-nutrition in intrauterine life and over-nutrition in early infancy, as both these factors have been associated with higher incidence of insulin resistance in later life [1]. Children and teenagers are the highest consumers of fructose [2, 3], with emerging evidence that this may be implicated in the development and severity of NAFLD [4]. This chapter will describe unique features of childhood NAFLD, compared to adults with focus on factors that could be responsible for the development of accelerated fibrosis and cirrhosis.

The evidence for long-term outcome for children with NAFLD is largely unknown. Though suspected to have a high prevalence in Western countries, affecting 5–10% of school-age children [5, 6] and 44–70% of obese children [7, 8], we know worryingly little about outcome and appropriately targeting management. A major question is whether the epidemic of NAFLD in school-age children will lead to a major increase in need for liver transplantation within the next decade. We do not have evidence for this currently, but the presence of bridging fibrosis secondary to NAFLD in prepubertal children demonstrates that this is a real concern.

There are very few long-term follow-up studies of children who were diagnosed with NAFLD in childhood. Thus, the real outcome of children with this condition is unknown. There is an argument that outcome in terms of liver disease for those affected earlier in life will be worse. The question of whether paediatric NAFLD, which is often histologically distinct from adult NAFLD, is the same disease or something different needs also to be addressed.

*Clinical Dilemmas in Non-Alcoholic Fatty Liver Disease*, First Edition. Edited by Roger Williams and Simon D. Taylor-Robinson.
© 2016 John Wiley & Sons, Ltd. Published 2016 by John Wiley & Sons, Ltd.

In particular, the question as to whether fibrosis has the potential to progress to cirrhosis in children more than in adults is an interesting one. Though other types of paediatric liver disease are rare, large numbers of those affected will require liver transplantation. The best example is biliary atresia in which only 20% will be alive with their native liver in their 20s [9] and if corrective surgery does not result in jaundice clearance, transplantation is required within the first 2 years of life. Other relatively common paediatric liver diseases, such as autoimmune hepatitis and Wilson disease, often progress very rapidly and may either present with decompensated cirrhosis in the first instance or may progress to end-stage liver disease during childhood.

## Developmental origins of paediatric NAFLD

The *in utero* transmission of the metabolic phenotype by obese mothers to their offspring has become a focus of interest. The 'priming' of a child's liver, even before birth, to injury, with lipid accumulation, increased oxidative stress, apoptosis and innate immune dysfunction may play a role in the development of NAFLD in these children. As 60% of mothers are now obese at the time of conception [10], this is an important epidemiological phenomenon. MRI findings demonstrate that maternal BMI predicts fetal intrahepatic lipid accumulation [11]. As deposition of adipose tissue does not occur until the third trimester, storage of the excess substrate that the fetus is exposed to during pregnancy appears to utilise the liver [12].

Mouralidarane et al. have clearly demonstrated *in utero* high-fat diet exposure results in lipid accumulation in addition to elevated levels of oxidative stress and impairment of innate immunity in a mouse model [13]. In this study, offspring mice were followed to 12 months following exposure to maternal obesity and a post-weaning high-fat diet. Both factors were independent risk factors for steatosis and at 12 months for steatohepatitis and fibrosis. There was a significant increase in liver injury in those exposed to both maternal obesity and a high-fat post-weaning diet [13]. Increased mRNA expression of inflammatory cytokines and fibrogenic enzymes were also found.

Taken together, this 'priming' of the liver, which may then be exposed to years of excess nutrition and sedentary behaviour, can result in a worse phenotype and/or more accelerated disease than would otherwise have been the case.

Interestingly, a macaque model of high-fat diet-fed macaques who were fed with a normal chow diet prior to breeding and during pregnancy produced offspring with substantially less steatosis than those who remained on the high-fat diet [14].

## Paediatric NAFLD: Histological evidence of early progression

Diagnosis of NAFLD on a histological basis is considerably less frequent than using non-invasive proxy measures (such as transaminases and liver ultrasound) to diagnose the condition in epidemiological studies. In order to qualify for liver biopsy, children may need considerably abnormal liver function tests and/or splenomegaly. Despite this relative referral bias, the prevalence of already significant fibrosis in large series of children with NAFLD including some reports of cirrhosis during childhood is of concern. This is, notwithstanding, relatively short exposure time to the environmental risk factors cited.

One of the earliest reports of children with NAFLD cirrhosis came from Molleston et al., with rapid progression of disease and decompensation of liver disease in childhood in one [15]. The first prospective series of children with NAFLD in 2000 also reported a 9-year-old with cirrhosis [16]. Similar findings have been reported in other large series since that time [15, 17–23].

The prevalence of significant fibrosis (generally taken as a fibrosis stage ≥ F2) at diagnosis varies across studies. There is, of course, an inherent bias in these figures as to merit a liver biopsy. There are generally some other markers present of more advanced disease. Nevertheless, the presence of significant liver damage in pre-teen children, in a disease that is thought to take years, if not decades, to develop, is concerning. The US NASH clinical research network (CRN) reported a prevalence of moderate or more severe fibrosis, including bridging and cirrhosis of 30% in children who were recruited [24]. In a UK paediatric series, 51% were staged as ≥ F2 [25] and an Italian paediatric series described advanced fibrosis (≥F3) in 15% [26].

## Paediatric NAFLD: A distinct disease?

Children may often have a different pattern of disease to adults with greater degree of steatosis, less prominent ballooning and portal, rather than pericentral accentuation of inflammation and fibrosis (type 2 NASH) [27]. In classical type 1 NASH, fibrosis occurs in the perisinusoidal region with a chicken wire pattern around hepatocytes [28]. The pattern of fibrosis in type 2 NAFLD is periportal. Schwimmer et al. reviewed the histological findings in a cohort of 100 children (2–18 years) with biopsy-proven NAFLD [17]. Type 1 NASH was present in 17% and type 2 NASH in 51% of the children. Sixteen per cent of biopsies had overlapping features of type 1 and 2 disease and the remaining 16% showed simple steatosis. Children with type 2 NASH were younger and had greater severity of obesity than in type 1 NASH. Boys and those of Asian, Native American and Hispanic ethnicities were more likely to have type 2 NASH. In contrast, in a study from Italy of 57 children with NASH, only 2.4% had type 1 NASH, and 28.6% were classified as type 2 NASH, whereas the majority (52.4%) had an overlap between the two (17% had simple steatosis) [18]. In a UK series of 45 children with NAFLD, 60% had type 2 NASH, 20% had mixed features, and no child was found to have classical type 1 NASH (20% had simples steatosis) [25]. Takahashi reports the presence of type 2 NASH in 9% of adult patients and 21% of paediatric patients studied in Japan [29]. The mechanism leading to the different phenotypes of NAFLD is not yet understood.

The NASH CRN reviewed the occurrence of portal inflammation as a distinct entity in NASH [30]. A study of biopsies from 728 adults and 205 children found that the presence of portal inflammation in adults was associated with older, female patients with a higher BMI and insulin resistance. There was a clear association with amount and location of steatosis, ballooning and advanced fibrosis. In the paediatric group, portal inflammation was associated with younger age, azonal location of steatosis and more advanced fibrosis (bridging). In both groups, it was associated with diagnosis of definitive NASH. There was no association with lobular inflammation in either group. It is not clear if this pattern is due to a separate pathophysiological mechanism, though it certainly seems to be a marker of more advanced NASH.

Varying patterns of fibrosis are found in different liver diseases. These differences may be due to a combination of the localisation of tissue damage and/or to the location of the different effector cells involved. Fibrosis in viral hepatitis follows a porto-central bridging pattern with interface hepatitis [31]. Biliary fibrosis follows more of a porto-portal pattern. In both, the ductular reaction (DR) has been found to be associated with severity of fibrosis [32]. The DR is a response to the activation of the proliferation of hepatic progenitor cells (HPCs), the secondary pathway of liver regeneration and repair. Normally in liver injury, hepatocyte replacement occurs by the regeneration of mature adjacent hepatocytes. The secondary pathway comes into effect when there is chronic or severe injury [33]. Biliary epithelial cells that contain HPCs appear in the periportal zone. HPCs are bipotent and can differentiate into both biliary epithelial cells and hepatocytes. In human liver disease, DR correlates with severity of fibrosis across a number of different liver diseases including hepatitis C [34], alcoholic liver disease, hereditary haemochromatosis [35] and recurrence of viral hepatitis post-liver transplantation [36], in addition to NAFLD. In cholestatic disorders, a florid DR often accompanies fibrosis [37]. The exact relationship between DR and fibrosis is not yet fully understood [38]. The level of portal inflammation has also been found to correlate with the DR and fibrosis.

## Ductular reaction, hedgehog signalling and advanced fibrosis

The portal activity in type 2 NASH mirrors that of the DR, which has been reported in NAFLD. The possible epithelial–mesenchymal transition of biliary cells in this process may relate to the pattern of fibrosis seen [39]. Richardson and colleagues reported that the extent of DR was associated with both fibrosis stage and NASH grade [39].

The question of why this pattern of injury differs in paediatric from adult livers is unknown. The susceptibility of the immature hepatocytes to various insults may be different and may be a contributing factor. In addition, the zonation of hepatocyte functions is well known. For example, enzymes, which are involved in the Krebs cycle, are found predominantly in zone 1, whereas p450 enzymes are preferentially located in zone 3. Children are actively growing and the pattern of disease seen may also reflect this in some way [40].

It is likely that the repair mechanism, or rather the propensity and vigour with which the liver regenerates, is different according to maturity and developmental stage. Fibroblast-specific protein (FSP) 100, a fibroblast marker, was greater in interlobular ductal cells in child-aged control (healthy) liver than adult control liver, demonstrating that ductal epithelial cells in children have a greater tendency to exhibit features of mesenchymal cells and implying epithelial–mesenchymal transition is more active within portal tracts in children [37].

Work undertaken by Diehl and colleagues over the last decade has explored the possible role of hedgehog (Hh) signalling in NAFLD [41]. The Hh pathway is a pivotal morphogenic signalling pathway central in organogenesis. The pathway becomes quiescent in the liver during adolescence and reactivates in the presence of injury. Thus, Hh signalling is involved in the activation of the regenerative pathway of liver. Healthy paediatric livers demonstrate more Hh signalling than healthy adult livers. Increased exposure to Hh ligands stimulated cells involved in wound healing. Normally these cells are tightly regulated however when deregulated, chronic inflammation, fibrosis and liver cancer may result. If children possess a proportionally greater number of Hh ligand-producing cells and Hh-responsive cells, then children may be at particular risk from insults that promote activation of the Hh pathway [42].

Guy et al. examined the association of portal fibrosis with the activation of the regenerative Hh signalling [41]. The number of Hh-responsive cells correlated closely with both portal injury and the severity of fibrosis in liver biopsies of adult's patients with NAFLD ($P < 0.0001$) supporting a relationship between Hh activation and liver damage [41]. For this study, immunohistochemistry for Hh ligand and Gli1 (Hh-responsive cells) was undertaken on 90 biopsies within the NASH CRN repository.

A follow-on study in children again demonstrated more Hh activation with good correlation of Hh ligand expression and Hh-responsive cells to liver injury and severity of disease [42].

## What do we know from other types of paediatric chronic liver disease?

It is not clear what makes children susceptible to fibrosis progression in some liver diseases and not in others. The nature of the insult may be relevant, but there is considerable heterogeneity within the same disease process. For example, in biliary atresia, the most common liver condition necessitating transplantation in childhood, there is huge variability in progression of fibrosis. This is even the case within cohorts where corrective surgery was undertaken at a young age and by the same experienced operator [43]. Similarly, though hepatitis C is widely regarded as a slowly progressive disease in childhood, there are reports of cirrhotic transformation in childhood. Autoimmune liver disease and Wilson disease frequently present as end-stage liver disease in childhood – again it is not clear why fibrosis progresses at such a rate in some and not in others. There is

likely to be both genetic and epigenetic factors involved in fibrosis progression in children with all types of chronic liver disease. To date, it has not been possible to distinguish rapid from slow 'fibrosers'. With the emergence of genome-wide association studies (GWAS), genetic profiling those who develop more rapid fibrosis has become of great interest. In the case of NAFLD, several GWAS have been published. The most consistent risk factor for both steatosis and fibrosis severity is homogeneity for the rs738409 GG genotype of PNPLA3. In an Italian cohort, the GG genotype was found in 32% of paediatric patients with NASH versus 1% of those without NASH giving an odds ratio (OR) of 52 for developing NASH. The number of children who had GG genotype only accounted for 16% of the entire cohort. The OR in an adult cohort from both Italy and the United Kingdom gave a lower OR of 1.7 for both NASH and fibrosis [44]. Again the prevalence of GG in the NAFLD group as a whole was 14%. It is clear that single genotypic variants cannot explain the majority of the heterogeneity in inflammation and fibrosis between patients. A combination of multiple genetic variations may be contributory however and is the subject of further study [45].

## What are the known risk factors for progression of fibrosis in NAFLD?

There are several well-described long-term studies in adult patients with NAFLD within which risk factors for progression of disease may be identified. In the absence of similar studies in paediatric patients, the findings from adult studies need to be considered. A consistent finding from adult studies is that simple steatosis without evidence of inflammation or fibrosis appears to have a benign course while NASH is a potentially serious condition, which can progress to cirrhosis. In a 10-year follow-up of 132 individuals with NAFLD, 22% of those with NASH versus 4% of those with simple steatosis went on to develop cirrhosis [46]. There was also a significantly higher liver-related mortality in the time period in the NASH group. Ekstedt et al. followed 129 patients over a mean period of 13.7 years and found progression of liver fibrosis in 44% [47]. All causes of mortality were higher in the NASH group versus those with simple steatosis, particularly from cardiovascular and liver-related deaths. Four hundred and twenty patients with NAFLD were followed in the Rochester Epidemiology Project, a population-based study. Liver-related mortality was the third leading cause of death in those with NAFLD [48]. Cirrhosis was present at follow-up in 5% of cohort. Adams et al.

reported a series of 103 patients with NAFLD with follow-up biopsy at a mean interval of 3.2 years and found that fibrosis progressed in 37%, remained stable in 34% and regressed in 29% [49]. A higher BMI and diabetes were associated with fibrosis progression. A systematic review of 10 studies including 221 patients with a mean follow-up of 5.6 years concluded that fibrosis progressed in 37.6% of those with NASH [50]. Musso et al. reported a further systematic review of 40 cohort studies examining the natural history of NAFLD in adults [51]. The authors found an overall and cause-specific pooled increase in mortality in those with NAFLD (OR 1.57 (1.18–2.1)) versus the general population. In those with a steatotic liver on ultrasound, the risk of mortality from cardiovascular disease was increased by an OR of 2.05, with an OR of 3.5 for the development of type 2 diabetes. With subgroup analysis patients with simple steatosis were found to have a similar mortality as the general population and those with NASH had an OR of 1.81 for overall mortality. The excess cause of death in this subgroup was mainly liver related with an incidence of 11–17% versus 1.7–2.7% in those with simple steatosis.

A systematic review of paired biopsy studies including 11 cohorts of 411 patients with biopsy-proven NAFLD demonstrated 33.6% fibrosis progression over 2145.5 person-years of follow-up. This meta-analysis suggested that patients with NAFL (steatosis) progressed through 1 stage of fibrosis in 14.3 years, whereas those with established NASH progressed over 7 years [52]. McPherson et al. challenge the dogma that those with simple NAFL rarely progress. In 108 patients over a median of 6.6 years, 42% progressed in terms of fibrosis and this was both in those with simple NAFL and NASH at baseline [53].

Aside from degree of fibrosis at baseline, no other consistent clinical risk factors for progression have been identified. Clearly time is an important factor and children in whom NAFLD is diagnosed have potentially another 60–70 years in which fibrosis may progress [54, 55].

Obviously the removal of the environmental trigger in this disease (obesity) and the improvement in metabolic parameters are the key to reversal of liver disease. However, we know that obese children are likely to become obese adults [56, 57].

## Conclusion

In children with incidental diagnosis of NAFLD, presence of simple steatosis is not a predictor of long-term outcome. On the other hand, the presence of bridging fibrosis at diagnosis is worrisome in that fibrosis has progressed despite a relatively short exposure to environmental factors (obesity and insulin resistance).

In the few cohort studies that exist of NAFLD in childhood, cirrhosis secondary to NASH has been reported in children as young as 10 years [15, 16]. Feldstein et al. describe the long-term outcome of 66 children with NAFLD followed for up to 20 years [20] with two children requiring liver transplantation for end-stage disease. Of five children who underwent follow-up biopsy, four showed progression of fibrosis. In common with adult studies [58], in children, severity of obesity and insulin resistance seem to be predictors of advanced fibrosis [59]. The difference between the natural history of type 1 and type 2 NASH has not yet been characterised and is an important subject for future research.

## References

1. Barker DJ. The developmental origins of insulin resistance. Horm Res 2005;64(Suppl 3):2–7.
2. Vos MB, Kimmons JE, Gillespie C, Welsh J, Blanck HM. Dietary fructose consumption among US children and adults: the Third National Health and Nutrition Examination Survey. Medscape J Med. 2008;10(7):160.
3. Sluik D, Engelen AI, Feskens EJ. Fructose consumption in the Netherlands: the Dutch national food consumption survey 2007–2010. Eur J Clin Nutr. 2015;69:475–81.
4. Vos MB, Lavine JE. Dietary fructose in nonalcoholic fatty liver disease. Hepatology. 2013;57(6):2525–31.
5. Schwimmer JB, Deutsch R, Kahen T, Lavine JE, Stanley C, Behling C. Prevalence of fatty liver in children and adolescents. Pediatrics. 2006;118(4):1388–93.
6. Fraser A, Longnecker MP, Lawlor DA. Prevalence of elevated alanine aminotransferase among US adolescents and associated factors: NHANES 1999–2004. Gastroenterology. 2007;133(6): 1814–20.
7. Sartorio A, Del Col A, Agosti F, Mazzilli G, Bellentani S, Tiribelli C, et al. Predictors of non-alcoholic fatty liver disease in obese children. Eur J Clin Nutr. 2007;61(7):877–83.
8. Nobili V, Svegliati-Baroni G, Alisi A, Miele L, Valenti L, Vajro P. A 360-degree overview of paediatric NAFLD: recent insights. J Hepatol. 2013;58(6):1218–29.
9. Shinkai M, Ohhama Y, Take H, Kitagawa N, Kudo H, Mochizuki K, et al. Long-term outcome of children with biliary atresia who were not transplanted after the Kasai operation: >20-year experience at a children's hospital. J Pediatr Gastroenterol Nutr. 2009;48(4):443–50.
10. Hinkle SN, Sharma AJ, Kim SY, Park S, Dalenius K, Brindley PL, et al. Prepregnancy obesity trends among low-income women, United States, 1999–2008. Matern Child Health J. 2012;16(7):1339–48.

11. Brumbaugh DE, Tearse P, Cree-Green M, Fenton LZ, Brown M, Scherzinger A, et al. Intrahepatic fat is increased in the neonatal offspring of obese women with gestational diabetes. J Pediatr. 2013;162(5):930–6.e1.

12. Brumbaugh DE, Friedman JE. Developmental origins of non-alcoholic fatty liver disease. Pediatr Res. 2014;75(1–2):140–7.

13. Mouralidarane A, Soeda J, Visconti-Pugmire C, Samuelsson AM, Pombo J, Maragkoudaki X, et al. Maternal obesity programs offspring nonalcoholic fatty liver disease by innate immune dysfunction in mice. Hepatology. 2013;58(1):128–38.

14. McCurdy CE, Bishop JM, Williams SM, Grayson BE, Smith MS, Friedman JE, et al. Maternal high-fat diet triggers lipotoxicity in the fetal livers of nonhuman primates. J Clin Invest. 2009;119(2):323–35.

15. Molleston JP, White F, Teckman J, Fitzgerald JF. Obese children with steatohepatitis can develop cirrhosis in childhood. Am J Gastroenterol. 2002;97(9):2460–2.

16. Rashid M, Roberts EA. Nonalcoholic steatohepatitis in children. J Pediatr Gastroenterol Nutr. 2000;30(1):48–53.

17. Schwimmer JB, Behling C, Newbury R, Deutsch R, Nievergelt C, Schork NJ, et al. Histopathology of pediatric nonalcoholic fatty liver disease. Hepatology. 2005;42(3):641–9.

18. Nobili V, Marcellini M, Devito R, Ciampalini P, Piemonte F, Comparcola D, et al. NAFLD in children: a prospective clinical-pathological study and effect of lifestyle advice. Hepatology. 2006;44(2):458–65.

19. Kinugasa A, Tsunamoto K, Furukawa N, Sawada T, Kusunoki T, Shimada N. Fatty liver and its fibrous changes found in simple obesity of children. J Pediatr Gastroenterol Nutr. 1984;3(3):408–14.

20. Feldstein AE, Charatcharoenwitthaya P, Treeprasertsuk S, Benson JT, Enders FB, Angulo P. The natural history of non-alcoholic fatty liver disease in children: a follow-up study for up to 20-years. Gut. 2009;58:1538–44.

21. Suzuki D, Hashimoto E, Kaneda K, Tokushige K, Shiratori K. Liver failure caused by non-alcoholic steatohepatitis in an obese young male. J Gastroenterol Hepatol. 2005;20(2):327–9.

22. Adams LA, Feldstein A, Lindor KD, Angulo P. Nonalcoholic fatty liver disease among patients with hypothalamic and pituitary dysfunction. Hepatology. 2004;39(4):909–14.

23. Rajindrajith S, Dassanayake AS, Hewavisenthi J, de Silva HJ. Advanced hepatic fibrosis and cirrhosis due to nonalcoholic fatty liver disease in Sri Lankan children: a preliminary report. Hepatol Int. 2008;2(2):209–12.

24. Molleston JP, Schwimmer JB, Yates KP, Murray KF, Cummings OW, Lavine JE, et al. Histological abnormalities in children with nonalcoholic fatty liver disease and normal or mildly elevated alanine aminotransferase levels. J Pediatr. 2014;164(4):707–13.e3.

25. Fitzpatrick E, Mitry RR, Quaglia A, Hussain M, Dhawan A. Serum levels of CK18 M30 and leptin are useful predictors of steatohepatitis and fibrosis in paediatric NAFLD. JPGN. 2010;51:500–6.

26. Alkhouri N, Mansoor S, Giammaria P, Liccardo D, Lopez R, Nobili V. The development of the pediatric NAFLD fibrosis score (PNFS) to predict the presence of advanced fibrosis in children with nonalcoholic fatty liver disease. PLoS One. 2014;9(8):e104558.

27. Carter-Kent C, Yerian LM, Brunt EM, Angulo P, Kohli R, Ling SC, et al. Nonalcoholic steatohepatitis in children: a multicenter clinicopathological study. Hepatology. 2009;50:1113–20.

28. Brunt EM. Pathology of fatty liver disease. Mod Pathol 2007;20(Suppl 1):S40–8.

29. Takahashi Y, Fukusato T. Pediatric nonalcoholic fatty liver disease: overview with emphasis on histology. World J Gastroenterol. 2010;16(42):5280–5.

30. Brunt EM, Kleiner DE, Wilson LA, Unalp A, Behling CE, Lavine JE, et al. Portal chronic inflammation in nonalcoholic fatty liver disease (NAFLD): a histologic marker of advanced NAFLD-Clinicopathologic correlations from the nonalcoholic steatohepatitis clinical research network. Hepatology. 2009;49(3):809–20.

31. Ishak K, Baptista A, Bianchi L, Callea F, De Groote J, Gudat F, et al. Histological grading and staging of chronic hepatitis. J Hepatol. 1995;22(6):696–9.

32. Ramm GA, Nair VG, Bridle KR, Shepherd RW, Crawford DH. Contribution of hepatic parenchymal and nonparenchymal cells to hepatic fibrogenesis in biliary atresia. Am J Pathol. 1998;153(2):527–35.

33. Pinzani M, Rombouts K. Liver fibrosis: from the bench to clinical targets. Dig Liver Dis. 2004;36(4):231–42.

34. Clouston AD, Powell EE, Walsh MJ, Richardson MM, Demetris AJ, Jonsson JR. Fibrosis correlates with a ductular reaction in hepatitis C: roles of impaired replication, progenitor cells and steatosis. Hepatology. 2005;41(4):809–18.

35. Wood MJ, Gadd VL, Powell LW, Ramm GA, Clouston AD. Ductular reaction in hereditary hemochromatosis: the link between hepatocyte senescence and fibrosis progression. Hepatology. 2014;59(3):848–57.

36. Prakoso E, Tirnitz-Parker JE, Clouston AD, Kayali Z, Lee A, Gan EK, et al. Analysis of the intrahepatic ductular reaction and progenitor cell responses in hepatitis C virus recurrence after liver transplantation. Liver Transpl. 2014;20(12):1508–19.

37. Omenetti A, Bass LM, Anders RA, Clemente MG, Francis H, Guy CD, et al. Hedgehog activity, epithelial-mesenchymal transitions, and biliary dysmorphogenesis in biliary atresia. Hepatology. 2011;53(4):1246–58.

38. Williams MJ, Clouston AD, Forbes SJ. Links between hepatic fibrosis, ductular reaction, and progenitor cell expansion. Gastroenterology. 2014;146(2):349–56.

39. Richardson MM, Jonsson JR, Powell EE, Brunt EM, Neuschwander-Tetri BA, Bhathal PS, et al. Progressive fibrosis in nonalcoholic steatohepatitis: association with altered regeneration and a ductular reaction. Gastroenterology. 2007;133(1):80–90.

40. Roberts EA. Non-alcoholic steatohepatitis in children. Clin Liver Dis. 2007;11(1):155–72, x.

41. Guy CD, Suzuki A, Zdanowicz M, Abdelmalek MF, Burchette J, Unalp A, et al. Hedgehog pathway activation parallels histologic severity of injury and fibrosis in human nonalcoholic fatty liver disease. Hepatology. 2012;55(6):1711–21.

42. Swiderska-Syn M, Suzuki A, Guy CD, Schwimmer JB, Abdelmalek MF, Lavine JE, et al. Hedgehog pathway and pediatric nonalcoholic fatty liver disease. Hepatology. 2013;57(5):1814–25.

43. Davenport M, De Ville de Goyet J, Stringer MD, Mieli-Vergani G, Kelly DA, McClean P, et al. Seamless management of biliary atresia in England and Wales (1999–2002). Lancet. 2004;363(9418):1354–7.

44. Valenti L, Al-Serri A, Daly AK, Galmozzi E, Rametta R, Dongiovanni P, et al. Homozygosity for the patatin-like phospholipase-3/adiponutrin I148M polymorphism influences liver fibrosis in patients with nonalcoholic fatty liver disease. Hepatology. 2010;51(4):1209–17.

45. Zimmer V, Lammert F. Genetics and epigenetics in the fibrogenic evolution of chronic liver diseases. Best Pract Res Clin Gastroenterol. 2011;25(2):269–80.

46. Matteoni CA, Younossi ZM, Gramlich T, Boparai N, Liu YC, McCullough AJ. Nonalcoholic fatty liver disease: a spectrum of clinical and pathological severity. Gastroenterology. 1999;116(6):1413–9.

47. Ekstedt M, Franzen LE, Mathiesen UL, Thorelius L, Holmqvist M, Bodemar G, et al. Long-term follow-up of patients with NAFLD and elevated liver enzymes. Hepatology. 2006;44(4):865–73.

48. Adams LA, Lymp JF, St Sauver J, Sanderson SO, Lindor KD, Feldstein A, et al. The natural history of nonalcoholic fatty liver disease: a population-based cohort study. Gastroenterology. 2005;129(1):113–21.

49. Adams LA, Sanderson S, Lindor KD, Angulo P. The histological course of nonalcoholic fatty liver disease: a longitudinal study of 103 patients with sequential liver biopsies. J Hepatol. 2005;42(1):132–8.

50. Argo CK, Northup PG, Al-Osaimi AM, Caldwell SH. Systematic review of risk factors for fibrosis progression in non-alcoholic steatohepatitis. J Hepatol. 2009;51(2):371–9.

51. Musso G, Gambino R, Cassader M, Pagano G. Meta-analysis: natural history of non-alcoholic fatty liver disease (NAFLD) and diagnostic accuracy of non-invasive tests for liver disease severity. Ann Med. 2011;43:617–49.

52. Singh S, Allen AM, Wang Z, Prokop LJ, Murad MH, Loomba R. Fibrosis progression in nonalcoholic fatty liver vs nonalcoholic steatohepatitis: a systematic review and meta-analysis of paired-biopsy studies. Clin Gastroenterol Hepatol. 2015;13:643–54.e1-9.

53. McPherson S, Hardy T, Henderson E, Burt AD, Day CP, Anstee QM. Evidence of NAFLD progression from steatosis to fibrosing-steatohepatitis using paired biopsies: implications for prognosis & clinical management. J Hepatol. 2015;62:1148–55.

54. Angulo P. Long-term mortality in nonalcoholic fatty liver disease: is liver histology of any prognostic significance? Hepatology. 2010;51(2):373–5.

55. Bhala N, Angulo P, van der Poorten D, Lee E, Hui JM, Saracco G, et al. The natural history of nonalcoholic fatty liver disease with advanced fibrosis or cirrhosis: an international collaborative study. Hepatology. 2011;54(4):1208–16.

56. Cunningham SA, Kramer MR, Narayan KM. Incidence of childhood obesity in the United States. N Engl J Med. 2014;370(17):1660–1.

57. Graversen L, Sorensen TI, Petersen L, Sovio U, Kaakinen M, Sandbaek A, et al. Preschool weight and body mass index in relation to central obesity and metabolic syndrome in adulthood. PLoS One. 2014;9(3):e89986.

58. Guha IN, Parkes J, Roderick PR, Harris S, Rosenberg WM. Non-invasive markers associated with liver fibrosis in non-alcoholic fatty liver disease. Gut. 2006;55(11):1650–60.

59. Schwimmer JB, Deutsch R, Rauch JB, Behling C, Newbury R, Lavine JE. Obesity, insulin resistance, and other clinico-pathological correlates of pediatric nonalcoholic fatty liver disease. J Pediatr. 2003;143(4):500–5.

# 5 Non-alcoholic fatty liver disease (NAFLD) as cause of cryptogenic cirrhosis

## Jay H. Lefkowitch

Department of Pathology and Cell Biology, College of Physicians and Surgeons, Columbia University, New York, NY, USA

## LEARNING POINTS

- A significant number of cases of cryptogenic cirrhosis today are due to late-stage NAFLD.

- Non-alcoholic steatohepatitis may progress to cirrhosis with eventual loss of fat.

- Important risk factors for NAFLD include obesity and diabetes, which show a higher association with cryptogenic cirrhosis when compared to other known causes of cirrhosis.

- Increased serum adiponectin levels are antisteatotic and, in combination with decreased vascular delivery to the liver of insulin and fatty acids due to portal hypertension, are important factors in fat loss from late-stage NAFLD-related cirrhosis.

- Late, inactive autoimmune hepatitis, occult hepatitis B and C viral infections, and chronic hepatitis E virus infection in immunosuppressed individuals are other possible causes of putative cryptogenic cirrhosis.

- Systems biology (genomics, transcriptomics, proteomics, and metabolomics) is likely to illuminate the etiology of residual cases of cryptogenic cirrhosis in the coming decades.

## Introduction

Most classifications of cirrhosis dating back 50 years or more have reserved the final entry on the list for the category "cryptogenic cirrhosis": *cirrhosis of unknown cause*. With each passing era, this category has been winnowed because of major advances in diagnostic methods and in our understanding of the etiopathogenesis of hepatobiliary diseases. Two prime examples are the identification of the hepatitis C virus (HCV) in 1989 and the seminal description of non-alcoholic steatohepatitis (NASH), published by Ludwig and colleagues at the Mayo Clinic in 1980 [1]. The discovery and, then, availability of serologic tests for HCV lifted the veil from many cases of cirrhosis thought to be cryptogenic or attributed to the viral agent non-A, non-B hepatitis. The impact of such discoveries is evident when comparing prevalence rates of cryptogenic cirrhosis in publications from nearly 35 years ago to current data. A relatively high prevalence rate of cryptogenic cirrhosis (35–59.6% of cases of cirrhosis) was reported in a 1981 20-year prospective study of cirrhosis from Birmingham, United Kingdom [2] (published before the identification of HCV and only 1 year after the description of NASH by Ludwig et al.). More recent estimates show a considerably lower prevalence of cryptogenic cirrhosis of 5–30% of cases [3], predominantly because of wider recognition and understanding of the clinicopathological features of NAFLD and NASH in a period of alarming growth of worldwide obesity and diabetes. Thus, at present, patients with newly diagnosed cirrhosis of uncertain cause will very likely be scrupulously assessed for risk factors for non-alcoholic fatty liver disease (NAFLD), and many will have a liver biopsy to confirm such a diagnosis. Recent data suggest that NAFLD and NASH are actually responsible for 30–70% of cryptogenic

*Clinical Dilemmas in Non-Alcoholic Fatty Liver Disease*, First Edition. Edited by Roger Williams and Simon D. Taylor-Robinson.

**TABLE 5.1** Causes of cirrhosis

**Well established**

Chronic hepatitis
 Hepatitis B virus (HBV)
 Hepatitis C virus (HCV)
 Autoimmune hepatitis (AIH)
 Alpha-1-antitrypsin deficiency
 Wilson's disease
Fatty liver disease (macrovesicular)
 Alcoholic (AFLD)
 Non-alcoholic (NAFLD)
Other metabolic disorders
 Hemochromatosis
Drug-induced liver injury (DILI)
Biliary tract disease
 Chronic large bile duct obstruction
 Primary biliary cirrhosis
 Primary sclerosing cholangitis
 Chronic ductopenic disorders
Hepatic venous outflow obstruction (e.g., Budd–Chiari syndrome)

**Possible**

Late, inactive autoimmune hepatitis
Occult viral hepatitis HBV or HCV
Antihepatitis viral therapy with sustained viral response (SVR)
"Posthepatitic" cirrhosis (following unknown viral infection or drug hepatitis)
Chronic hepatitis E virus (HEV) infection (immunosuppressed individuals)

**Unknown/rare ("cryptogenic")**

Mitochondriopathies
Keratin mutations
Short telomere syndromes
Metabolic/enzyme mutations

cirrhosis [4]. Thus, when considering individuals with cirrhosis at the present time (Table 5.1), after exclusion of the well-established causes and any clinicopathological evidence supporting NAFLD/NASH as a possible cause, the percentage of cases that can truly be deemed "cryptogenic" is likely to be of the order of only 5–10%. Schuppan and Afdahl in a recent review of cirrhosis [5] also provide a similar overall assessment: "the diagnosis of cirrhosis without apparent cause (cryptogenic cirrhosis) is rarely made." In the next decade or two, even this number will decline due to the advent of molecular and genomic diagnostics and application of the technologies that are currently referred to as "systems biology," as will be discussed later.

## Cryptogenic cirrhosis: Definition and characteristics

The term "cryptogenic cirrhosis" implies that no recognizable cause of cirrhosis has been found by clinical, pathological, serological, biochemical, or historical investigations [3]. For the clinician, the prototypic patient with cryptogenic cirrhosis is likely to be 60 years or older, often female, with obesity and diabetes and is discovered to have cirrhosis while asymptomatic and being evaluated for another condition, or will have recently presented with new ascites, variceal hemorrhage, encephalopathy, or hepatocellular carcinoma (HCC) [3]. Serum liver tests are usually nondiscriminating, with normal or slightly raised aminotransferases. Serum autoantibody evaluation to exclude autoimmune hepatitis (AIH) is usually negative, unless there is positivity (typically low titer) for antinuclear or antismooth muscle antibodies (a nonspecific/generic immune response that is seen in many individuals with NAFLD) [6].

For the pathologist, the "cryptogenic cirrhosis" found in liver biopsy, explant, or postmortem specimens is a "faceless" cirrhosis characterized by bland fibrous septa surrounding regenerative nodules without steatosis, cholestasis, or hemosiderin (Figure 5.1). The specific histological features associated with known etiologies will largely be absent (or potentially overlooked), including interface hepatitis (chronic hepatitis B and C and AIH); ground-glass hepatocellular inclusions (chronic hepatitis B); portal tract lymphoid aggregates (chronic hepatitis C and other causes of chronic hepatitis); bile duct damage, loss, or absence (primary biliary cirrhosis, primary sclerosing cholangitis); periductal onion-skin fibrosis (primary sclerosing cholangitis); copper and copper-binding protein positivity (Wilson's disease, chronic cholestatic diseases); and diastase-treated periodic acid–Schiff (DPAS) stain-positive globules within periportal hepatocytes (alpha-1-antitrypsin deficiency).

## Pathological recognition of NAFLD/NASH in cryptogenic cirrhosis

The range of histological findings that constitute NAFLD includes the spectrum from macrovesicular steatosis to steatohepatitis, cirrhosis, and HCC [7–11]. Although the diagnostic histological features of NASH have been the subject of many studies since its first description by Ludwig

(A)

(B)

(C)

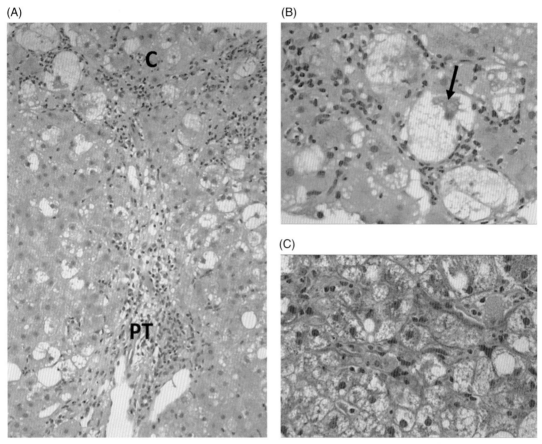

**FIG 5.1** Classical non-alcoholic steatohepatitis (NASH). (A) Steatosis, hepatocyte ballooning, and inflammation (the trio of changes representing the minimal histological criteria of steatohepatitis) are evident in the centrilobular region (C). (B) Hepatocyte ballooning and intracellular Mallory–Denk bodies (arrow) are shown at high magnification. (C) The characteristic pericellular/perisinusoidal "chicken-wire" pattern of fibrosis surrounding centrilobular hepatocytes is seen on this trichrome stain (A and B, hematoxylin and eosin stain; C: Masson trichrome stain). (*See insert for color representation of the figure.*)

and colleagues [1], many, if not all, of the hallmark changes may disappear once cirrhosis has developed, particularly steatosis (discussed later). NAFLD and NASH in adults chiefly affect centrilobular regions (acinar zone 3). In its fullest expression, the features of NASH include macrovesicular steatosis, hepatocyte ballooning, inflammation (lymphocytes and neutrophils), intrahepatocellular Mallory–Denk bodies [12], and perisinusoidal fibrosis surrounding hepatocytes in a characteristic "chicken-wire" pattern (Figure 5.1). The minimum criteria for a diagnosis of NASH include macrovesicular steatosis, hepatocyte ballooning, and inflammation [11], and these can be

evaluated semiquantitatively to determine the NAFLD activity score [13] (NAS) and the likelihood that NASH is present. Additional helpful diagnostic features may be seen, such as giant mitochondria [14, 15] and, in diabetic subjects, "glycogen nuclei" in periportal hepatocytes (Figure 5.2).

The fibrosis surrounding central veins in NASH eventually involves many or most central veins. Once established perivenular fibrosis extends through the hepatic lobules toward other central veins and, importantly, also toward portal tracts, thereby subdividing the lobular parenchyma into small units of hepatocytes. The process

(A)                                               (B)

(C)

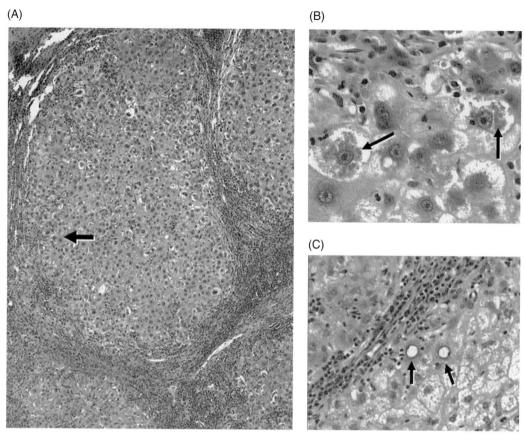

**FIG 5.2** "Cryptogenic cirrhosis" due to NAFLD. (A) Cirrhosis without fat is seen at low magnification. Portal tracts and fibrous septa contain mild to moderate chronic inflammatory cell infiltrates, rendering a superficial resemblance to chronic hepatitis. However, careful examination of the hepatocytes located at the periphery of the nodules (arrow) allows recognition of remaining NASH features (seen at high power in panel B). (B) High magnification of the parenchyma near the arrow in panel A. Hepatocytes are variably ballooned and there is robust Mallory–Denk body formation (arrows). (C): Occasional periportal/periseptal hepato-cytes show glycogenated nuclei (arrows) (A, B, and C: hematoxylin and eosin stain). (*See insert for color representation of the figure.*)

of central-to-portal bridging fibrosis in progressive NASH is associated with activation of periportal hepatic progenitor cells that form bile ductular structures (ductu-lar reaction), reflecting the impaired replication capacity of hepatocytes in NAFLD and NASH [16, 17]. In late NAFLD-related cirrhosis when fat is absent (or minimal and patchy), other features of NASH may be subtle and must be sought assiduously. Hepatocyte ballooning and Mallory–Denk bodies may be found microscopically in the peripheral regions of the cirrhotic nodules, near fibrous septa and portal tracts (Figure 5.2). Nonballooned

hepatocytes may contain Mallory–Denk bodies. Tri-chrome connective tissue stain may disclose residual foci of perisinusoidal/pericellular "chicken-wire" fibrosis. The predilection of NASH for centrilobular regions and central-to-central bridging fibrosis may spare some portal tracts that come to be localized in the centers of regenera-tive nodules, a process referred to as "reversed lobulation." The central-to-portal bridging fibrosis that often evolves from NASH may be remodeled to produce slender fibrous septa that are helpful regions for histological examination for residual hepatocyte ballooning and/or Mallory–Denk bodies. The hepatocytes near such slender septa may also show persistent immunostain positivity in adjacent hepatocytes for the urea cycle enzyme glutamine synthetase that is normally localized to centrilobular hepatocytes [18].

## Evidence for NAFLD as the cause of cryptogenic cirrhosis

Two landmark papers from the 1990s provided critical evidence for NAFLD/NASH as the etiology of many cases of cryptogenic cirrhosis. In 1990, Powell and colleagues [19] described a cohort of patients with NASH who transitioned to cirrhosis over a 5-year period with loss of fat and inflammation, thereby highlighting the potential for so-called "burnt-out" NAFLD. This was followed in 1999 by the study by Caldwell and colleagues [20] in which diabetes and obesity were found significantly more often in a cohort of subjects with cryptogenic cirrhosis in comparison to patients with primary biliary cirrhosis or chronic hepatitis C-related cirrhosis. These studies initiated a line of evidence that has been assembled during the subsequent decade that lends further support for NAFLD as the etiology of many, if not most, cases of cryptogenic cirrhosis. This evidence was reviewed by Caldwell and Crespo [4] and included (i) studies of explant livers from patients transplanted for cryptogenic cirrhosis who later developed posttransplantation NASH, with patchy steatosis, Mallory–Denk bodies, and hepatocyte ballooning [21]; (ii) correlative clinicopathological studies of individuals with cryptogenic cirrhosis in whom a cause was found in 85% (33% of which had features of NASH) [22]; and (iii) patients with cryptogenic cirrhosis and HCC in whom obesity and diabetes were significantly more common in comparison to matched controls [23].

## Loss of steatosis in late NAFLD/NASH with cirrhosis

NAFLD has eluded pathological detection as the cause of many cases of cryptogenic cirrhosis in large part due to the loss of large droplet steatosis from hepatocytes in the late cirrhotic stage (Figure 5.2). The pathogenesis of this fat loss has been the subject of several studies and hypotheses [24] (Table 5.2). Most hypotheses have addressed those physiological features of cirrhosis that would directly or

**TABLE 5.2** Possible causes of fat loss in late NAFLD-related cirrhosis

- Increased serum adiponectin levels cause reduction in hepatocyte steatosis
- Bile acids signal and bind to adipocytes in late cirrhosis and mediate increased adiponectin synthesis
- Catabolic state of cirrhosis
- Consumption of systemic fat stores for energy
- Aberrant portal venous drainage and/or portosystemic shunting of cirrhosis limits hepatocyte exposure to insulin and fatty acids
- Loss of sinusoidal fenestrations and acquisition of basement membrane material impair steatogenic molecule transfer across endothelium
- Senescent fatty hepatocytes have been repopulated by nonfatty hepatic progenitor cells

*Source:* See Ref. [24] for further discussion and study citations.

indirectly affect acquisition of triglyceride by hepatocytes, chiefly the altered vascular inflow patterns [25, 26] (and delivery of factors such as insulin and fatty acids) due to portal hypertension and abnormal sinusoidal access of steatogenic factors to underlying hepatocytes because of changes in the sinusoidal endothelium (abnormal fenestrae) or increased collagenous barriers located under the endothelium in the space of Disse ("capillarization" of the sinusoids in cirrhosis, with gains of basement membrane collagen) [27]. More recent work has focused on the antisteatotic effects of adiponectin on hepatocytes and the mechanisms whereby serum adiponectin becomes elevated in late NAFLD cirrhosis and mediates loss of fat [24]. Elevation of serum bile acids develops in many late forms of cirrhosis, including late NAFLD-related cirrhosis, and bile acid "cross talk" between adipocytes and hepatocytes and binding to bile acid receptors on adipocytes are among the pathways considered to be important in mediating elevation of serum adiponectin in late cirrhosis due to NAFLD.

## Other possible causes of cryptogenic cirrhosis and future directions

Conditions other than NAFLD can result in cryptogenic cirrhosis and should be considered in the differential diagnosis (Table 5.1). Late AIH without residual interface hepatitis and with only minimal or mild portal and septal lymphocytes and plasma cells is one such disorder. Occult or inactive HBV or HCV infection can also be included in this category. Antiviral treatment of an individual with HBV or HCV cirrhosis may result in a sustained viral response (SVR) status and a paradoxically bland-appearing cirrhosis with little or no inflammation. In immunosuppressed individuals, particularly liver transplant recipients, the possibility of developing posttransplantation cirrhosis due to chronic hepatitis E virus (HEV) infection also requires serologic exclusion [28–30].

Rarer conditions that may underlie cryptogenic cirrhosis include mitochondriopathies, keratin mutations, and short telomere syndromes. Mitochondriopathies comprise a variety of point mutations and/or deletions of mitochondrial DNA (mtDNA) resulting in defects of the respiratory chain [31]. Such defects can affect hepatocytes, muscles, and tissues of the nervous system, thereby causing multiorgan syndromes (e.g., neurohepatopathies) with cirrhosis in neonates, children, and adults. Loss of function mutations affecting the telomerase complex (which normally allows multiple generations of cell division and regeneration by adding successive TTAGGG sequences to the 3′ end of chromosomes) may cause an otherwise unexplained cirrhosis associated with idiopathic pulmonary fibrosis [32] or with dyskeratosis congenita [33]. Some cases of cryptogenic cirrhosis may be due to keratin 8 gene mutations [34].

In the coming decade, for the relatively small numbers of individuals for whom a cause of cirrhosis cannot be determined, it is likely that one or more systems biology techniques [35] will elucidate the etiology. These techniques, collectively referred to as "omics" (genomics, transcriptomics, proteomics, and metabolomics), allow identification of distinct moieties such as genomic sequences, proteins, and peptides within cells and tissues, which define or provide a "signature" of that individual's disease. NAFLD is an example where such techniques have already been broadly applied and have generated exceptionally useful data. Genomic studies assessing single nucleotide polymorphisms (SNPs) have demonstrated an important and consistent mutation in the *PNPLA3* gene in subjects with NAFLD that results in a nonsynonymous substitution of a methionine for an isoleucine at position 148 in the enzyme PNPLA3 and the accumulation of fat in hepatocytes [36]. PNPLA3 (patatin-like phospholipase domain-containing protein 3 or adiponutrin) is a triacylglycerol lipase that mediates triacylglycerol hydrolysis in adipocytes. Metabolomics (detecting small-sized molecules,

<1500 Da in size, by high-throughput nuclear magnetic resonance spectroscopy and/or mass spectrometry) in NAFLD has demonstrated a specific lipidomic signature that is associated with progressive disease [37, 38]. These are only several examples of the potential future uses of systems biology in clarifying the etiology of remaining cases of "cryptogenic" cirrhosis.

## Summary

Cryptogenic cirrhosis has, by definition, always been a diagnosis of uncertainty as far as its etiology is concerned. The past 30 years have shown an alarming growth in the prevalence of obesity, diabetes, metabolic syndrome, and NAFLD in developed countries and elsewhere. Outcomes data on the natural history of NAFLD have emerged and indicate that ~9–20% of individuals with NASH will later develop cirrhosis [39]. Many of these individuals with cirrhosis will retain sufficient clinical and pathological features of NAFLD and NASH to make the etiology clear, but there yet remain individuals with NAFLD who are diagnosed as having "cryptogenic cirrhosis," especially when major histological markers of NAFLD and NASH (particularly large droplet fat) have disappeared. Some 30–70% of cryptogenic cirrhosis cases today are believed to be due to NAFLD/NASH. Future investigations hold the promise of further winnowing the category of cryptogenic cirrhosis by identifying specific NAFLD/NASH genomic and/or metabolomic signatures and determining the presence of alternative unusual disorders by applying systems biology techniques (e.g., transcriptomics, genome-wide sequencing) to individual cases.

## References

1. Ludwig J, Viggiano TR, McGill DB, Oh BJ. Nonalcoholic steatohepatitis: Mayo Clinic experiences with a hitherto unnamed disease. Mayo Clin Proc 1980; 55: 434–438.
2. Saunders JB, Walters JRF, Davies P, Paton A. A 20-year prospective study of cirrhosis. Br Med J 1981; 282: 263–266.
3. Caldwell S. Cryptogenic cirrhosis: what are we missing? Curr Gastroenterol Rep 2010; 12: 40–48.
4. Caldwell SH, Crespo DM. The spectrum expanded: cryptogenic cirrhosis and the natural history of non-alcoholic fatty liver disease. J Hepatol 2004; 40: 578–584.
5. Schuppan D, Afdhal NH. Liver cirrhosis. Lancet 2008; 371: 838–851.

6. Loria P, Lonardo A, Leonardi F, et al. Non-organ-specific autoantibodies in nonalcoholic fatty liver disease: prevalence and correlates. Dig Dis Sci 2003; 48: 2173–2181.

7. Yeh MM, Brunt EM. Pathology of nonalcoholic fatty liver disease. Am J Clin Pathol 2007; 128: 837–847.

8. Hübscher SG. Histological assessment of non-alcoholic fatty liver disease. Histopathology 2006; 49: 450–465.

9. Tannapfel A, Denk H, Dienes H-P, et al. Histopathological diagnosis of non-alcoholic and alcoholic fatty liver disease. Virchows Arch 2011; 458: 511–523.

10. Brunt EM. Non-alcoholic fatty liver disease: what's new under the microscope? Gut 2011; 60: 1152–1158.

11. Yeh MM, Brunt EM. Pathological features of fatty liver disease. Gastroenterology 2014; 147: 754–764.

12. Zatloukal K, French SW, Stumptner C, et al. From Mallory to Mallory–Denk bodies: what, how and why? Exp Cell Res 2007; 313: 2033–2049.

13. Kleiner DE, Brunt EM, Van Natta M, et al. Design and validation of a histological scoring system for nonalcoholic fatty liver disease. Hepatology 2005; 41: 1313–1321.

14. Le TH, Caldwell SH, Redick JA, et al. The zonal distribution of megamitochondria with crystalline inclusions in nonalcoholic steatohepatitis. Hepatology 2004; 39: 1423–1429.

15. Lotowska JM, Sobaniec-Lotowska ME, Backowska SB, Lebensztejn DM. Pediatric non-alcoholic steatohepatitis: the first report on the ultrastructure of hepatocyte mitochondria. World J Gastroenterol 2014; 20: 4335–4340.

16. Richardson MM, Jonsson JR, Powell EE, et al. Progressive fibrosis in nonalcoholic steatohepatitis: association with altered regeneration and a ductular reaction. Gastroenterology 2007; 133: 80–90.

17. Gadd VL, Skoien R, Powell EE, et al. The portal inflammatory infiltrate and ductular reaction in human nonalcoholic fatty liver disease. Hepatology 2014; 59: 1393–1405.

18. Lefkowitch JH, Morawski JL. Late nonalcoholic fatty liver disease with cirrhosis: a pathologic case of lost or mistaken identity. Semin Liver Dis 2012; 32: 92–98.

19. Powell EE, Cooksley WGE, Hanson R, Searle J, Halliday JW, Powell LW. The natural history of nonalcoholic steatohepatitis: a follow-up study of forty-two patients for up to 21 years. Hepatology 1990; 11: 74–80.

20. Caldwell SH, Oelsner DH, Iezzoni JC, Hespenheide EE, Battle EH, Driscoll CJ. Cryptogenic cirrhosis: clinical characterization and risk factors for underlying disease. Hepatology 1999; 29: 664–669.

21. Conto MJ, Cales W, Sterling RK, et al. Development of nonalcoholic fatty liver disease after orthotopic liver transplantation for cryptogenic cirrhosis. Liver Transpl 2001; 7: 363–373.

22. Ayata G, Gordon FD, Lewis WD, et al. Cryptogenic cirrhosis: clinicopathologic findings at and after liver transplantation. Hum Pathol 2002; 33: 1098–1104.

23. Bugianasi E, Leone N, Vanni E, et al. Expanding the natural history of nonalcoholic steatohepatitis from cryptogenic cirrhosis to hepatocellular carcinoma. Gastroenterology 2012; 123: 134–140.

24. van der Poorten D, Samer CF, Ramezani-Moghadam M, et al. Hepatic fat loss in advanced nonalcoholic steatohepatitis: are alterations in serum adiponectin the cause? Hepatology 2013; 57: 2180–2188.

25. Matsui O, Kadoya M, Takahashi S, et al. Focal sparing of segment IV in fatty livers shown by sonography and CT: correlation with aberrant gastric venous drainage. Am J Roentgenol 1995; 164: 1137–1140.

26. Nosadini R, vogaro A, Mollo F, et al. Carbohydrate and lipid metabolism in cirrhosis. Evidence that hepatic uptake of gluconeogenic precursors and of free fatty acid depends on effective hepatic flow. J Clin Endocrinol Metab 1984; 58: 1125–1132.

27. Schaffner H, Popper H. Capillarization of the sinusoids. Gastroenterology 1963; 44: 339–342.

28. Kamar N, Selver J, Mansuy J-M, et al. Hepatitis E virus and chronic hepatitis in organ-transplant recipients. N Engl J Med 2008; 358: 811–817.

29. Kamar N, Mansuy J-M, Cointault O, et al. Hepatitis E virus-related cirrhosis in kidney-and kidney-pancreas-transplant recipients. Am J Transplant 2008; 8: 1744–1748.

30. Singh GKJ, Ijaz S, Rockwood N, et al. Chronic hepatitis E as a cause for cryptogenic cirrhosis in HIV. J Infect 2012; 66: 103–106.

31. Pesce V, Cormio A, Marangi LC, et al. Depletion of mitochondrial DNA in the skeletal muscle of two cirrhotic patients with severe asthenia. Gene 2012; 286: 143–148.

32. Carulli L, Dei Cas A, Nascimbeni F. Synchronous cryptogenic liver cirrhosis and idiopathic pulmonary fibrosis: a clue to telomere involvement. Hepatology 2012; 56: 2001–2003.

33. Calado RT, Brudno J, Mehta P, et al. Constitutional telomerase mutations are genetic risk factors for cirrhosis. Hepatology 2011; 53: 1600–1607.

34. Ku N-O, Gish R, Wright TL, Omary MB. Keratin 8 mutations in patients with cryptogenic liver disease. N Engl J Med 2001; 344: 1580–1587.

35. Mato JM, Martínez-Chantar ML, Lu SC. Systems biology for hepatologists. Hepatology 2014; 60: 735–743.

36. Daly AK, Ballestri S, Carulli L, Loria P, Day CP. Genetic determinants of susceptibility and severity in nonalcoholic fatty liver disease. Expert Rev Gastroenterol Hepatol 2011; 5: 253–263.

37. Barr J, Caballeria J, Martinez-Arranz I, et al. Obesity-dependent metabolic signatures associated with nonalcoholic fatty liver disease progression. J Proteome Res 2012; 1: 2521–2532.

38. Barr J, Vázquez-Chantada M, Alonso C, et al. Liquid chromatography-mass spectrometry-based parallel metabolic profiling of human and mouse model serum reveals putative biomarkers associated with the progression of nonalcoholic fatty liver disease. J Proteome Res 2010; 9: 4501–4512.

39. Starley BQ, Calcagno CJ, Harrison SA. Nonalcoholic fatty liver disease and hepatocellular carcinoma: a weighty connection. Hepatology 2010; 51: 1820–1832.

# 6 Is NAFLD different in absence of metabolic syndrome?

**Yusuf Yilmaz**

Department of Gastroenterology, School of Medicine, Marmara University, Istanbul, Turkey

## LEARNING POINTS

- A number of experimental and epidemiological studies convincingly suggest that the presence of the metabolic syndrome (MS) is the main risk factor for the development of non-alcoholic fatty liver disease (NAFLD).

- However, this association is not invariable and NAFLD can develop even in subjects without a formal diagnosis of the MS (metabolically normal NAFLD).

- There may be specific and underrecognized risk factors that modulate the likelihood that an individual without the MS will experience NAFLD.

- These include increased hemoglobin levels, iron overload, and genetic risk factors—all of which appear to be interrelated.

- Although a great deal of knowledge has been accrued on NAFLD and MS, there are ample opportunities for more to be learned in the future from metabolically normal NAFLD.

- Besides differing from traditional MS-associated NAFLD in terms of pathogenesis, metabolically normal NAFLD seems to be related to more favorable clinical outcomes.

- The complex interrelationships between hemoglobin, iron overload, and genetic risk factors for metabolically normal NAFLD are highly relevant for our future understanding of fatty liver overload and developing new groundbreaking therapies.

## Introduction

Non-alcoholic fatty liver disease (NAFLD) is a common disorder characterized by hepatic fat accumulation (steatosis) that is at or above 5% of liver weight in the absence of significant alcohol consumption (<20 g/day) and other viral, toxic, autoimmune, or rare causes of liver disease [1–3]. NAFLD and its progressive variant non-alcoholic steatohepatitis (NASH) are commonly considered as the hepatic manifestations of the metabolic syndrome (MS)—a pathophysiological construct where insulin resistance predisposes to the clustering of hyperglycemia, abdominal obesity, dyslipidemia, and hypertension [4–6]. The strong association between NAFLD and the MS is supported both by a pathophysiological and epidemiological standpoint. In terms of pathophysiology, NAFLD is associated with hepatic insulin resistance and an impaired ability of insulin to suppress hepatic glucose production [5]. This results in mild hyperglycemia and stimulation of insulin secretion, leading to hyperinsulinemia. Notably, insulin normally inhibits the production of very-low-density lipoproteins (VLDL) from the liver. Overproduction of VLDL and the defect in insulin suppression of VLDL production correlate with the amount of hepatic fat accumulation [7]. With regard to epidemiological evidence, liver fat content has been associated with the components of the MS independent of body mass index (BMI) [8]. Moreover, hepatic fat accumulation in subjects aged 20–65 years has been reported to be fourfold higher in subjects with the MS compared with those without [8]. As a result, MS is universally recognized as the main risk factor for NAFLD, and recent studies have advocated the inclusion of fatty liver into the diagnostic criteria for the MS [9].

Notwithstanding this evidence, puzzlingly enough, NAFLD and the MS do not appear to be inexorably linked [10–13]. In recent years, it has become apparent that only

*Clinical Dilemmas in Non-Alcoholic Fatty Liver Disease*, First Edition. Edited by Roger Williams and Simon D. Taylor-Robinson.

20–80% of all NAFLD patients actually meet the criteria for the MS [14, 15]. Conversely, there may be subjects who have a diagnosis of MS but will not develop NAFLD [14, 15]. Therefore, not all studies affirm an invariable association between NAFLD and the MS. In our seminal study [10], we sought to compare the general characteristics of biopsy-proven NAFLD patients with and without the MS. The results indicated that approximately 40% of NAFLD patients did not meet the diagnostic criteria for the MS and could be classified as "metabolically normal NAFLD." Compared with subjects with the MS, biopsy-proven NAFLD patients without the MS were younger and showed lower BMI and C-reactive protein levels, a higher prevalence of male subjects, a lower prevalence of gallstone disease, and significantly higher levels of hemoglobin (Hb). Importantly, increased Hb concentrations were the most important independent predictor of both NASH and severe fibrosis in metabolically normal NAFLD [10]. Besides Hb, genetic factors seem to play a key role in the pathogenesis of NAFLD in the absence of MS. In this regard, the rs738409 GG variant in the patatin-like phospholipase domain-containing family member A3 (*PNPLA3*) gene has been recently associated with an increased risk of NAFLD in the general population, especially in subjects without the MS, independent of dietary patterns and metabolic factors [16]. Such differences in risk factors seem to carry important clinical implications. In the National Health and Nutrition Examination Survey III (NHANES III) cohort, Younossi et al. [13] demonstrated that 305 of the 1448 study participants (21%) with ultrasound-diagnosed NAFLD did not meet the diagnostic criteria for the MS. Compared with metabolically normal NAFLD, subjects who met the criteria for the MS were more likely to be non-Hispanic white and older and have higher aminotransferase levels. Importantly, all-cause mortality and cardiovascular mortality were higher in NAFLD patients with MS than in those with metabolically normal NAFLD. Interestingly, mortality of subjects with NAFLD but without the MS was similar to the cohort without liver disease [13]. Because factors other than the MS may clearly play a role in the pathogenesis of NAFLD, the potential mechanisms underlying metabolically normal NAFLD are now critically discussed.

## Metabolically normal NAFLD, Hb, and iron

In NAFLD patients without a diagnosis of MS, Hb was identified as the main predictor of the severity of liver lesions (NASH and fibrosis) [10]. Specifically, an Hb level

>144 g/L had a sensitivity and specificity of 75.5 and 71.3% for a diagnosis of NASH in metabolically normal NAFLD, respectively. The area under the curves for Hb in the detection of advanced fibrosis was 0.850 by receiver operating characteristic analysis. Using 147 g/L as the optimal cutoff value, Hb showed a sensitivity and specificity for advanced fibrosis of 72.7 and 79.0%, respectively [10]. Notably, the potential role of Hb as a predictor of NAFLD has been confirmed by numerous independent investigations. Yu et al. [17] reported a stepwise increase in the risk of NAFLD for increasing Hb quintiles even after adjustment for potential confounders. Das et al. [18] subsequently confirmed that NAFLD patients have a significantly higher hematocrit than subjects without evidence of overt liver disease. In a recent study, Akahane and coworkers [19] reported that Hb levels are an independent predictor of NAFLD in Japanese women and are significantly associated with ferritin levels and insulin resistance. However, the exact mechanisms whereby increased Hb might lead to a higher risk of NAFLD especially in subjects without the MS are still unclear. One potential explanation is that higher Hb levels could lead to increased blood viscosity, thereby raising peripheral resistance and reducing liver perfusion [10, 11]. Notably, a reduced hepatic perfusion has been shown to accelerate hepatic fibrosis [20]. Another potential explanation is that Hb may simply serve as a proxy for body iron stores [21]. Accordingly, iron overload and elevated body iron stores have been proposed to be major risk factors for the development of NAFLD by increasing oxidative stress and promoting chronic parenchymal liver inflammation, ultimately resulting in profound hepatic architectural alterations [22, 23]. Concordantly, various parameters of iron metabolism such as transferrin saturation [24], ferritin [25], and hepcidin [26] have been associated with an increased risk of NAFLD. An indirect evidence of the pathogenic role played by iron in the pathogenesis of NAFLD has been recently provided by the usefulness of phlebotomy therapy (to achieve near-iron depletion, i.e., serum ferritin ≤50 μg/L or Hb 100 g/L) for improving liver histology in this clinical entity [27].

## Genetic factors and metabolically normal NAFLD

In recent years, the understanding of the genetic architecture of NAFLD has improved considerably [28]. Notably, there is evidence suggesting that certain genetic factors

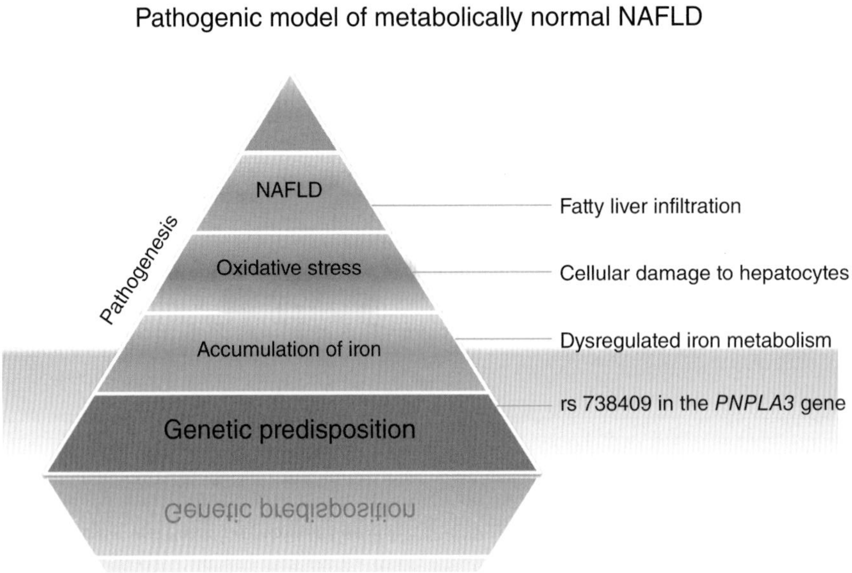

## Pathogenic model of metabolically normal NAFLD

**FIG 6.1** Interrelationship between the main variables that may influence the development of metabolically normal NAFLD.

may predispose to NAFLD even in the absence of MS. A genetic variant (rs738409, encoding I148M) in the patatin-like phospholipase domain-containing family member A3 (*PNPLA3*) gene has attracted much attention as a susceptibility factor for NAFLD [29]. The G allele of rs738409 in *PNPLA3*, changing the amino acid isoleucine to methionine at location 148 (I148M), has been repeatedly associated with NAFLD on a genome-wide significant level. In this regard, a meta-analysis of 16 studies enrolling a total of 2937 subjects has confirmed that the rs738409 variant in *PNPLA3* exerts a strong influence on liver fat accumulation, with the GG homozygotes having a 73% higher lipid fat content compared with the CC homozygotes [29]. In addition, carriers of the GG homozygous genotype have a 3.5-fold higher risk of developing NASH and 3.2-fold increased risk of developing fibrosis compared with the CC homozygotes [29]. Interestingly, although the association with hepatic fat content has been repeatedly validated [30, 31], the rs738409 variant does not seem to affect the components of the MS, including BMI, triglyceride levels, high- and low-density lipoprotein levels, or diabetes [32]. Accordingly, another study demonstrated that rs738409 GG genotype is associated with an increased risk of NAFLD in the general population, especially in the absence of the MS, independent of dietary patterns and metabolic factors [16]. Taken together, these results suggest that the mechanisms through which this polymorphism

influences interindividual differences in hepatic fat content and the risk of NAFLD are not mediated by the components of the MS. While the functional impact of the rs738409 variant remains unclear, Kawaguchi et al. [33] have shown a strong association between this polymorphism and iron deposition in the liver. This intriguing finding confirms the pathological involvement of iron accumulation and iron-related oxidative stress in the pathogenesis of metabolically normal NAFLD. An oxidative stress hypothesis has been suggested to be, at least in part, responsible for the accumulation of fat in the liver [34, 35]. Based on the available evidence, the pathogenic role of iron accumulation in NAFLD appears to be prominent in the absence of the MS. Figure 6.1 summarizes the interrelationship between the main variables that may influence the development of metabolically normal NAFLD.

### Prognostic implications of metabolically normal NAFLD

Although there has been a long-standing interest in identifying NAFLD, the natural history of this condition remains uncertain. In general, some patients seem to be characterized by an indolent course, whereas others develop advanced necroinflammation and liver fibrosis progressing to end-stage liver disease [36]. Patients with simple steatosis generally have a benign long-term prognosis without severe histological progression, whereas patients with NASH show a much more aggressive natural history with development of cirrhosis in up to 26% of the patients [37]. Importantly, the high frequency of NASH in patients with unexplained cirrhosis suggests a potential relationship between progressive NASH and cryptogenic cirrhosis [38]. Whether the presence of MS may influence the clinical course of NAFLD has recently become matter of investigation. The recent study by Younossi et al. [13] provides convincing evidence that the prognosis of subjects with metabolically normal NAFLD is significantly better than those of subjects with MS-associated NAFLD. Notably, there were no significant differences in terms of all-cause, liver-related, or cardiovascular mortality between subjects with metabolically normal NAFLD and those without evidence of fatty liver infiltration. From the authors' data, it was the presence of the MS—and not NAFLD per se—that was independently associated with overall mortality, liver-specific mortality, and cardiovascular mortality. These results are provocative and raise important questions about the clinical and prognostic relevance of ultrasound-diagnosed NAFLD per se, because the mortality figures in this study seem to be chiefly driven by the MS [13]. As recently highlighted by Angulo in an authoritative paper [39], a large study involving several hundreds of patients who underwent liver biopsy and have follow-up data for several years or decades is necessary to shed more light on the clinical impact of NAFLD on "hard" clinical endpoints (such as mortality). Currently, it seems that the presence and severity of liver fibrosis on histology (regardless of the pathologist' labeling of NASH or simple steatosis) are the most reliable evidence-based predictor of adverse long-term outcomes [39]. Assuming we can agree on the adverse prognostic significance of the MS [13], we should next ask what impact the absence of the MS will have on our clinical care of NAFLD patients. In other words, does metabolically normal NAFLD have specific implications in terms of clinical management?

## Does metabolically normal NAFLD require a specific treatment approach?

Low-calorie diets along with regular exercise are central to the management of MS-associated NAFLD [40, 41]. Indeed, all of the components of the MS and insulin resistance are improved by even modest amounts of weight loss achieved with diet and exercise [42]. Although lifestyle therapies are first-line interventions to reduce the metabolic risk factors, the ideal diet and form of exercise for the treatment of

NAFLD remain uncertain [43]. Owing to the absence of common metabolic risk factors, it is conceivable that metabolically normal NAFLD poses special therapeutic challenges. In particular, the convoluted nature of hepatic fat deposition in metabolically normal NAFLD hinders ready identification of therapeutic targets for pharmaceutical intervention. However, the potential involvement of Hb and iron theoretically provides a rationale for the development of iron-lowering strategies as viable new therapeutic strategies in this clinical entity. The idea of targeted iron removal in NAFLD is not new. Valenti et al. [44] demonstrated that iron depletion by venesection favors the normalization of insulin resistance and liver enzymes in nonhemochromatosis patients with NAFLD. In a recent phase II clinical trial, Beaton et al. [27] reported that iron reduction by phlebotomy resulted in a significant improvement in the NAFLD activity score, without significant effects in terms of fibrosis. As the knowledge of metabolically normal NAFLD will evolve, so will the understanding of the role of iron in its pathogenesis. Since the accumulation of iron in the liver presents a potential target for therapeutic intervention, future studies of iron chelators in NAFLD patients without the MS seem to be warranted.

## Conclusions

NAFLD is increasing in incidence and it currently represents a major public health issue. Although strong evidence suggests that insulin resistance and the related metabolic abnormalities are key risk factors for NAFLD, this association is not invariable and there can be a number of potential pathogenic factors that may influence the risk of developing NAFLD in the absence of a formal diagnosis of MS (e.g., increased Hb levels, iron overload, genetic risk factors). Clearly, these relationships warrant further investigation, particularly because they can serve as novel therapeutic targets for the prevention and treatment of NAFLD. In general, growing evidence suggests that NAFLD can develop—and even be common, even in subjects without overt metabolic abnormalities. Can specific iron-targeted interventions be developed for subjects with genetic risk factors for NAFLD even in the absence of the MS? Clearly, the relationship between Hb, iron overload, and the risk of NAFLD is highly relevant for both the current understanding of fatty liver overload and developing new groundbreaking therapies. Based on the current evidence, metabolically normal NAFLD seems to differ from traditional MS-associated NAFLD in terms of the key role played by

Hb, iron, and genetic factors in its pathogenesis, as well as with regard to more favorable clinical outcomes. Whether this entity should be targeted in a specific manner (especially with iron chelators) remains to be established.

## References

1. Masuoka HC, Chalasani N. Nonalcoholic fatty liver disease: an emerging threat to obese and diabetic individuals. Ann N Y Acad Sci 2013;1281:106–122.

2. Milić S, Stimac D. Nonalcoholic fatty liver disease/steatohepatitis: epidemiology, pathogenesis, clinical presentation and treatment. Dig Dis 2012;30:158–162.

3. Paredes AH, Torres DM, Harrison SA. Nonalcoholic fatty liver disease. Clin Liver Dis 2012;16:397–419.

4. Rahimi RS, Landaverde C. Nonalcoholic fatty liver disease and the metabolic syndrome: clinical implications and treatment. Nutr Clin Pract 2013;28:40–51.

5. Bugianesi E, Moscatiello S, Ciaravella MF, Marchesini G. Insulin resistance in nonalcoholic fatty liver disease. Curr Pharm Des 2010;16:1941–1951.

6. Kim CH, Younossi ZM. Nonalcoholic fatty liver disease: a manifestation of the metabolic syndrome. Cleve Clin J Med 2008;75:721–728.

7. Gaggini M, Morelli M, Buzzigoli E, et al. Non-alcoholic fatty liver disease (NAFLD) and its connection with insulin resistance, dyslipidemia, atherosclerosis and coronary heart disease. Nutrients 2013;5:1544–1560.

8. Kotronen A, Westerbacka J, Bergholm R, et al. Liver fat in the metabolic syndrome. J Clin Endocrinol Metab 2007;92:3490–3497.

9. Uchil D, Pipalia D, Chawla M, et al. Non-alcoholic fatty liver disease (NAFLD)—the hepatic component of metabolic syndrome. J Assoc Physicians India 2009;57:201–204.

10. Yilmaz Y, Senates E, Ayyildiz T, et al. Characterization of nonalcoholic fatty liver disease unrelated to the metabolic syndrome. Eur J Clin Invest 2012;42:411–418.

11. Yilmaz Y. NAFLD in the absence of metabolic syndrome: different epidemiology, pathogenetic mechanisms, risk factors for disease progression?. Semin Liver Dis 2012;32:14–21.

12. Yilmaz Y. Is nonalcoholic fatty liver disease the hepatic expression of the metabolic syndrome? World J Hepatol 2012;4:332–334.

13. Younossi ZM, Otgonsuren M, Venkatesan C, Mishra A. In patients with non-alcoholic fatty liver disease, metabolically abnormal individuals are at a higher risk for mortality while metabolically normal individuals are not. Metabolism 2013;62:352–360.

14. Chitturi S, Farrell GC. Etiopathogenesis of nonalcoholic steatohepatitis. Semin Liver Dis 2001;21:27–41.

15. Vanni E, Bugianesi E, Kotronen A, et al. From the metabolic syndrome to NAFLD or vice versa? Dig Liver Dis 2010;42:320–330.

16. Shen J, Wong GL, Chan HL, et al. PNPLA3 gene polymorphism accounts for fatty liver in community subjects without metabolic syndrome. Aliment Pharmacol Ther 2014;39:532–539.

17. Yu C, Xu C, Xu L, et al. Serum proteomic analysis revealed diagnostic value of hemoglobin for nonalcoholic fatty liver disease. J Hepatol 2012;56:241–247.

18. Das SK, Mukherjee S, Vasudevan DM, Balakrishnan V. Comparison of haematological parameters in patients with non-alcoholic fatty liver disease and alcoholic liver disease. Singap Med J 2011;52:175–181.

19. Akahane T, Fukui K, Shirai Y, et al. High hemoglobin level predicts non-alcoholic fatty liver disease in Japanese women. J Gastroenterol Hepatol 2013;2:623–627.

20. Leung TM, Tipoe GL, Liong EC, et al. Endothelial nitric oxide synthase is a critical factor in experimental liver fibrosis. Int J Exp Pathol 2008;89:241–250.

21. Houschyar KS, Lüdtke R, Dobos GJ, et al. Effects of phlebotomy-induced reduction of body iron stores on metabolic syndrome: results from a randomized clinical trial. BMC Med 2012;10:54.

22. Nelson JE, Klintworth H, Kowdley KV. Iron metabolism in nonalcoholic fatty liver disease. Curr Gastroenterol Rep 2012;14:8–16.

23. Fujita N, Takei Y. Iron overload in nonalcoholic steatohepatitis. Adv Clin Chem 2011;55:105–132.

24. Lee SH, Kim JW, Shin SH, et al. HFE gene mutations, serum ferritin level, transferrin saturation, and their clinical correlates in a Korean population. Dig Dis Sci 2009;54:879–886.

25. Utzschneider KM, Largajolli A, Bertoldo A, et al. Serum ferritin is associated with non-alcoholic fatty liver disease and decreased B-cell function in non-diabetic men and women. J Diabetes Complicat 2014;28:177–184.

26. Senates E, Yilmaz Y, Colak Y, et al. Serum levels of hepcidin in patients with biopsy-proven nonalcoholic fatty liver disease. Metab Syndr Relat Disord 2011;9:287–290.

27. Beaton MD, Chakrabarti S, Levstik M, et al. Phase II clinical trial of phlebotomy for non-alcoholic fatty liver disease. Aliment Pharmacol Ther 2013;37:720–729.

28. Anstee QM, Day CP. The genetics of NAFLD. Nat Rev Gastroenterol Hepatol 2013;10:645–655.

29. Sookoian S, Pirola CJ. Meta-analysis of the influence of I148M variant of patatin-like phospholipase domain containing 3 gene (PNPLA3) on the susceptibility and histological severity of non-alcoholic fatty liver disease. Hepatology 2011;53:1883–1894.

30. Romeo S, Kozlitina J, Xing C, et al. Genetic variation in PNPLA3 confers susceptibility to nonalcoholic fatty liver disease. Nat Genet 2008;40:1461–1465.

31. Rotman Y, Koh C, Zmuda JM, et al. The association of genetic variability in patatin-like phospholipase domain-containing protein 3 (PNPLA3) with histological severity of nonalcoholic fatty liver disease. Hepatology 2010;52:894–903.

32. Speliotes EK, Butler JL, Palmer CD, et al. PNPLA3 variants specifically confer increased risk for histologic nonalcoholic fatty liver disease but not metabolic disease. Hepatology 2010;52:904–912.

33. Kawaguchi T, Sumida Y, Umemura A, et al. Genetic polymorphisms of the human PNPLA3 gene are strongly associated with severity of non-alcoholic fatty liver disease in Japanese. PLoS One 2012;7:e38322.

34. Ahmed U, Latham PS, Oates PS. Interactions between hepatic iron and lipid metabolism with possible relevance to steatohepatitis. World J Gastroenterol 2012;18:4651–4658.

35. Messner DJ, Rhieu BH, Kowdley KV. Iron overload causes oxidative stress and impaired insulin signaling in AML-12 hepatocytes. Dig Dis Sci 2013;58:1899–1908.

36. Musso G, Gambino R, Cassader M, Pagano G. Meta-analysis: natural history of non-alcoholic fatty liver disease (NAFLD) and diagnostic accuracy of non-invasive tests for liver disease severity. Ann Med 2011;43:617–649.

37. Ong JP, Younossi ZM. Epidemiology and natural history of NAFLD and NASH. Clin Liver Dis 2007;11:1–16.

38. Caldwell SH, Lee VD, Kleiner DE, et al. NASH and cryptogenic cirrhosis: a histological analysis. Ann Hepatol 2009;8:346–352.

39. Angulo P. Long-term mortality in nonalcoholic fatty liver disease: is liver histology of any prognostic significance? Hepatology 2010;51:373–375.

40. Fan JG, Cao HX. Role of diet and nutritional management in non-alcoholic fatty liver disease. J Gastroenterol Hepatol 2013;28(Suppl 4):81–87.

41. Gerber LH, Weinstein A, Pawloski L. Role of exercise in optimizing the functional status of patients with nonalcoholic fatty liver disease. Clin Liver Dis 2014;18:113–127.

42. Fock KM, Khoo J. Diet and exercise in management of obesity and overweight. J Gastroenterol Hepatol 2013;28 (Suppl 4):59–63.

43. Xiao J, Guo R, Fung ML, Liong EC, Tipoe GL. Therapeutic approaches to non-alcoholic fatty liver disease: past achievements and future challenges. Hepatobiliary Pancreat Dis Int 2013;12:125–135.

44. Valenti L, Moscatiello S, Vanni E, et al. Venesection for non-alcoholic fatty liver disease unresponsive to lifestyle counselling—a propensity score-adjusted observational study. QJM 2011;104:141–149.

# 7 Occurrence of noncirrhotic HCC in NAFLD

**Dawn M. Torres[1] and Stephen A. Harrison[2]**

[1] Division of Gastroenterology, Department of Medicine, Walter Reed National Military Medical Center, Bethesda, MD, USA

[2] Division of Gastroenterology, Department of Medicine, San Antonio Military Medical Center, Fort Sam Houston, San Antonio, TX, USA

## LEARNING POINTS

- Liver cancer has been reported increasingly in noncirrhotic non-alcoholic fatty liver disease (NAFLD) patients.

- Obesity and diabetes are associated with increased rates of liver cancer in NAFLD populations.

- It is not feasible or recommended to screen all those with NAFLD with serial imaging for HCC, although it should be done for those with NASH cirrhosis.

- Stage 3 NASH patients or those with NAFLD and a strong family history of liver cancer can be considered for serial imaging.

- There is insufficient data to recommend metformin as chemoprophylaxis for liver cancer in NAFLD, although it may be considered in patients with coexisting diabetes.

The incidental finding of mildly elevated serum aminotransferases or hepatic steatosis on abdominal imaging often leads to the diagnosis of non-alcoholic fatty liver disease (NAFLD). NAFLD is by far the most common cause of chronic liver disease in the Western world with an estimated prevalence of 30–40% in the United States [1]. The most clinically relevant subset of patients with NAFLD are the approximately 5–20% who meet histopathologic criteria for non-alcoholic steatohepatitis (NASH) with its inherent risk for progression to cirrhosis. NASH is the second leading etiology of liver disease among adults awaiting liver transplantation in the United States with almost triple the number of adults with NASH awaiting liver transplant in 2013, compared to 2004 [2]. Independent of the complications of cirrhosis, such as hepatic encephalopathy or ascites, there is also a markedly increased risk for hepatocellular carcinoma (HCC), which has led the American Association for the Study of Liver Diseases (AASLD) to recommend biannual imaging as a screening modality for patients with cirrhosis from any etiology [3].

Currently, other causes of liver disease including chronic hepatitis C (CHC), chronic hepatitis B (CHB), and alcoholic liver disease are the most common causes of HCC, although this is expected to change with the increasing prevalence of NAFLD. The rate of HCC related to NASH-induced cirrhosis is a *lready* increasing. A recent retrospective cohort study using the United Network for Organ Sharing (UNOS) registry demonstrated a consistent rise in the rates of liver transplantation for NASH-related HCC from 8.3% in 2002 to 10.3% in 2007 to 13.5% in 2012 [4]. In 2012, NASH-related HCC was only second to CHC-related HCC.

Overall, HCC itself is a leading cause of cancer worldwide and is a major cause of cancer-related deaths [5]. With improved screening, cirrhotic patients are often diagnosed at an earlier stage where more treatment options are available. Resection, local regional therapy such as chemoembolization or radiofrequency ablation, and liver transplantation are increasingly more successful in cirrhotic patients who are incidentally found to have a small HCC on imaging.

While screening is an established practice to detect early HCC in NASH-related cirrhosis, the known phenomenon of HCC in the absence of cirrhosis in NAFLD presents a unique problem, as it is not feasible to image all NAFLD patients serially. Noncirrhotic HCC, arising on a background of NAFLD, has been reported throughout the world and appears to be on the rise. Clinical presentation is varied, and multiple risk factors associated with NAFLD that may also predispose toward HCC have been investigated including obesity, insulin resistance (IR), and iron overload. More recent research efforts have focused on HCC-associated genes and metabolites in NAFLD. This is an exciting area of study that offers hope that high-risk individuals can eventually be identified from the unwieldy 30–40% of the population with NAFLD. This discussion addresses the epidemiology as well as some potential mechanisms behind the occurrence of HCC in noncirrhotic NAFLD.

## The metabolic syndrome, NAFLD, and HCC

NAFLD as the hepatic manifestation of the metabolic syndrome (MS) is strongly associated with obesity, IR, and diabetes. Each of these risk factors for NAFLD has also been evaluated as independent risk factors for HCC.

One major association that has been evaluated in a number of different populations is the link between obesity and HCC. Obesity has also been associated with multiple other malignancies including the colon, endometrium, breast (postmenopausal), kidney, esophagus, pancreas, and gallbladder and hematological causes [6, 7]. The data in HCC populations mostly favor an association between obesity and higher rates of HCC. A systematic review of 10 cohort studies demonstrated 7 studies with an increased relative risk (RR) ranging from 1.4 to 4.1, two studies showing no association, and one study showing an inverse association [8]. Critics of these data noted that they relied on small numbers of HCC in the individual studies, as well as the utilization of body mass index (BMI) as a surrogate for obesity [9]. They described BMI as a somewhat arbitrary measure that classifies as obese or nonobese and rather advocate the use of hip-to-waist ratio. Recent data from the European Prospective Investigation into Cancer and Nutrition (EPIC) cohort showed a threefold increased HCC risk in subjects in the upper tertile of waist-to-hip ratio compared to the lowest

tertile and appears to substantiate the previous data using BMI as a surrogate for obesity [10].

Population attributable fraction (PAF) is another way to evaluate the association of obesity with HCC and takes into account the prevalence as well as the RR with the goal of predicting a percent reduction in the disease process if the risk factor was eliminated. Using this approach, data from US SEER-Medicare attributed 36.6% of HCC in US Medicare populations to diabetes and/or obesity [11]. Similarly, data from the EPIC attributed 16% of HCC to obesity [12]. These high PAFs may overestimate the relationship between obesity and HCC. El-Serag *et al.* argued that PAF estimates use assumptions to establish attributable risk leading to estimates that represent "worst-case scenarios." Despite the aforementioned limitations, obesity appears to be a risk factor for HCC. Further study is required to better understand what degree of obesity is highest risk, and if this affects outcomes, as suggested by an early study showing increased overall cancer mortality with increasing weight [13].

The connection between diabetes or IR and NAFLD is considered similar but distinct from the association of obesity and NAFLD. There is good evidence that diabetes is an independent risk factor for both NAFLD and HCC. An increased rate of HCC in diabetic patients was demonstrated in a large longitudinal study even after excluding patients with viral hepatitis, alcohol use, or fatty liver disease [14]. Similarly, an increased RR of HCC in diabetes was also shown in a large prospective cohort study where diabetic women had an RR of 1.4 (95% CI; 1.05–1.86) and diabetic men were even at an even greater RR of 2.26 (95%CI; 1.89–2.70) [15]. Two large meta-analyses—one with 13 case–control studies and a second with 17 case–control and 32 cohort studies—both confirmed an increased RR for HCC in diabetes with RR of 2 and 2.31, respectively [16, 17]. The association of diabetes and elevated serum fasting glucose with HCC was shown to be independent of cirrhosis in a Korean study, and glucose levels >125 mg/dL also showed increased overall cancer mortality [18]. In total, there is abundant evidence to support the association of diabetes and IR with HCC. By the same token, IR is essential in the pathogenesis of NAFLD and at least partially can explain the increased risk of HCC seen in NAFLD.

While there is abundant evidence linking diabetes to HCC, there are less data investigating how diabetes impacts outcomes in HCC. Recent study in a cohort of 505 patients with HCC (134 with DM, 371 without) suggested that while DM does not affect postoperative mortality or morbidity after curative hepatectomy, lower overall survival was seen in those with DM [19]. Previous studies in smaller retrospective cohorts demonstrate conflicting results with some showing increased mortality in diabetic HCC patients [20] and others showing no difference in long-term survivals or rates of HCC recurrence [21]. Further study is required to clarify the issue.

Obesity and hyperglycemia (DM) have been independently associated with HCC but remain individual components of the MS, as defined by the presence of 3 or more of the following: abdominal obesity, hypertriglyceridemia, low high-density lipoprotein (HDL), hypertension, and elevated fasting plasma glucose [22]. The MS as whole has been less studied compared to its individual components in terms of its association with HCC, but there is still evidence suggesting an increased risk for HCC in those patients that meet criteria for MS [23]. The strongest evidence to date comes from Italy where Turati et al. demonstrated increased incidence of HCC in patients with MS, when compared to those without MS. The risk for HCC was increased fourfold in those with ≥2 MS components, although it is notable that the only two independently associated components of the MS from the study were DM and obesity [24]. Thus, it is reasonable to associate MS as well as obesity and DM with HCC, but this cannot be extended to independent associations with abnormal lipids or hypertension.

## Pathogenesis linking HCC and NAFLD

While a complete understanding of the mechanisms that lead to both isolated fatty liver and steatohepatitis is not yet a reality, knowledge has grown from the original two-hit hypothesis to a complicated interplay of processes related both to intrinsic host factors and extrinsic environmental factors. The same can be said for the steps leading to hepatocarcinogenesis, where genetic and host factors as well as environmental conditions work in concert to cause tumor growth. A detailed discussion of both the pathogenesis of NAFLD and HCC is beyond the scope of this chapter, but the mechanisms that overlap will be highlighted here. See Figure 7.1.

As previously mentioned, IR is fundamental in the pathogenesis of NAFLD and appears to be important in the development of HCC, given the multiple epidemiologic studies showing increased RR for HCC with IR and/or DM. In NAFLD, elevated levels of insulin lead to increased production of insulin growth factor-1 (IGF-1), which in turn activates insulin receptor substrate-1 (IRS-1) [25]. Activation of IRS-1 promotes processes that induce cellular proliferation and inhibit apoptosis including p53, mitogen-activated protein kinase (MAPK), and phosphatidylinositol-3-kinase (P13K)/Akt and are important in the development of HCC [26]. P12K/Akt signaling is in turn regulated by phosphatase and tensin homolog (PTEN) [27]. Alterations in PTEN function in the mouse model have been shown to promote both NASH and HCC via P12k/Akt activation resulting in cell hyperproliferation and antiapoptosis [28].

Increased levels of tumor necrosis factor-α (TNF-α) and interleukin-6 (IL-6) are also seen in NASH as part of the proinflammatory cytokine release secondary to elevated insulin levels [29]. In mouse models of NASH, nuclear factor-κβ (NF-κβ) is activated by TNF-α and results in hepatocarcinogenesis when exposed to the carcinogen diethylnitrosamine (DEN) [30]. TNF-α and NF-κβ are involved in the aforementioned MAPK3 kinase pathway, as well as transforming growth factor-β (TGF-β)-activated kinase 1 (TAK1), both of which promote HCC [31]. The two cytokines also activate signal transducer and activator of transcription-3 (STAT3), yet another signaling protein that appears to be important in both NAFLD and HCC [32]. A particularly intriguing study in mice demonstrated hepatic steatosis in the setting of a single mutant STAT5 allele and steatosis and HCC in mice with two mutant STAT5 alleles [33].

Leptin is a peptide that is produced in excess in obesity by adipose tissue and can also activate TFG-β as well as the JAK–STAT pathway, which is thought to promote fibrinogenesis [34]. Although there are conflicting data in NASH populations with some studies showing elevated leptin in NASH while others do not, leptin has generally been shown to be increased in HCC. Some of this association may be from the promotion of hepatic fibrosis with other studies demonstrating that leptin induces hepatic angiogenesis, which is also thought to be important in HCC development [35]. The role of adiponectin as an anti-inflammatory cytokine produced by adipocytes is equally complicated with decreased levels of adiponectin being associated with IR, elevated BMI, and early NASH but lower levels seen in advanced NASH and HCC [36, 37]. Further study is required of both leptin and adiponectin to better understand their likely roles in both NAFLD and HCC.

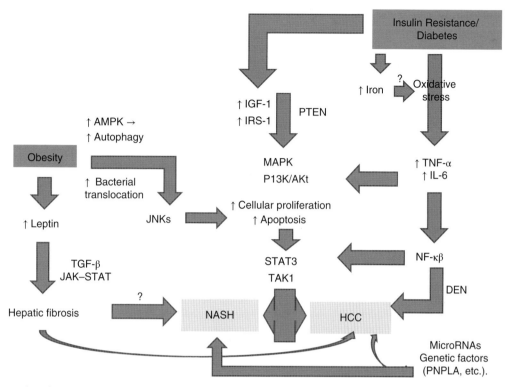

**FIG 7.1** Shared pathways in the pathogenesis of NAFLD and HCC. AMPK, adenosine monophosphate-activated protein kinase; DEN, diethylnitrosamine; IGF-1, insulin growth factor-1; IRS-1, insulin receptor substrate-1; JNK, c-Jun amino-terminal kinases; MAPK, mitogen-activated protein kinase; NF-κβ, nuclear factor kappa beta; P13K, phosphatidylinositol-3-kinase/Akt=protein kinase B; PTEN, phosphatase and tensin homolog; TAK1, transforming growth factor-β-activated kinase 1; TGF-β, transforming growth factor beta; TNF-α, tumor necrosis factor-alpha.

Lipotoxicity is another common pathway thought to be important in both the pathogenesis of NAFLD as well as HCC and refers to the generation of reactive oxygen species from increased free fatty acid (FFA) metabolism in sites of fat accumulation such as the liver [38]. In NAFLD, c-Jun amino-terminal kinases (JNKs) mediate lipoapoptosis in the presence of abundant FFAs resulting in the development of NASH [39]. JNKs are activated in the setting of IR and downregulated when there is weight loss [40].

JNKs have also been shown to be involved in hepatocarcinogenesis with multiple animal and human studies linking JNK to the phosphorylation of genes important in cellular proliferation [41]. One study demonstrated that ~70% of HCC tissue immunostained for phosphorylated JNK was positive compared to background negative controls [42]. In the mouse model using DEN as a carcinogen, c-Jun mediates hepatocarcinogenesis via activation of JNK [43], and DEN-treated mice have higher rates of liver

cancer with JNK1 activation [44]. In total, the evidence suggests that JNK activation in the setting of IR and obesity promotes NAFLD, NASH, and HCC.

JNK activation can also occur via another distinct pathway involving adenosine monophosphate-activated protein kinase (AMPK) that has been implicated in both the pathogenesis of NAFLD and HCC [45]. AMPK1 is an essential mediator of autophagy, which provides vital housekeeping throughout the body removing everything from damaged proteins and organelles to microorganisms and even lipid droplets in hepatocytes in the setting of NASH [46]. Autophagy is also vital in preventing tumor growth and reducing systemic inflammation [47]. Inhibition of AMPK1 and downregulation of autophagy occur in the setting of obesity, which both promotes the development of hepatic steatosis and allows for unabated cell growth as seen in hepatocarcinogenesis [48]. Interference with autophagy has led to spontaneous HCC development in the mouse model [49]. AMPK is also important in the mammalian target of rapamycin (mTOR) pathway, where it normally suppresses tumor growth and increases cellular apoptosis [50]. As previously mentioned, AMPK is inhibited in the settings of obesity marked by a relative lack of adiponectin and represents another potential avenue for tumor growth [51]. Interestingly, metformin has been shown to suppress JNK-mediated NF-κB-dependent pathway [52] and upregulate AMP kinase with a potential inhibitory effect on HCC [53].

Increased hepatic iron stores are another metabolic consequence of the IR and hepatic inflammation that is seen in both NAFLD and HCC populations [54]. Increased hepatic iron stores have been associated with increase hepatic fibrosis in NASH populations [55], and in NASH cirrhotics, increased hepatic iron has been shown to be a risk factor for the development of HCC [56]. The exact mechanism for this link is undetermined, but one author hypothesized that dysregulation of hepcidin transcription resulting in the iron overload is associated with the IR seen in NAFLD [57]. Further study is certainly required as phlebotomy has been shown to improve IR in NAFLD patients with hyperferritinemia [58] and represents a potential therapeutic intervention that could be employed should a cause and effect relationship between iron overload and HCC be confirmed.

The composition of the intestinal microbiome is also thought to be important in the pathogenesis of NAFLD and potentially HCC. Alterations in gut flora in the setting of obesity appear to increase bacterial translocation leading to activation of Toll-like receptors (TLRs), which in turn activate macrophage and dendritic cells as part of the innate immune system [59, 60].

Activation of TLRs ultimately results in another pathway, leading to the activation of NF-κβ and JNK, which as previously described is important in the pathogenesis of NAFLD. In the mouse NASH model, mice lacking the TLR4 receptor had less intracellular lipid accumulation [61], and from an HCC perspective, TLR4-deficient mice were shown to have fewer, smaller, and less frequent DEN-induced tumors when compared to mice with intact TLR4 receptors [62]. Another intriguing animal study demonstrated that antibiotics or gut sterilization reduced hepatic levels of TNF-α as well as few and smaller tumors [63].

The relationship of microRNAs (miRNAs) to both NAFLD and HCC is an active area of research as these small noncoding RNAs are important in transcription regulation for numerous products essential in maintaining cellular homeostasis. For example, the high-fat diet given to promote NASH in the mouse model has been shown to promote expression of miR-155, which in turn promoted hepatocarcinogenesis [64]. Further study in a mouse model demonstrated that increased activity of NF-κβ, seen in NASH, upregulates the oncogenic miR-155 as well as increasing levels of another miRNA, miR-21 [65]. miR-21 has been described as an upstream regulator of PTEN, which, as previously discussed, is known to participate in tumorigenesis in NASH. Another miRNA of interest is the hepatocyte-specific miR-122 that has been shown to have decreased expression in NASH patients [66], as well as downregulation in HCC tissue [67].

One final and new frontier of research is the study of candidate genes common to NAFLD and liver cancer. One recent meta-analysis looked at the patatin-like phospholipase (PNPLA) 3 rs738409 single nucleotide polymorphism that has previously been shown to promote hepatic steatosis and NASH [68] and investigated its association with HCC [69]. Intriguingly, PNPLA3 was associated with an increased risk of hepatic fibrosis among patients with a variety of liver disease. In NASH populations specifically, PNPLA3 was shown to be an independent risk factor for HCC with an OR 1.67 (95% CI 1.27–3.21). Limitations of this meta-analysis were that most patients were Caucasian and the association was not seen in all of the 24 studies, but rather in subgroup analysis. Additional genome-wide analysis of candidate gene loci associated with NAFLD and HCC is required and may provide the ability to predict who is at risk of developing NASH and HCC in the future.

## Conclusions

The occurrence of noncirrhotic HCC in a background of NAFLD presents a unique dilemma. If HCC is diagnosed early, there are numerous therapeutic options, but if HCC is not picked up until the patient is symptomatic, the options are limited and the outcomes are poor. Our current screening algorithm for cirrhotic patients including 6–12-month imaging is not practical to apply to 30–40% of the Western world who meets criteria for NAFLD. Patients with known NASH with advanced fibrosis (stage 3 or greater) or a family history of liver cancer along with NAFLD do seem reasonable to consider serial imaging. While no chemoprophylaxis exists, there are preliminary positive data from two studies that showed metformin use was associated with reduced risk for HCC [70, 71]. The data are inadequate to recommend the universal use of metformin, but certainly it would be a good medication for those diabetic patients with NAFLD who required oral hypoglycemic therapy. It is predicted that NAFLD will become the leading indication for liver transplantation in the United States in the next 10–20 years [72], independent of the phenomenon of HCC in noncirrhotic NAFLD. Substantial efforts need to be directed at better understanding the factors leading to HCC in NAFLD and ways to risk stratifying from the large NAFLD population as a whole. In the interim continuing to address obesity and sedentary lifestyles in our clinics remains the only weapon to combat this and other obesity-associated malignancies.

## References

1. Williams CD, Stengel J, Asike M et al. Prevalence of nonalcoholic fatty liver disease and nonalcoholic steatohepatitis among a largely middle-aged population utilizing ultrasound and liver biopsy: a prospective study. Gastroenterology 2011;140(1):124–131.

2. Wong RJ, Aguilar M, Cheung R et al. Nonalcoholic steatohepatitis is the second leading etiology of liver disease among adults awaiting liver transplantation in the United States. Gastroenterology 2015;148:547–555.

3. Bruix J, Sherman M. Management of hepatocellular carcinoma: an update. Hepatology 2011;53(3):1020–1022.

4. Wong RJ, Cheung R, Ahmed A. Non-alcoholic steatohepatitis is the most rapidly growing indication for liver transplantation in the patients with hepatocellular carcinoma in the U.S. Hepatology 2014;59:2188–2195.

5. Venook AP, Papandreou C, Furuse J, de Guevara LL. The incidence and epidemiology of hepatocellular carcinoma: a global and regional perspective. Oncologist 2010;15 Suppl 4:5–13.

6. Vucenik I, Stains JP. Obesity and Cancer risk: evidence, mechanisms, and recommendations. Ann N Y Acad Sci 2012;1271:37–43.

7. Lichtman MA. Obesity and the risk for a hematological malignancy: leukemia, lymphoma, or myeloma. Oncologist 2011;15:1083–1101.

8. Saunders D, Seidel D, Allison M, Lyratzopoulous G. Systematic review: the association between obesity and hepatocellular carcinoma—epidemiological evidence. Aliment Pharmacol Ther 2010;31:1051–1063.

9. El-Serag HB, Kanwal F. Obesity and hepatocellular carcinoma: hype and reality. Hepatology 2014;60(3):779–781.

10. Schleisinger S, Aleksandrova K, Pischon T et al. Abdominal obesity, weight gain during adulthood and risk of liver and biliary tract cancer in a European cohort. Int J Cancer 2013;132:645–657.

11. Welzel TM, Graubard BI, Quraishi S et al. Population-attributable fractions of risk factors for hepatocellular carcinoma in the United States. Am J Gastroenterol 2013;108:1314–1321.

12. Trichopoulos D, Bamia C, Lagiou P et al. Hepatocellular carcinoma risk factors and disease burden in a European cohort: a nested case-control study. J Natl Cancer Inst 2011;103:1686–1696.

13. Calle EE, Rodriguez C, Walker-Thurmond K, Thun MJ. Overweight, obesity, and mortality from cancer in a prospectively studied cohort of US adults. N Engl J Med 2003;348(17):1625–1638.

14. El-Serag HB, Tran T, Everhart JE. Diabetes increases the risk of chronic liver disease and hepatocellular carcinoma. Gastroenterology 2004;126(2):460–468.

15. Campbell PT, Newton CC, Patel AV et al. Diabetes and cause-specific mortality in a prospective cohort of one million U.S. adults. Diabetes Care 2012;35:1835–1844.

16. El-Serag HB, Hampel H, Javadi F. The association between diabetes and hepatocellular carcinoma: a systematic review of epidemiologic evidence. Clin Gastroenterol Hepatol 2006;4(3):369–380.

17. Wang P, Kang D, Cao W et al Diabetes mellitus and risk of hepatocellular carcinoma: a systemic review and meta-analysis. Diabetes Metab Res Rev 2012;28:109–122.

18. Jee SH, Ohrr H, Sull JW et al. Fasting serum glucose level and cancer risk in Korean men and woman. JAMA 2005;293(2):194–202.

19. Wang YY, Huang S, Zhong JH. Impact of diabetes mellitus on the prognosis of patients with hepatocellular carcinoma after curative hepatectomy. PLoS One 2014;9(12):e113858.

20. Ikeda Y, Shimada M, Hasegawa H et al. Prognosis of hepatocellular carcinoma with diabetes mellitus after hepatic resection. Hepatology 1998;27:1567–1571.

21. Poon RT, Fan ST, Wong J. Does diabetes mellitus influence the perioperative outcome or long term prognosis after resection of hepatocellular carcinoma? Am J Gastroenterol 2002;97:1480–1488.

22. Ford ES, Giles WH, Dietz WH. Prevalence of the metabolic syndrome among US adults: findings from the third National Health and Nutrition Examination Survey. JAMA 2002;287: 356–359.

23. Duan XF, Tang P, Li Q et al. Obesity, adipokines and hepatocellular carcinoma. Int J Cancer 2012;133:1776–1783.

24. Turati F, Talamini R, Pelucchi C et al. Metabolic syndrome and hepatocellular carcinoma risk. Br J Cancer 2013;108:222–228.

25. Yu J, Shen J, Sun TT, Xiang Z, Wong N. Obesity, insulin resistance, NASH, and hepatocellular carcinoma. Semin Cancer Biol 2013;23P:483–491.

26. Page JM, Harrison SA. NASH and HCC. Clin Liver Dis 2009;13:631–647.

27. Peyrou M, Bourgoin L, Foti M. PTEN in non-alcoholic fatty liver disease/non-alcoholic steatohepatitis and cancer. Dig Dis 2010;28(1):236–246.

28. Watanabe S, Horie Y, Kataoka E et al. Non-alcoholic steato-hepatitis and hepatocellular carcinoma in hepatocyte specific phosphatase and tensin homolog (PTEN)-deficient mice. J Gastroenterol Hepatol 2007;22(Suppl 1); S96–S100.

29. Hashimoto E, Tokushige K. Hepatocellular carcinoma in nonalcoholic steatohepatitis: growing evidence of an epidemic. Hepatol Res 2012;42(1):1–14.

30. Wang Y, Ausman LM, Greenberg AS et al. Nonalcoholic steatohepatitis induced by a high-fat diet promotes diethyl-nitrosamine-initiated early hepatocarcinogenesis in rats. Int J Canter 2009;124(3):540–546.

31. Betterman K, Vucur M, Haybaeck J et al. TAK1 suppresses a NEMO-dependent but NF-β-independent pathway to liver cancer. Cancer Cell 2010;17(5):481–496.

32. He G, Yu GY, Temkin V et al. Hepatocyte IKKbeta/NF-kappaB inhibits tumor promotion and progression by prevention oxidative stress-driven STAT3 activation. Cancer Cell 2010;17(3):286–297.

33. Mueller KM, Kornfeld JW, Friedbichler K et al. Impairment of hepatic growth hormone and glucocorticoid receptor signaling causes steatosis and hepatocellular carcinoma in mice. Hepatology 2011;54(4):1398–1409.

34. Ikejima K, Honda H, Yoshikawa M et al. Leptin augments inflammatory and profibrogenic responses in the murine liver induced by hepatotoxic chemicals. Hepatology 2001;34:288–297.

35. Alzahrani B, Iseli TJ, Hebbard LW. Non-viral causes of liver cancer: does obesity led inflammation play a role? Cancer Lett 2014;345:223–229.

36. Jarrar MH, Baranova R, Collantes B et al. Adipokines and cytokines in nonalcoholic fatty liver disease. Aliment Pharmacol Ther 2008;27:412–421.

37. Chen MJ, Yeh YT, Lee KT et al. The promoting effects of adiponectin in hepatocellular carcinoma. J Surg Oncol 2012;106:181–187

38. Vanni E, Bugianesi E. Obesity and liver cancer. Clin Liv Dis 2014;18:191–203.

39. Wree A, Kahraman A, Gerken G, Canby A. Obesity affects the liver—the link between adipocytes and hepatocytes. Digestion 2011;83(1–2):124–133.

40. Solinas G, Karin M. JNK1 and IKKbeta: molecular links between obesity and metabolic dysfunction. FASEB J 2010;24(8):2596–2611.

41. Maeda S. NF-kB, JNK, and TLR signaling pathways in hepa-tocarcinogenesis. Gastroenterol Res Pract 2010;367694.

42. Chang Q, Zhang Y, Beezhold KJ et al. Sustained JNK1 acti-vation is associated with altered histone H3 methylations in human liver cancer. J Hepatol 2009;50(2)323–333.

43. Eferl R, Ricci R, Kenner L et al. Liver tumor development. C-Jun antagonizes the proapoptotic activity of p53. Cell 2003;112(2):181–192.

44. Sakurai T, Maeda S, Chang L, Karin M. Loss of hepatic NF-kappa B activity enhances chemical hepatocarcinogenesis through sustain c-Jun N-terminal kinase 1 activation. Proc Natl Acad Sci U S A 2006;103(28)10544–10551.

45. Torres DM, Harrison SA. Nonalcoholic steatohepatitis and noncirrhotic hepatocellular carcinoma: fertile soil. Semin Liver Dis 2012;32:30–38.

46. Singh R, Kaushik S, Wang Y et al. Autophagy regulates lipid metabolism. Nature 2009;458(7242):1131–1135.

47. Dikic I, Johansen T, Kirkin V. Selective autophagy in cancer development and therapy. Cancer Res 2010;70(9):3431–3434.

48. Chan EY. mTORC1 phosphorylates the ULK-mAtg13-FIP200 autophagy regulatory complex. Sci Signal 2009;2:51.

49. Takamura A, Komatsu M, Hara T et al. Autophagy-deficient mice develop multiple liver tumors. Genes Dev 2011;25(8): 795–800.

50. Luo Z, Saha AK, Xiang X et al. AMPK, the metabolic syn-drome and cancer. Trends Pharmacol Sci 2005;26(2):69–76.

51. Karagozian R, Derdak Z, Baffy G. Obesity-associated mech-anisms of hepatocarcinogenesis. Metabolism 2014;63: 607–617.

52. Hsieh SC, Tsai JP, Yang SF et al. Metformin inhibits the inva-sion of human hepatocellular carcinoma cells and enhances the chemosensitivity to sorafenib through a downregulation of the ERK/JNK-mediated NF-kB-dependent pathway that reduces uPA and MMP-9 expression. Amino Acids 2014; 46:2809–2822.

53. Cheng J, Huang T, Li Y et al. AMP-activated protein kinase suppresses the in vitro and in vivo proliferation of hepato-cellular carcinoma. PLoS One 2014;9:e93256.

54. Mendler Mh, Turlin B, Moirand R et al. Insulin resistance-associated hepatic iron overload. Gastroenterology 1999; 117(5):1155–1163.

55. George DK, Goldwurm S, Macdonald GA et al. Increased hepatic iron concentration in nonalcoholic steatohepatitis is associated with increased fibrosis. Gastroenterology 1998; 114(2):311–318.

56. Sorrentino P, D'Angelo S, Ferbo U, Micheli B et al. Liver iron excess in patients with hepatocellular carcinoma developed on non-alcoholic steatohepatitis. J Hepatol 2009;50:351–357.

57. Kew MC. Hepatic iron overload and hepatocellular carci-noma. Liver Cancer 2014;3:31–40.

58. Valenti L, Fracanzani AL, Dongiovanni P, Bugianesi E et al. Iron depletion by phlebotomy improves insulin resistance in patients with nonalcoholic fatty liver disease and

hyperferritinemia: evidence from a case-control study. Am J Gastroenterol 2007;102:1251–1258.

59. Starley BQ, Calcagno CJ, Harrison SA. Nonalcoholic fatty liver disease and hepatocellular carcinoma: a weighty connection. Hepatology 2010. 51:1820–1832.

60. Takeuchi O, Akira S. Toll-like receptors: their physiological role and signal transduction system. Int Immunopharmacol 2001;1(4):625–635.

61. Rivera CA, Adegboyega P, van Rooijen N et al. Toll-like receptor 4 signaling and Kupffer cells play pivotal roles in the pathogenesis of nonalcoholic steatohepatitis. J Hepatol 2007;47(4)571–579.

62. Seki E, Brenner DA. Toll-like receptors and adaptor molecules in liver disease: update. Hepatology 2008;48(1): 322–335.

63. Stickel F, Hellerbrand C. Non-alcoholic fatty liver disease as a risk factor for hepatocellular carcinoma: mechanisms and implications. Gut 2010;59:1303–1307.

64. Wang B, Majumder S, Nuovo G et al. Role of microRNA-155 at early stages of hepatocarcinogenesis induced by choline-deficient and amino acid-defined diet in C578BL/6 mice. Hepatology 2009;50(4):1152–1161.

65. Wong VW, Wong GL, Tsang SW et al. Metabolic and histological features of nonalcoholic fatty liver disease patients with different serum alanine aminotransferase levels. Aliment Pharmacol Ther 2009;29:387–396.

66. Cheung O, Puri P, Eicken C et al. Nonalcoholic steatohepatitis is associated with altered hepatic MicroRNA expression. Hepatology 2008;48:1810–1820.

67. Zeng C, Wang R, Li D et al. A novel GSK-3 beta-C/EBP alpha-miR-122-insulin-like growth factor 1 receptor regulatory circuitry in human hepatocellular carcinoma. Hepatology 2010;52:1702–1712.

68. Sookoian S, Pirola CJ. Meta-analysis of the influence of I148M variant of patatin-like phospholipase domain containing 3 gene (PNPLA3) on the susceptibility and histological severity of nonalcoholic fatty liver disease. Hepatology 2011;53:883–894.

69. Singal AG, Manjunaath H, Yopp AC et al. The effect of PNPLA3 on fibrosis progression and development of hepatocellular carcinoma: a meta-analysis. Am J Gastroenterol 2014;109:324–334.

70. Lai SW, Chen PC, Liao KF et al. Risk of hepatocellular carcinoma in diabetic patients and risk reduction associated with anti-diabetic therapy: a population based cohort study. Am J Gastroenterol 2012;107:46–52.

71. Donadon V, Balbi M, Mas MD et al. Metformin and reduced risk of hepatocellular carcinoma in diabetic patients with chronic liver disease. Liver Int 2010;30:750–758.

72. Charlton MR, Burns JM, Pedersen RA et al. Frequency and outcomes of liver transplantation for nonalcoholic steatohepatitis in the United States. Gastroenterology 2011;141: 1249–1253.

# PART II
# Factors in Disease Progression

# 8  Fibrosis progression: Putative mechanisms and molecular pathways

## Wing-Kin Syn[1] and Anna Mae Diehl[2]

[1] Foundation for Liver Research, The Institute of Hepatology, London, UK
[2] Division of Gastroenterology, Department of Medicine, Duke University, Durham, NC, USA

---

### LEARNING POINTS

- Non-alcoholic steatohepatitis (NASH) is a more advanced stage of non-alcoholic fatty liver disease, and individuals with NASH are at a higher risk of disease progression and developing complications such as liver cirrhosis, liver failure and hepatocellular carcinoma.

- The proliferation of liver progenitors (stem cells) and activation of hepatic stellate cells occur as part of liver repair (constitute the ductular reaction) and in response to autocrine, paracrine and endocrine signals. Liver fibrosis develops when this repair response become deregulated.

- Hepatic and extra-hepatic signals such as those from adipose tissue, the gut microbiota, circulating hormones and hypoxia from sleep apnoea play an integrated role in regulating liver fibrogenesis.

- The Hedgehog signalling pathway and Osteopontin are emerging core mediators of liver fibrosis.

---

## Introduction

The presence of hepatocyte injury and death is the hallmark of non-alcoholic steatohepatitis (NASH), and individuals with NASH are at a much higher risk of developing progressive liver disease (i.e. fibrosis – cirrhosis – cancer) compared with those with simple steatosis [1, 2]. The pathogenic mechanisms that drive non-alcoholic fatty liver disease (NAFLD) progression to NASH and NASH fibrosis are complex, but the prevailing dogma suggests that multiple hits ensuing from oxidative stress and immune, cytokine and hormonal

deregulation overwhelm homeostatic mechanisms within a fatty hepatocyte; cellular injury and death trigger a repair response [3, 4]. Scar tissue deposition and accumulation occur when the repair response becomes excessive or deregulated.

Tissue repair involves the concerted efforts of multiple cell types (hepatic stellate cells (HSC) or liver pericytes, liver progenitor cells, endothelial cells and immune cells). During an acute injury (such as following acute drug injury or liver resection), expansion of liver progenitors and pericytes occurs to replace dying epithelial cells (hepatocytes and cholangiocytes), while the sinusoidal endothelium regulates the trafficking of immune cell subsets in the liver to remove cellular debris that further stimulates regeneration of new epithelial cells [5]. Recovery occurs when the insult is removed, and dying cells are replaced by functioning new epithelial cells. By contrast, such 'restorative' repair does not occur during chronic liver injury; sustained activation of liver pericytes and aberrant reprogramming of liver progenitors lead to excess collagen deposition and accumulation (i.e. fibrosis). Fibrogenic outcomes are perpetuated or even amplified by the preferential recruitment of 'effector–pro-fibrogenic' immune cells rather than 'fibrosis-resolving' subsets [6]. Recent studies show that liver repair is normally tightly regulated by multiple molecular signals and that the dichotomy in liver outcomes (i.e. restorative repair vs. deregulated repair) may be explained in part by perturbations in these signalling pathways.

---

*Clinical Dilemmas in Non-Alcoholic Fatty Liver Disease*, First Edition. Edited by Roger Williams and Simon D. Taylor-Robinson.
© 2016 John Wiley & Sons, Ltd. Published 2016 by John Wiley & Sons, Ltd.

In this chapter, we first introduce the concept of liver repair and then summarise putative mechanisms. We will focus on three 'emerging' molecular pathways and their potential as anti-fibrotic targets. Although this chapter is NASH focused, many of these molecular signals are likely to be relevant to other liver diseases and tissues outside the liver.

## The concept of liver repair

The presence of dying and ballooned hepatocytes distinguishes NASH from simple steatosis [7, 8]. Mechanistically, excessive free fatty acid influx, de novo lipogenesis and impaired fatty acid oxidation lead to the development of steatosis. Sustained insults from subsequent oxidative, cytotoxic and immune stresses lead to hepatocyte injury and death. Fat-laden hepatocytes that remain are unable to replicate to replace the lost hepatocytes. Instead, an expansion of the liver progenitors (or stem cell) occurs, in an attempt to restore architecture and function [9, 10]. This liver progenitor cell response is termed the 'ductular reaction' in humans, is a harbinger of fibrosis and is characteristic of progressive liver disease [11].

### Cell death

Gores and colleagues first reported an increased number of apoptotic hepatocytes in patients with NASH [7] and showed that the magnitude of apoptosis positively correlated with disease grade and stage [12]. Mice deficient in caspase-2 (an initiator caspase responsible for long-chain fatty acid-induced cell death) exhibited reduced hepatocyte apoptosis and developed significantly less fibrosis when fed the high-fat (a model of steatosis and early NASH) or the methionine–choline-deficient diet (a model of advanced NASH fibrosis) [13]. Pharmacologic approaches using a pan-caspase inhibitor similarly resulted in decreased active caspase-3, cell death and fibrosis [14]. These studies in animal models and in humans show that hepatocyte death is intricately linked to NASH progression.

### Tissue repair and fibrogenesis

The loss of functioning hepatocytes is accompanied by a compensatory proliferation of liver progenitors (i.e. liver stem cells) located in the Canals of Hering. These liver progenitors are surrounded by liver pericytes (referred to as HSC), portal fibroblasts and an extracellular matrix enriched with endothelial cells forming neovasculature. Liver progenitors, liver pericytes, stromal cells and extracellular matrix collectively constitute the progenitor niche [15, 16].

For many individuals with chronic liver disease, fibrosis (i.e. deregulated repair) is the general outcome. Although the reasons for this remain poorly understood, animal studies show that factors stimulating the progenitor response are pro-fibrogenic and progenitor cells themselves are highly reactive and secrete high levels of pro-inflammatory and pro-fibrogenic cytokines. Fate mapping and immunohistochemistry studies demonstrate that liver progenitors may be directly reprogrammed, from an epithelial to a mesenchymal (and possibly fibrogenic) phenotype [17, 18], and recently liver pericytes were identified as multipotent progenitors capable of secreting collagen matrix as well as giving rise to new epithelial progenitors (i.e. mesenchymal to epithelial phenotype) [19, 20]. In addition, the progenitor-derived 'secretome' can act on neighbouring immune and endothelial cells to perpetuate and amplify fibrogenic outcomes [21]. Thus, the resultant ductular reaction observed during chronic injury should be considered a fibrogenic repair response (i.e. fibrosis promoting).

'Restorative' repair (where progenitors differentiate into new functioning epithelial cells) occurs when the injury and pro-fibrogenic/pro-inflammatory stimuli are removed.

## Mechanisms of liver fibrogenesis

### The link between hepatocyte injury/death and repair

Despite ample evidence showing that cell death triggers fibrogenesis, the mechanistic link remains poorly understood. Previously, it was proposed that phagocytosis of apoptotic hepatocytes by macrophages and HSC led to secretion of pro-fibrogenic mediators [22]. In turn, these promoted HSC activation and fibrosis (an indirect mechanism). More recently, injury-associated inflammasome activation and release of damage-associated molecular patterns (DAMPs) were reported to promote disease progression [23]. Inflammasome activation and DAMP release trigger immune cell recruitment, and RAGE, a receptor for high-mobility group box 1 (HMGB1; an example of DAMP), is required for progenitor cell proliferation [24].

Despite this, there is no convincing evidence for DAMPs directly activating HSC.

Recent studies suggest that soluble mediators released by injured and dying hepatocytes are major regulators of repair. Using cell culture and *in vivo* models, investigators showed that stressed or dying hepatocytes release Hedgehog (Hh) ligands, a morphogen normally responsible for orchestrating tissue development and cell fate [25]. Hh ligands directly stimulate liver progenitors and HSC (i.e. fibrogenic repair) [26, 27], provoke secretion of chemokines that lead to the recruitment of inflammatory cells (i.e. repair-associated inflammation) [28] and promote capillarisation of liver sinusoidal endothelium [29] – features characteristic of progressive liver disease. Importantly, the level of Hh pathway activation correlated with the amount of injury and fibrosis [27, 30], suggesting that targeting the

Hh pathway could be beneficial in the treatment of fibrosis (Figure 8.1).

## Local regulation of fibrogenesis

Liver disease outcomes are dictated by the prevailing microenvironment (Figure 8.2). For example, an upregulation of pro-fibrogenic molecules would promote scar deposition and accumulation, while an excess of matrix-degrading enzymes could facilitate resolution of fibrosis:

a.  *Cytokines and growth factors* are small soluble proteins secreted by immune cells, progenitor and ductular cells (cholangiocytes), liver pericytes and endothelial cells and are responsible for mediating cellular crosstalk (cell-to-cell communication) and regulating tissue metabolic responses. Transforming

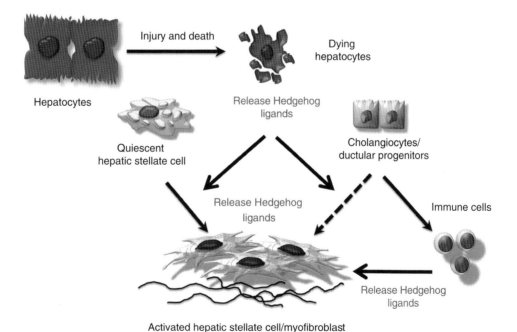

Activated hepatic stellate cell/myofibroblast

**FIG 8.1** Link between cell death and fibrogenic liver repair. Liver cell injury or death from lipotoxicity, oxidative stress and immune imbalance leads to the release of signalling factors (such as Hedgehog ligands), which promote the proliferation of ductular progenitors and liver pericytes (hepatic stellate cells) as part of the repair response. Stimulated hepatic stellate cells transition into collagen-producing myofibroblasts, and ductular progenitor cells secrete high levels of cytokines and growth factors that recruit immune cells into the liver. In turn, recruited immune cells secrete even more cytokines and growth factors that perpetuate the inflammatory and fibrogenic response. Ductular progenitors may also undergo direct differentiation into scar-producing myofibroblasts. (*See insert for color representation of the figure.*)

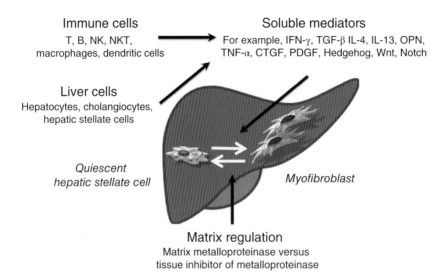

**FIG 8.2** Local factors regulating liver fibrogenesis. Hepatic stellate cell activation occurs in the presence of pro-fibrogenic factors. Cytokines (e.g. IFN-γ, TNF-α, TGF-β, IL4, IL13, OPN), growth factors (PDGF, CTGF) and morphogens (Hedgehog, Wnt, Notch) are secreted by resident liver cells, as well as recruited immune cells (T cells, NK cells, NKT cells, T regulatory cells, γδT cells, monocytes and macrophages). Matrix composition is dynamically regulated by endopeptidases (matrix metalloproteinase (MMP)) responsible for matrix degradation. In turn, MMPs are inhibited by extracellular tissue inhibitors of metalloproteinases (TIMPs), which bind to active MMPs to inhibit enzymatic activity. The relative expressions of MMPs and TIMPs modulate rate and pattern of matrix degradation and influence fibrosis outcomes.

growth factor-beta (TGF-β), for example, is the prototypical pro-fibrogenic cytokine that is upregulated during chronic liver disease and promotes progenitor and pericyte proliferation and activation [31]. In the next section, we will highlight novel mediators (Hh and Osteopontin (OPN)) responsible for driving NASH progression.

b. *The extracellular matrix* is dynamically regulated, even during progressive fibrogenesis. The deposition of fibrillar collagens (especially collagen type 1), elastin and matrix proteins by liver pericytes is matched by activities of matrix metalloproteinases (MMPs) (endopeptidases responsible for matrix degradation) produced by inflammatory cells and pericytes. MMPs in turn are inhibited by extracellular tissue inhibitors of metalloproteinases (TIMPs), which bind to active MMPs to inhibit their enzymatic activities [32, 33]. The balance between MMPs and TIMPs alters the rate and pattern of matrix degradation, allowing for the fine regulation of matrix turnover. As an example, mice overexpressing TIMP1 developed more fibrosis and failed to remodel the matrix during the fibrosis resolution

phase, while rats overexpressing MMP8 developed less fibrosis [34].

c. Chronic liver injury is often associated with the *recruitment of immune subsets* (*chronic inflammation*) into the liver [35]. Activated T and B cells, T regulatory cells, natural killer and natural killer T (NKT) cells, monocyte–macrophage subsets and dendritic and innate lymphoid cells together constitute the innate and adaptive arms of the immune response. Collectively, these cells are responsible for maintaining liver tolerance on one hand and for defence on the other (patrolling and clearance of cellular debris). Trafficking of immune cells into the liver is tightly regulated by chemokines (chemotactic cytokines), as well as expression of specific adhesion molecules on the liver sinusoidal endothelial surface [36]. During NASH, upregulation of adhesion molecules (ICAM1 and VCAM1) and chemokines (CXCL16, CXCL9, CXCL10, CXCL11) promotes accumulation of liver NKTs, which then secrete high levels of pro-fibrogenic factors (IL-13, Osteopontin (OPN) and Hh) [37, 38]. Mice genetically deficient in NKT cells, on the other hand, are protected from NASH fibrosis. Macrophages

(Kupffer cells) not only promote fibrosis but also are major sources of MMPs. Recent studies show that the Ly6C intermediate–low phenotype macrophage subset is a key source of MMPs during fibrosis resolution [39]. Thus, inhibiting recruitment of the 'pro-fibrogenic' subset could prevent fibrosis development, while increasing recruitment of the 'pro-resolution' subset could enhance fibrosis resolution through secretion of MMP12 and MMP13.

## Non-liver factors

Signals from the brain, gut and adipose tissue are important co-regulators of repair (Figure 8.3):

a.  *Gut–liver*

    The human intestine normally harbours a diverse community of microbes that promotes metabolism and digestion in a symbiotic relationship with the host. Cumulative evidence shows that changes to the

intestinal microbiota (dysbiosis) lead to adverse liver outcomes. For example, compositional changes may increase energy extraction from food and result in the development of NAFLD [40]. Feeding mice with a high-fat diet and inducing dysbiosis (by reducing the ratio between *Bacteroidetes* and *Firmicutes* while increasing Gram-negative proteobacteria) accelerate fibrogenesis [41]. Mechanistically, dysbiosis causes intestinal inflammation, a loss of intestinal barrier and the translocation of microbial products (such as lipopolysaccharides (LPS)). These lead to activation of pattern recognition receptors such as Toll-like receptors (TLR)4 and perturbations in choline and bile acid metabolism. Interestingly, altered interactions between microbiota and inflammasome sensing may also govern the rate of NAFLD progression. To date, most of these data arise from animal experiments; better designed, longitudinal studies in humans are needed.

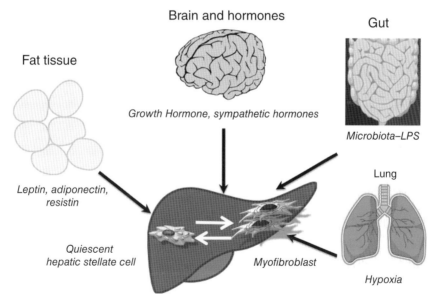

**FIG 8.3** Non-hepatic regulators of liver fibrogenesis. **Gut**: changes to the gut microbiota (dysbiosis) lead to loss of intestinal barriers and increase translocation of lipopolysaccharides (LPS) into the portal circulation. Binding of LPS to Toll-like receptor 4 (TLR4) on liver immune cells enhances secretion of pro-fibrogenic TNF-α and TGF-β. **Adipose tissues**: secrete multiple cytokines (adipokines) including leptin, adiponectin and resistin. Leptin is a pro-fibrogenic cytokine that directly activates hepatic stellate cells and potentiates TGF-β effects. Adiponectin is hepatoprotective and is anti-fibrotic. **Brain and hormones**: (i) in the autonomic nervous system, norepinephrine and acetylcholine induce HSC fibrogenesis. (ii) Growth hormone (GH) resistance is common among individuals with liver fibrosis, and impaired GH signalling leads to increased levels of oxidative stress and hepatocyte cell death. **Lung**: obstructive sleep apnoea is common among individuals with NAFLD and is associated with an increased risk of NASH and advanced fibrosis. Nocturnal hypoxia induces VEGF expression in HSC via hypoxia-inducible factor (HIF)-1α; VEGF, in turn, activates HSC.

**b.** *Adipose–liver*

The adipose tissue is a metabolically active 'cytokine factory'. The vast majority of individuals with NAFLD are overweight or obese, and in these individuals, the adipose tissue is enriched with immune infiltrates and secretes high levels of pro-inflammatory, pro-fibrogenic cytokines including leptin and tumour necrosis factor alpha (TNF-α) [42]. Serum leptin levels are significantly upregulated in patients with NASH and have been shown to directly activate HSC and potentiate TGF-β-mediated effects [43, 44]. By contrast, adiponectin levels are inversely correlated with fat mass and are suppressed in patients with NASH. Adiponectin exerts hepatoprotective and anti-fibrogenic effects, and mice with adiponectin deficiency developed more severe liver fibrosis after the high-fat diet [45].

*Other contributory factors*

**c.** *Hormonal regulation of repair/brain–liver crosstalk:* There is increasing evidence of pituitary and endocrine (hormonal) regulation of NAFLD and/or fibrosis outcomes.

*Growth hormone (GH):* Patients with hypopituitarism and GH deficiency are at increased risk of developing NAFLD (and NASH) [46]. Restoring GH levels in rats rescued mitochondria function and reduced oxidative stress, leading to the resolution of NASH. While GH deficiency per se is rare among those with (NAFLD) fibrosis and cirrhosis, GH (or GH signalling) resistance is common. Compared with GH–GH receptor intact mice, mice deficient in GH receptors expressed significantly lower hepatocyte protective factors (hepatocyte nuclear factor 6 and epidermal growth factor receptor), displayed increased levels of oxidative stress and hepatocyte apoptosis and developed more advanced liver fibrosis [47].

*Sympathetic and parasympathetic hormones:* Emerging data in animal models show that the autonomic nervous system influences liver repair [48]. The liver pericyte expresses adrenoceptors, contains catecholamine biosynthetic enzymes and secretes norepinephrine. Treating HSC in cell cultures with acetylcholine and norepinephrine markedly stimulates HSC proliferation and induces fibrogenesis, while blockade with prazosin (a α1-adrenoceptor antagonist) inhibits this. Interestingly, norepinephrine is leptin regulated. ob/ob mice, with leptin deficiency (and reduced norepinephrine), do not develop NASH fibrosis, but treating

ob/ob mice with norepinephrine induced HSC proliferation, upregulated TGF-β and increased liver fibrosis [49].

**d.** *Hypoxia and obstructive sleep apnoea*

Obstructive sleep apnoea (OSA) is common among obese individuals with NAFLD. Recent studies show that nocturnal hypoxia, a hallmark of OSA, is independently associated with an increased risk of NAFLD (OR: 2.37), NASH (OR: 2.16) and advanced fibrosis (2.30) [50]. This holds true even among those without obesity; the presence of OSA with daytime sleepiness is associated with NASH and fibrosis. The mechanisms that link OSA to NASH and fibrosis remain unclear but are likely to be related to angiogenic factors. Angiogenesis occurs in parallel with fibrosis development in both patients and in animal models of liver injury, and high levels of vascular endothelial growth factor (VEGF, a pro-angiogenic factor) are often detected in the chronically injured liver and in association with HSC. Cell culture studies show that HSC respond to hypoxia by upregulating VEGF in a hypoxia-inducible factor (HIF)-1α-dependent way; VEGF, in turn, stimulates HSC proliferation and promotes collagen deposition [51].

## Key molecular pathways

Distinct mechanisms and multiple signals from liver cells, immune cells and extra-hepatic tissues are integrated to generate a coherent repair response. We will highlight three molecular pathways currently being evaluated as targets for anti-fibrotic treatments.

### Hedgehog (Hh) signalling

The Hh pathway is critical for tissue development and cellular responses including proliferation, apoptosis and differentiation [52, 53]. Excessive activation of the Hh pathway during development leads to childhood cancers such as medulloblastoma, while inactivity impairs wound healing.

### Components of the Hh pathway

The binding of Hh ligands (Sonic Hh or Indian Hh) to cognate receptor Patched (Ptc) on cell surface membranes leads to the depression of a co-receptor Smoothened (Smo). Depressed Smo is responsible for the transduction of signals downstream and leads to the nuclear translocation of glioblastoma (Gli1, Gli2, Gli3) transcription factors and expression of Hh target genes (i.e. canonical Hh signalling). Ptc/Smo-independent activation of the Hh pathway has also been described (i.e. non-canonical Hh signalling).

### Relationship between Hh and other pro-fibrogenic factors

The regulation of the Hh signalling pathway is complex, and future studies will be needed to fully understand the effects of canonical versus non-canonical pathways on liver outcomes. Interestingly, leptin and PDGF effects are mediated by increased secretion of Hh ligands (canonical signalling) [54], while TGF-β and insulin-like growth factor enhances non-canonical Hh signalling [55]. TGF-β induces Gli transcription and Gli protein stabilisation, while insulin-like growth factor inhibits Gli phosphorylation by glyogen synthase kinase-3β (GSK-3β), preventing its proteasomal degradation (i.e. more pathway activation). More recently, Hh signalling has also been shown to be a regulator of the LPS response and links hypoxia with fibrosis via HIF1α.

### Summary of Hh actions

Injured (endoplasmic reticulum stress) or dying hepatocytes (pro-apoptotic stimuli) produce high levels of Hh ligands that act on surrounding liver progenitors, liver pericytes, sinusoidal endothelial cells and immune cells (i.e. Hh-responsive cells) [25, 56]:

i.   Hh ligands stimulate HSC proliferation and promote their transition into collagen-producing myofibroblasts. In turn, HSC and myofibroblasts secrete additional Hh ligands that amplify fibrogenesis [26, 54].

ii.  Hh ligands induce proliferation of liver progenitors and promote reprogramming of epithelial progenitors into mesenchymal (fibrogenic) phenotype [27]. They also stimulate the secretion of chemokines such as CXCL16, which recruit inflammatory T and NKT cell subsets into the liver [28].

iii. Infiltrating immune cells are Hh responsive, and activated T cells, NKT cells and macrophages secrete Hh ligands that perpetuate liver injury [37, 57, 58].

iv.  Activation of the Hh pathway activates sinusoidal endothelial cells, upregulates expression of key adhesion molecules and induces capillarisation of sinusoidal endothelium [29].

### Evidence of the Hh pathway in human liver disease

There is minimal Hh pathway activity in a healthy adult liver. By contrast, Hh pathway activation occurs in chronic liver diseases (ALD, NAFLD, PBC and chronic viral hepatitis), and the activity of the Hh pathway parallels liver fibrosis stage [27, 30, 59–61].

### Modulating the Hh pathway in vivo

Activation of the Hh pathway also occurs in models of liver fibrosis (chronic carbon tetrachloride, bile duct ligation, methionine–choline-deficient diet (NASH), alcohol-induced injury and genetic models of biliary fibrosis or NAFLD), and mice genetically engineered to exhibit greater Hh pathway activation developed more liver fibrosis than wild-type mice [27, 60–62]. Inhibiting the Hh pathway by pharmacological (i.e. cyclopamine or GDC-0449; both Smo antagonists) or genetic approaches (i.e. conditional deletion of the Smo gene) prevents fibrosis progression [17, 18, 27].

### Clinical relevance

The aggregate data in humans and mice suggest that the Hh pathway is a key regulator and integrator of fibrogenic signals (such as LPS/TLR4, leptin, TGF-β and HIF1α). Hh pathway inhibitors such as vismodegib (GDC-0449) are already licensed for use in patients with advanced skin and haematological cancers and should be evaluated as antifibrotic agents.

## Osteopontin

OPN is both a pro-inflammatory (Th1) cytokine and a matrix protein and is highly upregulated at sites of inflammation, repair and malignancy [63]. Mice deficient in OPN exhibit poor wound healing (i.e. less fibrosis) and are protected from cancers, while the overexpression of OPN leads to excess fibrosis and spontaneous tumour development [64, 65].

OPN is expressed and/or secreted by liver progenitors, liver pericytes, sinusoidal endothelial cells and immune cells (macrophages, dendritic cells, T and B cells, NKT cells), and its expression is modulated by pro-inflammatory cytokines (TNF-α, IL-6), growth factors (PDGF), morphogens (Hh, Wnt signals), adipokines (leptin) and sympathetic hormones (epinephrine) [63]. Its pleiotropic functions can be explained by the ability of the OPN molecule to bind to multiple integrins ($\alpha_v$, $\alpha_4$, $\alpha_9$) and CD44.

Recent studies further show that OPN exists as multiple isoforms (including intracellular and extracellular OPN), thus increasing the complexity of its regulation and function [66].

### Summary of OPN actions

i. OPN stimulates HSC proliferation and activation, and the loss of OPN by RNA interference or OPN-neutralising antibody inhibits this [21, 67]. Preliminary studies further support a role for OPN in modulating MMP–TIMP balance.

ii. OPN promotes liver progenitor cell proliferation and wound healing by enhancing TGF-β signalling: OPN neutralisation represses phospho-Smad2/3 levels (indicative of reduced TGF-β activation) and maintains levels of transcriptional co-repressors, Ski and SnoN [21].

iii. Immune cells are OPN responsive and secrete OPN that amplify the inflammatory response [68].

iv. OPN activates the liver sinusoidal endothelium, upregulates adhesion molecules and chemokines and modulates leucocyte trafficking (*personal communications*).

### Evidence of OPN in human liver diseases

Liver and plasma levels of OPN are significantly upregulated in ALD, NASH, PBC/PSC and chronic viral hepatitis [21, 67, 69]. Recent studies show that OPN is Hh regulated and is a downstream effector of Hh signalling [67]. Thus, OPN is co-expressed by Hh-responsive cells, and expression of OPN parallels Hh pathway activity and liver fibrosis stage.

### Targeting OPN in vivo

Multiple studies to date have utilised small animal models genetically deficient in OPN. These studies do not necessarily reflect the role of OPN *in vivo* because genetic silencing of the OPN gene leads to loss of both intracellular and extracellular OPN isoforms [21]. On the other hand, neutralising extracellular OPN using OPN antibodies and OPN specific aptamers resulted in a significant reduction of liver injury and fibrosis in NASH.

### Clinical relevance

Outside of the liver, accumulating evidence further suggests that OPN is a key effector of metabolic outcomes [70]. OPN is significantly increased in inflamed adipose tissues and in inflamed vascular endothelium and is upregulated in patients with ischaemic heart disease and type 2 diabetes mellitus. Mice genetically deficient in OPN also exhibit improved peripheral insulin sensitivity and metabolic profiles (improved lipid and glucose handling).

The aggregate (cell culture, animal and human) data support the concept that targeting OPN may be beneficial in patients with advanced (NASH) fibrosis.

### TGF-β

TGF-β is the most potent pro-fibrogenic cytokine that induces fibrosis by direct activation of HSC and liver progenitors, stimulating the synthesis of extracellular matrix and inhibiting matrix degradation through the production of TIMPs [31]. TGF-β is secreted as an inactivated protein bound to a latency-associated peptide; when activated, TGF-β then signals through its cognate receptors (i.e. activin-like kinase, ALK5), leading to the phosphorylation and nuclear translocation of its transcription factors, Smad2/3.

The overexpression of TGF-β promotes fibrosis, while deletion of TGF-β and Smad3 protects against fibrosis. Therefore, targeting this pathway appears to be attractive, and multiple approaches include antisense oligonucleotides (which inhibit TGF-β mRNA), specific neutralising antibodies (that interfere with ligand binding), natural TGF-β antagonists (such as Smad7) and TGF-β receptor kinase blockers. However, as TGF-β signalling is also important for tumour suppression, immune regulation and cell differentiation, strategies that selectively target excess matrix deposition and accumulation will need to be developed. In a recent study, investigators described the selective delivery of an ALK5 inhibitor by coupling the compound to mannose-6-phosphate human serum albumin (M6PHSA), which allows selective uptake by HSC (the main liver cell type responsible for matrix deposition) [71]. In another, specific blockade or loss of HSC-expressing αv integrins (by pharmacologic and genetic approaches, respectively) inhibited TGF-β activation and fibrogenesis [72].

### Clinical relevance

Pirfenidone (Esbriet) is an anti-fibrotic that inhibits TGF-β expression and function. It has been licensed to treat patients with advanced idiopathic pulmonary fibrosis and is currently being evaluated as a treatment of liver fibrosis [73].

## Conclusions and future

The mechanisms and molecular pathways that regulate liver repair are complex and involve multiple local (liver) and non-liver factors (gut, brain and adipose tissue). This suggests that no one mechanism or pathway is 'more important' than another. It is likely that various pathways interact and signals integrate to formulate a common fibrogenic response. Thus, identifying and targeting these 'core or common' mediators (such as Hh, OPN and TGF-β) that regulate fibrosis may be more clinically useful than targeting any one of the final effector pathways.

## Acknowledgements

WKS is funded by The Foundation for Liver Research, The Polkemmet Trust, EASL and CORE. AMD is funded by the US National Institutes of Health R37 AA010154 and R01 DK077794.

## References

1. Adams, L.A., et al., The natural history of nonalcoholic fatty liver disease: a population-based cohort study. Gastroenterology, 2005. 129(1): p. 113–21.

2. Matteoni, C.A., et al., Nonalcoholic fatty liver disease: a spectrum of clinical and pathological severity. Gastroenterology, 1999. 116(6): p. 1413–9.

3. Day, C.P. and O.F. James, Steatohepatitis: a tale of two "hits"? Gastroenterology, 1998. 114(4): p. 842–5.

4. Fan, Y. and A. Bergmann, Apoptosis-induced compensatory proliferation. the cell is dead. Long live the cell! Trends Cell Biol, 2008. 18(10): p. 467–73.

5. Diehl, A.M. and J. Chute, Underlying potential: cellular and molecular determinants of adult liver repair. J Clin Invest, 2013. 123(5): p. 1858–60.

6. Holt, A.P., et al., Immune interactions in hepatic fibrosis. Clin Liver Dis, 2008. 12(4): p. 861–82, x.

7. Feldstein, A.E., et al., Hepatocyte apoptosis and fas expression are prominent features of human nonalcoholic steatohepatitis. Gastroenterology, 2003. 125(2): p. 437–43.

8. Wieckowska, A., et al., In vivo assessment of liver cell apoptosis as a novel biomarker of disease severity in nonalcoholic fatty liver disease. Hepatology, 2006. 44(1): p. 27–33.

9. Yang, S., et al., Oval cells compensate for damage and replicative senescence of mature hepatocytes in mice with fatty liver disease. Hepatology, 2004. 39(2): p. 403–11.

10. Roskams, T. and V. Desmet, Ductular reaction and its diagnostic significance. Semin Diagn Pathol, 1998. 15(4): p. 259–69.

11. Richardson, M.M., et al., Progressive fibrosis in nonalcoholic steatohepatitis: association with altered regeneration and a ductular reaction. Gastroenterology, 2007. 133(1): p. 80–90.

12. Feldstein, A.E., et al., Cytokeratin-18 fragment levels as noninvasive biomarkers for nonalcoholic steatohepatitis: a multicenter validation study. Hepatology, 2009 Oct. 50(4): p. 1072–8.

13. Machado, M.V., et al., Reduced lipoapoptosis, hedgehog pathway activation and fibrosis in caspase-2 deficient mice with non-alcoholic steatohepatitis. Gut 2014 Jul 22. doi: 10.1136/gutjnl-2014-307362.

14. Witek, R.P., et al., Pan-caspase inhibitor VX-166 reduces fibrosis in an animal model of nonalcoholic steatohepatitis. Hepatology, 2009 Nov. 50(5): p. 1421–30.

15. Santoni-Rugiu, E., et al., Progenitor cells in liver regeneration: molecular responses controlling their activation and expansion. APMIS, 2005. 113(11–12): p. 876–902.

16. Roskams, T., Relationships among stellate cell activation, progenitor cells, and hepatic regeneration. Clin Liver Dis, 2008. 12(4): p. 853–60, ix.

17. Michelotti, G.A., et al., Smoothened is a master regulator of adult liver repair. J Clin Invest, 2013. 123: p. 2380–94.

18. Swiderska-Syn, M., et al., Myofibroblastic cells function as progenitors to regenerate murine livers after partial hepatectomy. Gut, 2014 Aug. 63(8): p. 1333–44

19. Kordes, C., et al., Stellate cells from rat pancreas are stem cells and can contribute to liver regeneration. PLoS One, 2012. 7(12): p. e51878.

20. Kordes, C., et al., Hepatic stellate cells contribute to progenitor cells and liver regeneration. J Clin Invest, 2014 Dec 1. 124(12): p. 5503–15.

21. Coombes, J., et al., Osteopontin neutralisation abrogates the liver progenitor cell response and fibrogenesis in mice. Gut, 2014 Jun 5. doi: 10.1136/gutjnl-2013-306484.

22. Canbay, A., et al., Kupffer cell engulfment of apoptotic bodies stimulates death ligand and cytokine expression. Hepatology, 2003. 38(5): p. 1188–98.

23. Wree, A., et al., NLRP3 inflammasome activation results in hepatocyte pyroptosis, liver inflammation, and fibrosis in mice. Hepatology, 2014 Mar. 59(3): p. 898–910.

24. Pusterla, T., et al., Receptor for advanced glycation endproducts (RAGE) is a key regulator of oval cell activation and inflammation-associated liver carcinogenesis in mice. Hepatology, 2013 Jul. 58(1): p. 363–73.

25. Jung, Y., et al., Signals from dying hepatocytes trigger growth of liver progenitors. Gut, 2010. 59(5): p. 655–65.

26. Choi, S.S., et al., Hedgehog pathway activation and epithelial-to-mesenchymal transitions during myofibroblastic transformation of rat hepatic cells in culture and cirrhosis. Am J Physiol Gastrointest Liver Physiol, 2009. 297(6): p. G1093–106.

27. Syn, W.K., et al., Hedgehog-mediated epithelial-to-mesenchymal transition and fibrogenic repair in nonalcoholic fatty liver disease. Gastroenterology, 2009. 137(4): p. 1478–1488 e8.

28. Omenetti, A., et al., Repair-related activation of hedgehog signaling promotes cholangiocyte chemokine production. Hepatology, 2009. 50(2): p. 518–27.

29. Xie, G., et al., Hedgehog signalling regulates liver sinusoidal endothelial cell capillarisation. Gut, 2013. 62(2): p. 299–309.

30. Pereira Tde, A., et al., Viral factors induce Hedgehog pathway activation in humans with viral hepatitis, cirrhosis, and hepatocellular carcinoma. Lab Invest, 2010. 90(12): p. 1690–703.

31. Dooley, S. and P. ten Dijke, TGF-beta in progression of liver disease. Cell Tissue Res, 2012. 347(1): p. 245–56.

32. Iredale, J.P., et al., Human hepatic lipocytes synthesize tissue inhibitor of metalloproteinases-1. Implications for regulation of matrix degradation in liver. J Clin Invest, 1992. 90(1): p. 282–7.

33. Arthur, M.J., et al., Secretion of 72 kDa type IV collagenase/gelatinase by cultured human lipocytes. Analysis of gene expression, protein synthesis and proteinase activity. Biochem J, 1992. 287(Pt 3): p. 701–7.

34. Garcia-Bañuelos, J., et al., Cirrhotic rat livers with extensive fibrosis can be safely transduced with clinical-grade adenoviral vectors. Evidence of cirrhosis reversion. Gene Ther, 2002 Jan. 9(2): p. 127–34.

35. Lalor, P.F. and D.H. Adams, The liver: a model of organ-specific lymphocyte recruitment. Expert Rev Mol Med, 2002. 4(2): p. 1–16.

36. Shetty, S., et al., Lymphocyte recruitment to the liver: molecular insights into the pathogenesis of liver injury and hepatitis. Toxicology, 2008 Dec 30. 254(3): p. 136–46.

37. Syn, W.K., et al., NKT-associated hedgehog and osteopontin drive fibrogenesis in non-alcoholic fatty liver disease. Gut, 2012. 61(9): p. 1323–9.

38. Syn, W.K., et al., Accumulation of natural killer T cells in progressive nonalcoholic fatty liver disease. Hepatology, 2010. 51(6): p. 1998–2007.

39. Ramachandran, P., et al., Differential Ly-6C expression identifies the recruited macrophage phenotype, which orchestrates the regression of murine liver fibrosis. Proc Natl Acad Sci U S A, 2012 Nov 13. 109(46): p. E3186–95.

40. Bäckhed, F., et al., The gut microbiota as an environmental factor that regulates fat storage. Proc Natl Acad Sci U S A, 2004 Nov 2. 101(44): p. 15718–23.

41. De Minicis, S., et al., Dysbiosis contributes to fibrogenesis in the course of chronic liver injury in mice. Hepatology, 2014 May. 59(5): p. 1738–49.

42. Klaus, S., Adipose tissue as a regulator of energy balance. Curr Drug Targets, 2004. 5(3): p. 241–50.

43. Choi, S.S., et al., Leptin promotes the myofibroblastic phenotype in hepatic stellate cells by activating the hedgehog pathway. J Biol Chem, 2010. 285(47): p. 36551–60.

44. Bataller, R. and D.A. Brenner, Liver fibrosis. J Clin Invest, 2005. 115(2): p. 209–18.

45. Kumar, P., et al., Adiponectin modulates focal adhesion disassembly in activated hepatic stellate cells: implication for reversing hepatic fibrosis. FASEB J, 2014 Dec. 28(12): p. 5172–83.

46. Nishizawa, H., et al., Nonalcoholic fatty liver disease in adult hypopituitary patients with GH deficiency and the impact of GH replacement therapy. Eur J Endocrinol, 2012 Jul. 167(1): p. 67–74.

47. Stiedl, P., et al., Growth hormone resistance exacerbates cholestasis-induced murine liver fibrosis. Hepatology, 2014 Sep 1. doi: 10.1002/hep.27408.

48. Oben, J.A., et al., Sympathetic nervous system regulation of liver repair. Anat Rec A Discov Mol Cell Evol Biol, 2004 Sep. 280(1), 874–83.

49. Li, Z., et al., Norepinephrine regulates hepatic innate immune system in leptin-deficient mice with nonalcoholic steatohepatitis. Hepatology, 2004. 40(2): p. 434–41.

50. Pulixi, E.A., et al., Risk of obstructive sleep apnea with daytime sleepiness is associated with liver damage in non-morbidly obese patients with nonalcoholic fatty liver disease. PLoS One, 2014 Apr 24. 9(4): p. e96349.

51. Nath, B., et al., Hypoxia and hypoxia inducible factors: diverse roles in liver diseases. Hepatology, 2012 Feb. 55(2): p. 622–33.

52. Hirose, Y., T. Itoh, and A. Miyajima, Hedgehog signal activation coordinates proliferation and differentiation of fetal liver progenitor cells. Exp Cell Res, 2009. 315(15): p. 2648–57.

53. Briscoe, J., et al., The mechanisms of Hedgehog signalling and its roles in development and disease. Nat Rev Mol Cell Biol, 2013 Jul. 14(7): p. 416–29.

54. Yang, L., et al., Sonic hedgehog is an autocrine viability factor for myofibroblastic hepatic stellate cells. J Hepatol, 2008. 48(1): p. 98–106.

55. Yoo, Y.A., et al., Sonic hedgehog signaling promotes motility and invasiveness of gastric cancer cells through TGF-beta-mediated activation of the ALK5-Smad 3 pathway. Carcinogenesis, 2008. 29(3): p. 480–90.

56. Rangwala, F., et al., Increased production of sonic hedgehog by ballooned hepatocytes. J Pathol, 2011. 224(3): p. 401–10.

57. Syn, W.K., et al., Role for hedgehog pathway in regulating growth and function of invariant NKT cells. Eur J Immunol, 2009. 39(7): p. 1879–92.

58. Pereira, T.A., et al., Macrophage-derived Hedgehog ligands promotes fibrogenic and angiogenic responses in human schistosomiasis mansoni. Liver Int, 2013. 33(1): p. 149–61.

59. Guy, C.D., et al., Hedgehog pathway activation parallels histologic severity of injury and fibrosis in human nonalcoholic fatty liver disease. Hepatology, 2012. 55(6): p. 1711–21.

60. Omenetti, A., et al., Hedgehog signaling regulates epithelial-mesenchymal transition during biliary fibrosis in rodents and humans. J Clin Invest, 2008. 118(10): p. 3331–42.

61. Jung, Y., et al., Accumulation of hedgehog-responsive progenitors parallels alcoholic liver disease severity in mice and humans. Gastroenterology, 2008. 134(5): p. 1532–43.

62. Omenetti, A., et al., Hedgehog-mediated mesenchymal-epithelial interactions modulate hepatic response to bile duct ligation. Lab Invest, 2007. 87(5): p. 499–514.

63. Uede, T., Osteopontin, intrinsic tissue regulator of intractable inflammatory diseases. Pathol Int, 2011. 61(5): p. 265-80.

64. Liaw, L., et al., Altered wound healing in mice lacking a functional osteopontin gene (spp1). J Clin Invest, 1998. 101(7): p. 1468–78.

65. Rangaswami, H., A. Bulbule, and G.C. Kundu, Osteopontin: role in cell signaling and cancer progression. Trends Cell Biol, 2006. 16(2): p. 79–87.

66. Inoue, M., et al., Intracellular osteopontin (iOPN) and immunity. Immunol Res, 2011 Apr 49(1–3): p. 160–72.

67. Syn, W.K., et al., Osteopontin is induced by hedgehog pathway activation and promotes fibrosis progression in nonalcoholic steatohepatitis. Hepatology, 2011. 53(1): p. 106–15.

68. Ashkar, S., et al., Eta-1 (osteopontin): an early component of type-1 (cell-mediated) immunity. Science, 2000. 287(5454): p. 860–4.

69. Patouraux, S., et al., The osteopontin level in liver, adipose tissue and serum is correlated with fibrosis in patients with alcoholic liver disease. PLoS One, 2012. 7(4): p. e35612.

70. Kiefer, F.W., et al., Neutralization of osteopontin inhibits obesity-induced inflammation and insulin resistance. Diabetes, 2010. 59(4): p. 935–46.

71. van Beuge, M.M., et al., Enhanced effectivity of an ALK5-inhibitor after cell-specific delivery to hepatic stellate cells in mice with liver injury. PLoS One, 2013. 8(2): p. e56442.

72. Henderson, N.C., et al., Targeting of αv integrin identifies a core molecular pathway that regulates fibrosis in several organs. Nat Med, 2013 Dec. 19(12): p. 1617–24.

73. King, T.E. Jr., et al., A phase 3 trial of pirfenidone in patients with idiopathic pulmonary fibrosis. N Engl J Med, 2014 May 29. 370(22): p. 2083–92.

# When is it NAFLD and when is it ALD?: Can the histologic evaluation of a liver biopsy guide the clinical evaluation?

**Elizabeth M. Brunt[1] and David E. Kleiner[2]**

[1] Department of Pathology and Immunology, Washington University School of Medicine, St. Louis, MO, USA
[2] Laboratory of Pathology, National Cancer Institute, National Institutes of Health, Bethesda, MD, USA

## LEARNING POINTS

- Although alcoholic and non-alcoholic liver disease share many features, there are differences that would support one etiology over another.

- The unique zone 1 borderline injury pattern of pediatric fatty liver disease does not have a corresponding injury pattern in alcoholic liver disease.

- Diffuse microvesicular steatosis, bilirubinostasis, neutrophilic satellitosis of Mallory–Denk body-containing balloon cells, and dense networks of perisinusoidal fibrosis in the lobules are more likely in alcoholic than non-alcoholic steatohepatitis.

- Only alcoholic hepatitis shows a significant incidence of veno-occlusive lesions and the related finding of sclerosing hyaline necrosis.

- Canalicular cholestasis may be found in alcoholic hepatitis but when identified in cases of NAFLD or NASH should raise questions about unrelated etiologies.

## Introduction

Most pathology literature and nearly all clinical literature related to fatty liver disease comment that alcoholic and non-alcoholic fatty liver disease are indistinguishable histologically. In fact, this was the basis for the appellation of fatty liver disease related to obesity in patients without significant alcohol consumption, an unfortunate "non-"term. This may be true of steatosis and of mild forms of steatohepatitis, but

pathologists have noted features that may distinguish the two, particularly in the severe form of ALD [1, 2]. These include lesions to the outflow veins described from the earliest work in ALD [3], as well as canalicular cholestasis [4], a lesion included in a new scoring system for alcoholic hepatitis [5], but not a feature of NASH.

In this chapter, we review the primary lesions of both alcoholic and non-alcoholic fatty liver diseases as well as features that may be unique or more common in one compared to the other. A review of the literature of comparative studies summarized conclusions of investigators that the shared lesions are often more "severe" in the severe forms of ALD [2]. Further, clinical context is essential in biopsy interpretation. Finally, grading systems for both have been published [6, 7]; the former was developed primarily for comparing lesions for clinical trials, while the latter was for prognostication for alcoholic hepatitis. The lesions utilized in these systems are a reflection of significant features, and therefore both shared and different histopathologic features of these entities can be regarded as differing histologic manifestations. Table 9.1 shows a summary of shared and differing lesions of ALD and NAFLD, most of which are summarized in the following.

## Steatosis

### Macrovesicular

Macrovesicular steatosis is the form of lipid storage most often observed in ALD and NAFLD. In its simplest form, the hepatocyte contains a single large vacuole of lipid that

*Clinical Dilemmas in Non-Alcoholic Fatty Liver Disease*, First Edition. Edited by Roger Williams and Simon D. Taylor-Robinson.
© 2016 John Wiley & Sons, Ltd. Published 2016 by John Wiley & Sons, Ltd.

**TABLE 9.1** Similarities and differences between ALD and NAFLD

**Features that are common to both ALD and NAFLD**

| | |
|---|---|
| Steatosis, macrovesicular | Both may have variable amounts of steatosis in a zone 3 to panacinar distribution |
| Inflammation, lobular | In general, parenchymal inflammation is commonly seen, particularly with respect to mononuclear foci |
| Inflammation, portal | Mononuclear portal inflammation is common, particularly as fibrosis progresses |
| Ballooning | Ballooning is a characteristic feature of both alcoholic hepatitis and NASH. There is significant overlap in the character, location, and number of balloon cells |
| Mallory–Denk bodies | MDBs may be found in both alcoholic hepatitis and NASH |
| Fibrosis | In both ALD and adult NAFLD, early fibrosis is characterized by perisinusoidal fibrosis that involves zone 3; periportal and bridging fibrosis develop later, with eventual progression to cirrhosis |
| Apoptotic hepatocytes | May be observed in both ALD and NAFLD |
| Megamitochondria | May be observed in both ALD and NAFLD |

**Features that may help to differentiate ALD from NAFLD**

| | ALD | NAFLD |
|---|---|---|
| Steatosis, macrovesicular | Steatosis is not a required feature of alcoholic hepatitis | Some degree of steatosis is required; zone 1 steatosis distribution in children |
| Steatosis, microvesicular | Diffuse microvesicular steatosis may be seen (alcoholic foamy degeneration) | Microvesicular steatosis usually limited to single cells or small patches in NASH |
| Inflammation, lobular | Neutrophilic inflammation common in active ALD, particularly satellitosis around hepatocytes with MDB | Neutrophilic inflammation is uncommon |
| Inflammation, portal | Neutrophilic infiltrates may be seen, particularly in association with ductular reaction and in active ALD | Neutrophilic infiltrates rarely seen |
| Mallory–Denk bodies | MDBs may be more numerous, better formed, and more often associated with satellitosis by neutrophils | MDBs are often thin and poorly formed, rarely attracting neutrophils |
| Fibrosis | Perisinusoidal fibrosis may be dense and may extend to involve the whole lobule. Thick perivenular fibrosis may be present and associated with occlusive fibrosis of the vein (sclerosing hyaline necrosis). Portal hypertension may develop prior to true cirrhosis due to this extensive fibrosis | Children may develop periportal fibrosis without the zone 3 perisinusoidal fibrosis |
| Ductular reaction | May be prominent in portal areas and may extend into perivenular region | Usually mild, particularly in precirrhotic NAFLD |
| Canalicular cholestasis | May be seen in alcoholic hepatitis; may raise consideration of pancreatitis or biliary obstruction | Never seen in NAFLD or NASH—presence should raise the consideration of a second process or ALD |
| Iron | Hepatocellular iron deposition may be heavy, particularly in cirrhosis | Hepatocellular iron deposition is usually mild, if found at all |

fills nearly the entire cell, and both indents and displaces the nucleus to the periphery of the cell. The lipid droplet is mainly composed of triglyceride that is metabolically dynamic. Hepatocytes may be enlarged beyond their normal size by the lipid droplet, and marked macrovesicular steatosis can be accompanied by hepatomegaly. Multiple lipid vacuoles of varied sizes may also be seen in macrovesicular steatosis. In this situation, one or more vacuoles may be present, ranging in size from less than a micron to

larger than the hepatocyte nucleus. This change may be differentiated from microvesicular steatosis, in which the hepatocyte cytoplasm has a foamy appearance due to innumerable tiny vacuoles less than a micron in size. The type of steatosis with intermediate-sized vacuoles is referred to as "mediovesicular" steatosis by some authors or mixed small and large droplet macrosteatosis by others, but since it likely represents a form of macrovesicular steatosis, we would assess it as such. The point is not to confuse the smaller droplets with true microvesicular steatosis, which may, in fact, carry a different meaning.

In both ALD and NAFLD, macrovesicular steatosis may be present as the only significant histological finding or as a component of alcoholic hepatitis or NASH. The character and distribution of the steatosis are similar. Macrovesicular steatosis is usually most prominent in acinar zone 3, particularly in early or mild disease [8, 9]. As the steatosis increases, it spreads to involve all of the acinar zones. With the development of advanced fibrosis and NASH, the distribution of steatosis in NAFLD may become uneven and is no longer in a zonal distribution [9]. It is likely that this is true of ALD as well, although it has not been specifically studied.

For the most part there is no difference in the character or distribution of macrovesicular steatosis between ALD and NAFLD. Steatosis is not required to diagnose alcoholic hepatitis [8], whereas some degree of steatosis (usually stated as 5%) is required for a diagnosis of NASH [10, 11]. The reason for this difference is that in ALD, the steatosis is very responsive to cessation of drinking, such that a patient with alcoholic hepatitis who has stopped drinking for several weeks prior to biopsy may no longer have much steatosis but may still have the other features of injury. In both ALD and NAFLD, the degree of steatosis may decrease as cirrhosis develops.

One notable exception to the zone 3-centered distribution of steatosis occurs in children with NAFLD. Pre- and peripubertal children may have macrovesicular steatosis in a zone 1-centered distribution [12, 13]. This zone 1 steatosis may be associated with increased portal inflammation and periportal fibrosis rather than zone 3 perisinusoidal fibrosis. Ballooning injury is typically absent or poorly defined, and Mallory–Denk bodies are not seen. This pattern of NAFLD has been dubbed the "zone 1 borderline pattern" of NAFLD because it shows some features of a progressive fatty liver disease but does not fulfill criteria for NASH [11, 13]. In a large cohort of US children, 28% were classified as having the zone 1 borderline pattern [13], while the same group found this pattern in only 1% of adults when pathologists were blinded to the age of the patient [14].

The natural history of macrovesicular steatosis in ALD and NAFLD does seem to vary by etiology. In NAFLD, macrovesicular steatosis without inflammation or fibrosis is generally deemed to have a good prognosis, with very little evidence of disease progression. In comparable patients with ALD who continue to drink, risk of progression remains. One early study followed 88 patients with alcoholic fatty liver and found that 10% progressed to cirrhosis after a median follow-up of 10.5 years [15]. In another classic study, 22% of alcoholic patients progressed from fatty liver with little or no fibrosis to cirrhosis after a median follow-up time of 12.8 years [16]. Patients with severe steatosis in this latter study were more likely to progress than those with less steatosis. There is recent data to suggest that fatty liver is not entirely benign in NAFLD. Pais et al. reported that 16 of 25 patients with non-alcoholic steatosis alone developed steatohepatitis over a mean of 3.7 years, with 6 developing bridging fibrosis [17]. The factors that separate patients with non-alcoholic steatosis who progress from those who do not are an area that remains under investigation. In ALD, continued drinking is one of the most significant drivers of disease progression.

### Microvesicular

Microvesicular steatosis is defined as a foamy change to the cytoplasm of hepatocytes in which the normal granular eosinophilic cytoplasm is replaced by innumerable tiny vacuoles; typically, the nucleus retains a central location. In toxic injuries, microvesicular steatosis has been linked to mitochondrial injury and is usually present in the majority of hepatocytes. In NAFLD, microvesicular steatosis is found in isolated but nonzonal hepatocytes and/or small patches. The finding of microvesicular steatosis has been studied in a large cohort of US patients [18]. Biopsies with microvesicular steatosis tended to have more severe disease, with more steatosis, more ballooning injury, more Mallory–Denk bodies, and more fibrosis. There was no difference in the clinical findings, including age, sex, body mass index, diabetes prevalence, or aminotransferase levels. Diffuse microvesicular steatosis has not been reported in NAFLD, although a form of diffuse microvesicular steatosis is described in ALD known as alcoholic foamy degeneration.

Alcoholic foamy degeneration is a form of ALD that does not appear to have a parallel in NAFLD. It is characterized by microvesicular steatosis in a zone 3 predominant distribution with few, if any, other features of alcoholic hepatitis [19]. The pattern is rare, comprising only 2.3% of ALD biopsies in a large series [20]. Macrovesicular steatosis may be seen but is typically in only a minority of hepatocytes. Most patients are jaundiced and have high serum aminotransferase levels and may present with acute liver failure. Bile accumulation in hepatocytes and canaliculi is observed microscopically. Perisinusoidal fibrosis may be seen, but the stage is usually not advanced and Mallory–Denk bodies are rare. By electron microscopy there is evidence of mitochondrial injury with matrix disorganization, loss of cristae, and massive enlargement. Megamitochondria are often noted at the light microscopic level. Cholestasis, as discussed later, is not feature of NASH or NAFLD and should raise concerns for other causes of liver injury (including alcohol).

## Inflammation

Inflammation can be broadly subdivided into lobular and portal compartments. Both ALD and NAFLD, in all stages, may show varying degrees of portal inflammation. Chronic inflammation is the most common form [21, 22] and has been noted to increase with advanced fibrosis in both [23, 24]. In NAFLD, Gadd et al. studied immune subtypes; macrophages are present in the earliest stages and precede even lobular inflammation. Further, in their study, all chronic inflammatory cells were more common in portal tracts/unit area than in the lobules/unit area and were in proximity to the periportal ductular reaction, whereas inflammatory cells within the lobules had no correlation with portal fibrosis or ductular reaction [22]. Macrophage populations are present but not readily appreciated without special stains, as noted in the following. Thus, portal chronic inflammation is not a discriminating feature in fatty liver disease evaluation. Lipogranulomas in the portal tracts have been noted as a feature of past alcohol use [25], but these lipid accumulations surrounded by macrophages are seen in NAFLD as well.

On the other hand, marked numbers of polymorphonuclear leukocytes (neutrophils, PMNs) in conjunction with ductular reaction in portal tracts are more common in ALD than in NAFLD; in addition, the periportal region may show angulated ductular profiles and fibrosis [26]. A differential diagnosis to suggest is pancreatitis [27] and/or choledocholithiasis, particularly when zone 3 canalicular cholestasis is also present. These findings would be unusual in the non-alcoholic setting.

Lobular inflammation is common to both ALD and NAFLD, but the nature of the infiltrates may vary. Chronic infiltrates comprised of mononuclear cells, and macrophages are commonly detected [22, 28]; lipogranulomas of varying sizes may occur near terminal hepatic venules

(THV) and may be surrounded by wispy collagen. Mild, moderate, or even severe aggregates of chronic inflammatory infiltrates may be present in NAFLD; when aggregated in zone 3 near a THV and a lobular artery [29], there may be confusion for a ductless portal tract. On the other hand, while occasional PMN's may occur in NAFLD, it is not common to see several foci of true satellitosis, a lesion of PMN's surrounding (or infiltrating into) Mallory–Denk body-containing hepatocytes, be they ballooned or acidophilic. This is likely one of the most distinguishing and common lesions associated with "alcoholic hepatitis," the clinical syndrome with a poor outcome. A recently proposed scoring system in alcoholic hepatitis found independent correlation with better outcome with neutrophilic infiltrates [7].

Multiple small foci of mononuclear, predominantly lymphocytic inflammation are commonly observed in the lobules of both ALD [27] and NAFLD, except pure steatosis [11]. The macrophage infiltrates of both ALD and NAFLD are rarely as recognizable on hematoxylin and eosin-stained sections as they are on special stains such as PAS with diastase or immunohistochemistry. By these stains, it is apparent cells of the macrophage lineage are numerous.

## Hepatocellular injury

Required for a diagnosis of steatohepatitis and therefore common to both ALD and NAFLD is a form of hepatocyte injury known as ballooning. Prior to architectural remodeling, ballooning is noted in acinar zone 3. The most typical features of ballooned hepatocytes are enlargement and alteration of the cytoplasm resulting in rarefaction or flocculent change. The cell may contain a lipid droplet, and often, the nucleus is hyperchromatic. If Mallory–Denk bodies are present, these are the same cells in which they will be found. In NAFLD, they are exclusively present within ballooned hepatocytes, but in ALD, as alluded to in Section "Inflammation," MDB may also be seen in hepatocytes that have undergone apoptosis. Mallory–Denk bodies are comprised of clumped keratins 8 and 18, as well as p62 and ubiquitin. These ropy intracytoplasmic inclusions may be detected by trichrome staining, but more sensitive and specific immunostains include the K8/18, p62, or ubiquitin probes. It has been written that MDB in ALD are better formed than in NAFLD [30], but this would not likely be a reproducible discriminator in some cases of severe NASH.

However, the presence of numerous MDB and multiple foci of satellitosis may be considered to favor ALD over NAFLD [31].

The second most common form of cell injury in fatty liver disease is apoptosis. Histologically, brightly eosinophilic, rounded cytoplasmic aggregates are noted extruded from the hepatic cords. Fragments of hyperchromatic nuclear material may be present but are not required for a diagnosis. This form of cell death is common to both ALD and NAFLD and would not be a histologic discriminator.

Necrosis is very unusual in NAFLD since jejunal–ileal bypass surgery is no longer done. Nanki et al. described a single case of liver failure with bridging necrosis following prednisolone therapy for lupus in 1999 [32], and Caldwell et al. reported five subjects with subacute liver failure in the setting of cryptogenic cirrhosis, two of whom had "necrosis" by histologic evaluation of liver tissue in 2002 [33]. On the other hand, necrosis can be a marker of chronic and severe ALD; most commonly, this is in the form of "sclerosing hyaline necrosis." The lesion was first described by Edmondson et al. in 1963 [3] but is still seen today. Steatosis is often absent; THV are typically obliterated by dense connective tissue, and it may require special stains to observe the remnant perivenular sheath. Numerous MDB are seen in adjacent hepatocytes.

## Fibrosis

The overall development and progression are similar between ALD and NAFLD. Early stages of fibrosis require connective tissue stains for detection. In NAFLD, the earliest evidence of fibrosis is found in zone 3, with the deposition of delicate strands of collagen in the space of Disse. This perisinusoidal fibrosis extends outward in a network extending from the central vein, trapping hepatocytes singly and in small clusters. In ALD, perivenular fibrotic thickening is thought to be the earliest fibrotic lesion, defined as a layer of collagen at least 4 µm thick extending around most of the circumference of a central vein [34]. This lesion is closely associated with the same kind of perisinusoidal fibrosis seen in cases of NAFLD. Perisinusoidal fibrosis interferes with the normal exchange of proteins and other macromolecules between the hepatocytes and the sinusoidal space and leads to "capillarization" of the endothelial cells. In ALD, this earliest stage of fibrosis may be observed in cases with steatosis alone, and patients with steatosis and early fibrosis are more likely to progress to advanced fibrosis and cirrhosis than patient with steatosis without fibrosis [35]. In NAFLD, the early stages of fibrosis are almost always observed in association with other changes of NASH [14, 36]. While the diagnosis of NASH does not require the presence of fibrosis [11], the original WHO definition of alcoholic hepatitis required evidence of perisinusoidal fibrosis [8].

Periportal fibrosis follows the zone 3 perisinusoidal fibrosis in both ALD and NAFLD. The edge of the limiting plate is disrupted by thin extensions of collagen between hepatocytes. The portal area becomes enlarged and takes on a more stellate appearance. The exception to this progression occurs in the zone 1 borderline pattern of NAFLD seen in young children. In these cases, periportal fibrosis occurs initially, and there is no evidence of perivenular or perisinusoidal fibrosis in zone 3 [12, 13]. Bridging fibrosis develops mainly between central veins and portal areas in ALD and NAFLD or between central veins. Bridging fibrosis can appear initially as an extension of the perisinusoidal fibrosis with a basket weave appearance of fibrotic connections. As trapped hepatocytes are lost, wide fibrotic bridges form. Children with the zone 1 borderline pattern can develop portal to portal bridging fibrosis that mimics the fibrosis progression of chronic hepatitis. In the final stage of cirrhosis, most of the major vascular structures are incorporated into the fibrotic bands, leaving behind micronodules of hepatocytes without veins or portal areas. Many of the specific features of ALD and NAFLD may be lost or difficult to recognize in cirrhotic livers, leading to classification of many cases as "cryptogenic." However, careful examination of biopsies can often lead to identification of characteristic ballooning injury or Mallory–Denk bodies, which can allow for correct classification of a patient's disease as having derived from fatty liver disease.

Fibrosis is staged in NAFLD/NASH according to now-standardized criteria [6, 37, 38]. Five main stages are identified that follow the sequence outlined previously: no fibrosis, perisinusoidal or periportal fibrosis, perisinusoidal and periportal fibrosis, bridging fibrosis, and cirrhosis with some minor variations between systems. There are no parallel staging systems that have been incorporated into clinical practice with ALD biopsies, but most pathologists either adapt a NAFLD/NASH system or use a descriptive approach that mirrors the stages described in the preceding when appropriate. The development of fibrosis has been recognized as a poor prognostic factor in both NAFLD and ALD [34, 35, 39].

Although the broad outlines of fibrosis progression are similar between ALD and NAFLD, there are some nuances that can help distinguish these etiologies, particularly with respect to ALD. In ALD, the perivenular fibrosis can be particularly severe and associated with necrosis or dropout of perivenular hepatocytes. This lesion is further discussed in the following. In addition, in ALD there may be extensive networks of dense perisinusoidal fibrosis that involve the entire acinus and obliterate the sinuses. This appearance seems to be unique to ALD and may be associated with significant portal hypertension. Recently, a proposed scoring system for prognosis in alcoholic hepatitis has included "lobular fibrosis" (presence and zonal extent); this is the first system to do so and highlights the recognition of a finding unique to ALD [7].

## Other lesions

### Cholestasis

Acute cholestasis, that is, accumulation of visible bile or bilirubinostasis, may occur in severe ALD but is rare enough in NAFLD (except in decompensated cirrhosis) to raise a concern of either overlapping ALD or another additional process. Bilirubinostasis is also included in the recently proposed scoring system for alcoholic hepatitis [7], where the type correlated with bacterial infection. In ALD, bile plugs can be seen in hepatocyte canaliculi in zone 3 or cholestatic rosettes in the lobules. In sepsis, bile stasis may occur in dilated periportal cholangioles, a lesion known as "cholangitis lenta." Obstruction from pancreatitis or stones may result in either form of bile stasis.

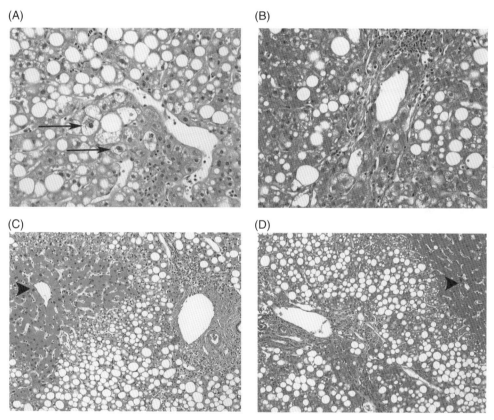

**FIG 9.1** Non-alcoholic fatty liver disease. Examples of the zone 3 and zone 1 injury patterns. (A) Typical steatohepatitis with perivenular inflammation and ballooning (arrows). (B) Masson trichrome stain from the same case showing delicate zone 3 perisinusoidal fibrosis. (C) Zone 1 borderline pattern with periportal steatosis and portal inflammation. No injury is seen around the terminal hepatic venule (arrowhead). (D) Masson trichrome stain from the same case showing periportal fibrosis but no perivenular fibrosis (arrowhead). (*See insert for color representation of the figure.*)

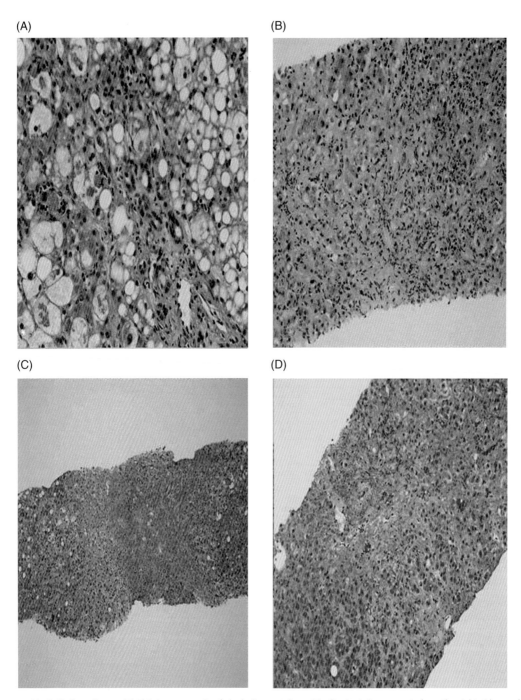

**FIG 9.2** Alcoholic liver disease. (A) This is an example of alcoholic steatohepatitis. Steatosis is apparent along the right side; marked ballooning and Mallory–Denk bodies are noted in hepatocytes along the left. Satellitosis is also seen as well as ductular reaction. (B–D) These figures are from a patient who presented with signs and symptoms of venous outflow obstruction. (B) In this example of several alcoholic hepatitis, there is very little steatosis, and one can appreciate near obliteration of all vascular (terminal hepatic venule and portal tract) structures. The primary component of the cellular infiltrate is neutrophils. With close inspection, Mallory–Denk bodies can be seen, as well as bile-stained hepatocytes. This is an example of sclerosing hyaline necrosis and would not be seen in NAFLD/ NASH. (C) A low-power trichrome stain shows obliterative fibrosis of a centrilobular region; this extent and type of fibrotic response are not described in NAFLD/NASH. (D) The high-power view of the Masson trichrome highlights the remnant of a terminal hepatic venule centrally and dense sinusoidal fibrosis in the lobules. Capillarization to this extent in alcoholic liver disease results in portal hypertension without the classic histologic features of cirrhosis. (*See insert for color representation of the figure.*)

Findings of chronic cholestasis are not seen in ALD or NAFLD and should raise consideration of separate disease processes.

## Lesions of THV

As noted, sclerosing hyaline necrosis is limited to ALD. Other lesions in ALD occur in the THV and sublobular veins [8]; these include subendothelial fibrosis [40], perivenular fibrosis or phlebosclerosis [41, 42], and perivenular fibrosis with dense perisinusoidal fibrosis extending into the parenchyma [43]. These are not lesions described in NAFLD.

## Megamitochondria

Megamitochondria are common to both ALD [44] and NAFLD [45]; their significance in both is unclear. In ALD, they may be an indication of chronicity [46], or milder disease [47]. They may be seen in hepatocytes with microvesicular steatosis. In pure steatosis of ALD, Teli et al. showed the combination of mixed steatosis and megamitochondria was associated with progression to fibrosis [15]. In the aforementioned scoring system for prognosis in alcoholic hepatitis, megamitochondria correlated with better outcome [7]. Studies in NAFLD have not correlated megamitochondria with outcome.

## Glycogenated nuclei

This lesion of nuclear vacuolization has long been associated with NAFLD and initially potentially a "marker" of abnormal glucose metabolism [48]. It is a commonly noted feature in NAFLD and has been noted as more common than in ALD [26].

## Grading and staging: ALD and NAFLD

Grading and staging are mentioned for two reasons. As was stated in the introduction, for a meaningful method, only the lesions of significance for a given disease process are included in a final scoring system. Thus, methods derived for chronic hepatitis or a chronic cholestatic liver disease cannot be superimposed on either ALD or NAFLD or vice versa. Likewise, it is apparent that while there is overlap of many lesions within the spectrum of fatty liver disease, that is, steatosis, and milder forms of steatohepatitis, that is not necessarily the case in all forms of ALD, and methods of scoring derived for

alcoholic hepatitis will not necessarily conform to those derived for non-alcoholic fatty liver disease. Thus a pathologist should not feel confined by lesions for scoring. Finally, just as a score for chronic hepatitis cannot be "translated" into a diagnosis, neither can a "score" for steatohepatitis be translated into either a diagnosis or an etiology. However, it is apparent that a combination of lesions and severity of injury may occur that raise a concern of ALD. For a diagnostic pathologist, the best and most straightforward diagnosis to provide in a case in question is "steatohepatitis." One's comment may readily give the clinical team the information needed for further management.

Figures 9.1 and 9.2 demonstrate examples of NAFLD and ALD, respectively. The former includes a comparison of adult and pediatric NAFLD, and the latter highlights discussed lesions of severe disease in ALD.

## References

1. Diehl AM. Alcoholic liver disease: natural history. Liver Transpl Surg. 1997;3:206–11.
2. Brunt EM. Alcoholic and nonalcoholic steatohepatitis. Clin Liver Dis. 2002;6:399–420.
3. Edmondson HA, Peters RL, Reynolds TB, Kuzma OT. Sclerosing hyaline necrosis in the liver of the chronic alcoholic. A recognizable lesion. Ann Intern Med. 1963;59:646–73.
4. MacSween RNM, Burt AD. Histologic spectrum of alcoholic liver disease. Semin Liver Dis. 1986;6:221–32.
5. Altamirano J, Miquel R, Katoonizadeh A, Abraldes JG, Duarte-Rojo A, Louvet A, et al. A histologic scoring system for prognosis of patients with alcoholic hepatitis. Gastroenterology. 2014 May;146(5):1231–9.
6. Kleiner DE, Brunt EM, Van Natta M, Behling C, Contos MJ, Cummings OW, et al. Design and validation of a histological scoring system for nonalcoholic fatty liver disease. Hepatology. 2005 Jun;41(6):1313–21.
7. Altamarino J, Miquel R, Katoonizadeh A, Duarte-Rojo A, Smyrk TC, Michelena J, et al. Development and validation of a novel histological classification with prognostic value for alcoholic hepatitis. Hepatology. 2011;54:968A.
8. Baptista A, Bianchi L, de Groote J. Alcoholic liver disease: morphological manifestations. Review by an international group. Lancet. 1981;1:707–11.
9. Chalasani N, Wilson L, Kleiner DE, Cummings OW, Brunt EM, Unalp A, et al. Relationship of steatosis grade and zonal location to histological features of steatohepatitis in adult patients with non-alcoholic fatty liver disease. J Hepatol. 2008;48:829–34.

10. Sanyal AJ, Brunt EM, Kleiner DE, Kowdley KV, Chalasani N, Lavine JE, et al. Endpoints and clinical trial design for nonalcoholic steatohepatitis. Hepatology. 2011 Jul;54(1):344–53.

11. Kleiner DE, Brunt EM. Nonalcoholic fatty liver disease: pathologic patterns and biopsy evaluation in clinical research. Semin Liver Dis. 2012;32(1):3–13.

12. Schwimmer JB, Behling C, Newbury R, Deutsch R, Nievergelt C, Schork NJ, et al. Histopathology of pediatric nonalcoholic fatty liver disease. Hepatology. 2005;42:641–9.

13. Patton HM, Lavine JE, Van Natta ML, Schwimmer JB, Kleiner D, Molleston J. Clinical correlates of histopathology in pediatric nonalcoholic steatohepatitis. Gastroenterology. 2008 Dec;135(6):1961–71.

14. Neuschwander-Tetri BA, Clark JM, Bass NM, Van Natta ML, Unalp-Arida A, Tonascia J, et al. Clinical, laboratory and histological associations in adults with nonalcoholic fatty liver disease. Hepatology. 2010;52(3):913–24.

15. Teli MR, Day CP, Burt AD, Bennett MJ, James OF. Determinants of progression to cirrhosis or fibrosis in pure alcoholic fatty liver. Lancet. 1995;346:987–90.

16. Dam-Larsen S, Franzmann MB, Christoffersen P, Larsen K, Becker U, Bendtsen F. Histological characteristics and prognosis in patients with fatty liver. Scand J Gastroenterol. 2005 Apr;40(4):460–7.

17. Pais R, Charlotte F, Fedchuk L, Bedossa P, Lebray P, Poynard T, et al. A systematic review of follow-up biopsies reveals disease progression in patients with non-alcoholic fatty liver. J Hepatol. 2013;59(3):550–6.

18. Tandra S, Yeh MM, Brunt EM, Vuppalanchi R, Cummings OW, Unalp-Arida A, et al. Presence and significance of microvesicular steatosis in nonalcoholic fatty liver disease. J Hepatol. 2011 Sep;55(3):654–9.

19. Uchida T, Kao H, Quispe-Sjogren M, Peters RL. Alcoholic foamy degeneration—a pattern of acute alcoholic injury of the liver. Gastroenterology. 1983;84:683–92.

20. Montull S, Pares A, Bruguera M, Caballeria J, Uchida T, Rodes J. Alcoholic foamy degeneration in Spain. Prevalence and clinico-pathological features. Liver. 1989 Apr;9(2):79–85.

21. Colombat M, Charlotte F, Ratziu V, Poynard T. Portal lymphocytic infiltrate in alcoholic liver disease. Hum Pathol. 2002;33(12):1170–4.

22. Gadd VL, Skoien R, Powell EE, Fagan KJ, Winterford C, Horsfall L, et al. The portal inflammatory infiltrate and ductular reaction in human nonalcoholic fatty liver disease. Hepatology. 2014 Apr;59(4):1393–405.

23. Brunt EM, Kleiner DE, Wilson LA, Unalp A, Behling CE, Lavine JE, et al. Portal chronic inflammation in nonalcoholic fatty liver disease (NAFLD): a histologic marker of advanced NAFLD-Clinicopathologic correlations from the nonalcoholic steatohepatitis clinical research network. Hepatology. 2009;49:809–20.

24. Rakha EA, Adamson L, Bell E, Neal K, Ryder SD, Kaye PV, et al. Portal inflammation is associated with advanced histological changes in alcoholic and non-alcoholic fatty liver disease. J Clin Pathol. 2010 Sep;63(9):790–5.

25. Yip WW, Burt AD. Alcoholic liver disease. Semin Diagn Pathol. 2006;23:149–60.

26. Itoh S, Yougel T, Kawagoe K.Comparison between nonalcoholic steatohepatitis and alcoholic hepatitis. Am J Gastroenterol. 1987;82(7):650–4.

27. Lefkowitch JH. Morphology of alcoholic liver disease. Clin Liver Dis. 2005 Feb;9(1):37–53.

28. Lee J, French B, Morgan T, French SW. The liver is populated by a broad spectrum of markers for macrophages. In alcoholic hepatitis the macrophages are M1 and M2. Exp Mol Pathol. 2014;96(1):118–25.

29. Gill RM, Belt P, Wilson L, Bass NM, Ferrell LD. Centrizonal Arteries and Microvessels in Nonalcoholic Steatohepatitis. Am J Surg Pathol. 2011;35(9):1400–4.

30. Ludwig J, McGill DB, Lindor KD. Nonalcoholic steatohepatitis. J Gastroenterol Hepatol. 1997 May;12(5):398–403.

31. Diehl AM, Goodman Z, Ishak KG. Alcohollike liver disease in nonalcoholics. A clinical and histologic comparison with alcohol-induced liver injury. Gastroenterology. 1988;95:1056–62.

32. Nanki T, Koike R, Miyasaka N. Subacute severe steatohepatitis during prednisolone therapy for systemic lupus erythematosus (Letter to editor). Am J Gastroenterol. 1999;94(11):3379.

33. Caldwell SH, Hespenheide EE. Subacute liver failure in obese women. Am J Gastroenterol. 2002;97:2058–62.

34. Nasrallah SM, Nassar VH, Galambos JT. Importance of terminal hepatic venule thickening. Arch Pathol Lab Med. 1980 Feb;104(2):84–6.

35. Worner TM, Lieber CS. Perivenular fibrosis as precursor lesion of cirrhosis. JAMA. 1985 Aug 2;254(5):627–30.

36. Gramlich T, Kleiner DE, McCullough AJ, Matteoni CA, Boparai N, Younossi ZM. Pathologic features associated with fibrosis in nonalcoholic fatty liver disease. Hum Pathol. 2004;35:196–9.

37. Brunt EM, Janney CG, Di Bisceglie AM, Neuschwander-Tetri BA, Bacon BR. Nonalcoholic steatohepatitis: a proposal for grading and staging the histological lesions. Am J Gastroenterol. 1999 Sep;94(9):2467–74.

38. Bedossa P, Poitou C, Veyrie N, Bouillot J-L, Basdevant A, Paradis V, et al. Histopathological algorithm and scoring system for evaluation of liver lesions in morbidly obese patients. Hepatology. 2012;56(5):1571–9.

39. Matteoni CA, Younossi ZM, Gramlich T, Boparai N, Liu YC, McCullough AJ. Nonalcoholic fatty liver disease: a spectrum of clinical and pathological severity. Gastroenterology. 1999 Jun;116(6):1413–19.

40. Goodman ZD, Ishak KG. Occlusive venous lesions in alcoholic liver disease. A study of 200 cases. Gastroenterology. 1982 Oct;83(4):786–96.

41. Burt AD, MacSween RNM. Hepatic vein lesions in alcoholic liver disease: retrospective biopsy and necropsy study. J Clin Pathol 1986;39:63–7.

42. Brunelli E, Macarri G, Jezequel AM, Orlandi F. Diagnostic value of the fibrosis of the terminal hepatic venule in fatty liver and chronic hepatitis due to ethanol or other aetiology. Liver. 1985 Oct;5(5):261–6.

43. Savolainen V, Perola M, Lalu K, Penttila A, Virtanen I, Karhunen PJ. Early perivenular fibrogenesis–precirrhotic lesions among moderate alcohol consumers and chronic alcoholics. J Hepatol. 1995 Nov;23(5):524–31.

44. Porta EA, Bergman BJ, Stein AA. Acute Alcoholic Hepatitis. Am J Pathol. 1965 Apr;46:657–89.

45. Caldwell SH, Swerdlow RH, Khan EM, Iezzoni JC, Hespenheide EE, Parks JK, et al. Mitochondrial abnormalities in non-alcoholic steatohepatitis. J Hepatol. 1999 Sep;31(3):430–4.

46. Hall PDLM. Alcoholic liver disease. In: MacSween RNM, Burt AD, Portmann BC, Ishak KG, Scheuer PJ, Anthony PP, editor. Pathology of the Liver. 4th ed. London: Churchill Livingstone; 2002. p. 273–311.

47. Chedid A, Mendenhall CL, Tosch T, Chen T, Rabin L, Garcia-Pont P, et al. Significance of megamitochondria in alcoholic liver disease. Gastroenterology. 1986;90(6): 1858–64.

48. Ludwig J, Viggiano TR, McGill DB, Oh BJ. Nonalcoholic steatohepatitis: Mayo Clinic experiences with a hitherto unnamed disease. Mayo Clin Proc. 1980;55(7):434–8.

# 10  Of men and microbes: Role of the intestinal microbiome in non-alcoholic fatty liver disease

**Mohammad Bilal Siddiqui[1], Mohammad Shadab Siddiqui[2], and Arun J. Sanyal[2]**

[1] Department of Internal Medicine, University of Texas Medical School, Houston, Texas, USA
[2] Virginia Commonwealth University, Richmond, VA, USA

## LEARNING POINTS

- To understand the role of gut microbiome in human physiology
- To understand the relationship between gut microbiome and obesity
- To understand the role of gut microbiome in non-alcoholic fatty liver disease (NAFLD)

## Introduction

NAFLD affects a third of the US population with increased prevalence among obese or diabetic individuals [1–4] and is closely associated with other metabolic disorders including obesity, insulin resistance (IR), hypertension, dyslipidemia, and obstructive sleep apnea [5, 6]. The higher incidence of cardiovascular disease, extrahepatic malignancies, and progression to cirrhosis is largely responsible for the decreased long-term survival seen in patients with NAFLD [5, 7, 8]. The disease burden from NAFLD is projected to mirror the rise in other metabolic disorders and will be the leading listing diagnosis for progression to cirrhosis and liver transplantation [9].

NAFLD is characterized by intrahepatic fat accumulation in the absence of excessive alcohol consumption (<20 g/day in women and <30 g/day in men) and exclusion of secondary causes of hepatic steatosis [10–13]. NAFLD represents a histopathologic spectrum ranging from simple hepatic steatosis to steatohepatitis characterized by hepatic steatosis with necroinflammatory changes. Non-alcoholic steatohepatitis (NASH) is associated with increased risk of progression to advanced fibrosis and cirrhosis [5, 14, 15].

Although NAFLD is commonly seen in conjunction with other features of the metabolic syndrome, an independent epidemiological association between IR and NAFLD has been confirmed in nondiabetic patients [16, 17]. Patients with steatohepatitis are more likely to have higher total insulin secretion and lower insulin sensitivity than controls even in the absence of overt diabetes. Fasting insulin levels are the best predictor of hepatic steatosis, and IR is an independent risk factor for development of NASH, irrespective of body mass index (BMI). In patients with NAFLD and normal alanine aminotransferase (ALT) values, IR has been independently associated with the presence of advanced fibrosis [18]. Emerging data implicates intestinal microbiome as an integral component in pathogenesis of metabolic disorders, particularly obesity and diabetes. The focus of the current review will be to explore the relationship between intestinal microbiome and NAFLD and its link to obesity and IR.

## Intestinal microbiome

The human gut contains $>10^{14}$ microorganisms and is collectively referred to as the intestinal or gut microbiota [19]. The intestinal microbiota is important in the maturation of the human immune system, strengthening of the host

*Clinical Dilemmas in Non-Alcoholic Fatty Liver Disease*, First Edition. Edited by Roger Williams and Simon D. Taylor-Robinson.

defenses, vitamin synthesis, and absorption and fermentation of polysaccharides [20–22]. Already implicated in the pathogenesis of obesity and diabetes, emerging data suggest a causal link between intestinal microbiome and NAFLD [23–28].

## Obesity, IR, and the intestinal microbiome

Diet is an important determinant of the composition of the intestinal microbiome, and indigestible polysaccharides are the main substrate available to the intestinal microbiome. The metabolism of polysaccharides by intestinal microbiome results in short-chain fatty acids (SCFAs) and other metabolites that play a key role in bacterial–host interaction. The role of intestinal microbiome in weight regulation was initially demonstrated in animal studies [20, 29]. Compared to conventionally raised mice, germfree mice had reduced adiposity and weight gain despite increased food consumption [29]. Furthermore, transplantation of cecal-derived microbial species from conventionally raised mice into germfree mice, a process known as conventionalization, led to a dramatic increase in body weight and adiposity that was independent of chow diet consumption or energy expenditure [29, 30]. Using 16S RNA pyrosequencing, the obese phenotype was associated with a decrease in the *Bacteroides* species and a concurrent increase in Firmicutes species [30, 31]. These findings were corroborated in human studies that showed that weight loss proportionally correlated with the extent of restoration of the *Bacteroidetes* population [32]. Similarly, dietary intake of high-fat diets has been shown to alter the intestinal microbiome by promoting the relative concentrations of Firmicutes and Proteobacteria [33, 34]. Although the mechanism of weight gain due to changes in intestinal microbiome remains an area of ongoing investigation, several microbial processes have been identified that favor an obesogenic phenotype. For instance, in the presence of excess polysaccharides, *Bacteroides thetaiotaomicron* upregulates glycoside hydrolases thereby increasing fermentation of otherwise indigestible polysaccharides into short-chain fatty acids (SCFA) that are more readily absorbed by the host [21, 35]. Additionally, the microbiome induces host monosaccharide transporters to further enhance host utilization of liberated polysaccharides and allow more efficient caloric extraction from dietary intake. Butyrate, a SCFA, has been shown to stimulate leptin production and GLP-1 secretion thereby promoting an obesinogenic phenotype, while propionate is used for gluconeogenesis and lipogenesis by the hepatocytes [36].

The intestinal microbiome also regulates weight by affecting fasting-induced adipose factor (*Fiaf*), a circulating lipoprotein lipase (LPL) inhibitor that is produced in the small intestines, liver, and adipocytes. Elevated *Fiaf* levels protect against weight gain by inhibiting adipocyte LPL and thereby decreasing available free fatty acids necessary for adipose tissue expansion [20]. Conventionalization of germfree mice leads to significant reduction in *Fiaf* and increase in body weight and adiposity [20]. *Fiaf*-null germfree mice had the same amount of weight gain and increase in adiposity as the conventionally raised mice reaffirming the role of intestinal microbiome in *Fiaf* regulation.

Expansion of adipose tissue depots (Figure 10.1) as a result of weight gain leads to infiltration of overloaded adipose tissue by activated macrophages leading to low-grade chronic inflammation, which is an important cause of IR [37]. Gut-derived endotoxins, dietary fats, relative hypoxia, and hormones have all been implicated in adipose tissue inflammation [38]. Macrophage infiltration of the adipose tissue promotes production and secretion of proinflammatory cytokines by adipocytes characterized by high levels of tumor necrosis factor alpha (*TNF-α*) and interleukin-6 (*IL-6*) and a decrease in adiponectin levels [39, 40]. This proinflammatory metabolic milieu leads to further deterioration of IR. Additionally, these adipocyte-secreted cytokines (adipokines) enter the portal circulation and are sensed by the liver, which releases additional cytokines (i.e., hs-CRP) as part of the acute phase reaction. These cytokines promote endothelial dysfunction, promote atherogenesis, promote thrombosis, impair fibrinolysis, impair the metabolic clearance of glucose, and lead to hepatic steatosis.

## NAFLD and the intestinal microbiome

The portal vein receives 70% of its blood flow from the intestinal circulation and serves as a direct link between the intestinal microbiome and the liver by facilitating hepatic exposure to gut-derived microbial products. Patients with NAFLD have an increased prevalence of small intestinal bacterial overgrowth (SIBO), which augments the interaction between the microbiome and the liver by altering paracellular intestinal permeability [41, 42]. Normally, the integrity of the paracellular tight junctions is maintained by the interaction between transmembrane proteins occludins and claudins, which bind to membrane proteins zona occludens-1 and 2 (ZO-1 and ZO-2) [43–45]. SIBO disrupts the function of the tight junction protein ZO-1, increasing

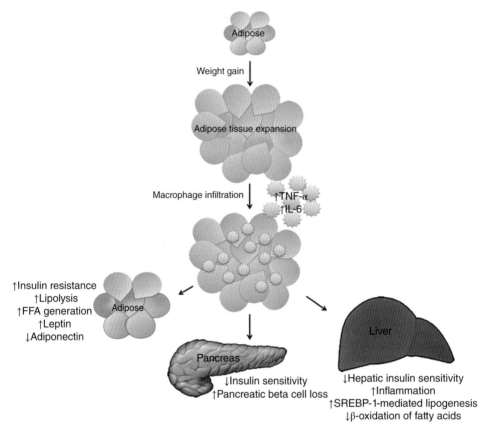

**FIG 10.1** Weight gain leads to adipose tissue expansion and inflammation, which results in a proinflammatory state. These adipokines worsen adipose tissue and hepatic and systemic insulin resistance. The deterioration in insulin sensitivity leads to pancreatic β-cell loss, de novo lipogenesis, and hepatic steatosis. (*See insert for color representation of the figure.*)

intestinal permeability and ultimately facilitating the increased absorption of microbial endotoxins into the portal circulation [42, 43] (Figure 10.2). Additionally, the association between intestinal permeability and the degree of steatosis is independent of other features of metabolic syndrome and SIBO, suggesting that the gut–liver axis is an important driver of hepatic steatosis [42].

## Interaction between liver and intestine via bile acids

Bile acids, produced as glycine or taurine conjugates from cholesterol in the liver and secreted into the small intestine, facilitate the cross talk between the liver and intestine. Bile acids have a direct bacteriostatic effect, and in animal models of cirrhosis, admiration of conjugated bile acids reduced bacterial overgrowth and translocation [46]. In intestinal epithelial cells, conjugated bile acids bind to farnesoid X

receptor (FXR), which increases production of antimicrobial proteins angiogenin 1 and ribonuclease family receptor member, thereby preventing bacterial overgrowth and promoting epithelial cell integrity [47]. Additionally, bile acid metabolism was disrupted in animal models of NASH potentially due to underlying hepatic inflammation and injury [48]. Corroborating the animal data, a recent phase 2 clinical trial of the FXR agonist obeticholic acid in patients with type 2 diabetes and NAFLD, showed significantly improved markers of inflammation and fibrosis [49].

## Intestinal microbiome and chronic inflammation

In addition to the recruitment of adipokines, the microbiome also contributes to chronic inflammation through the production of endotoxins. Endotoxins are key constituents of the microbial cell wall that illicit an immune response upon

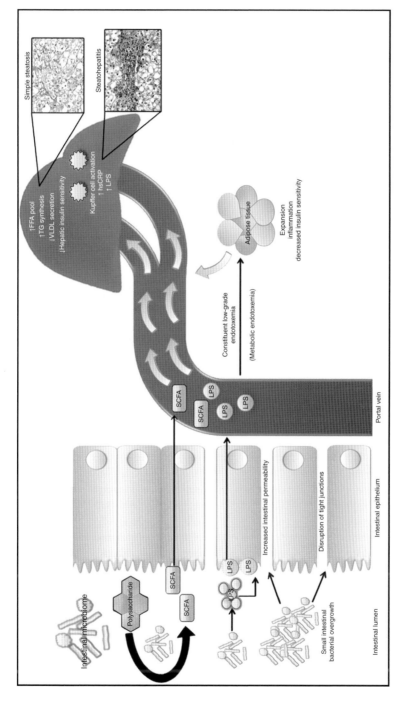

**FIG 10.2** NAFLD is associated with an increase in small intestinal bacterial overgrowth (SIBO). The intestinal microbiome breaks down polysaccharides into short-chain fatty acids (SCFAs), and increased bacterial productions (i.e., LPS) are then readily absorbed into the portal circulation. These by-products of digestion and intestinal microbiome subsequently influence insulin resistance and hepatic triglyceride synthesis and impair hepatic triglyceride synthesis leading to hepatic steatosis. (*See insert for color representation of the figure.*)

their release into the host. Lipopolysaccharide (LPS) is an active component of endotoxins. Food intake impacts serum endotoxin levels, which normally increase during the fed state and decline with fasting. However, a high-fat diet disrupts these cyclic changes in serum endotoxin levels and leads to chronic endotoxemia, which can be seen in as little as 3 days after initiation of the high-fat feeding (Figure 10.2) [26, 31]. Additionally, the proportion of LPS-expressing bacteria also increases with a high-fat diet [28]. Serum endotoxin levels in this chronic low-grade endotoxemia or metabolic endotoxemia are usually 10–50-folds lower than is normally seen in septicemia or infections and have been implicated in the pathogenesis of metabolic disorders including hepatic steatosis [28, 50]. LPS binds to LPS binding protein (LBP), which subsequently binds to CD-14 and activates toll-like receptor-4 (TLR-4). TLRs are pattern recognition receptors that recognized highly conversed microbial molecules termed pathogen-associated molecular patterns (PAMPs). LPS-mediated activation of TLRs in Kupffer results in increased expression of proinflammatory cytokines and hepatic injury [28]. Importance of CD-14 and TLR-4 in propagating the host response to LPS-mediated hepatotoxicity was confirmed in CD-14 and TLR-4 null mice that had a blunted response to high-fat diets [28, 51, 52].

The inducible proinflammatory state seen with metabolic endotoxemia in the liver and visceral adipose tissue is characterized by increased levels of $TNF-\alpha$, $IL-1\beta$, $IL-6$, and plasminogen activator inhibitor-1 (PAI-1) [27, 53–55]. These proinflammatory cytokines interfere with insulin signaling and lead to deterioration of both hepatic and systemic insulin sensitivities [40]. Metabolic endotoxemia also promotes hepatic triglyceride synthesis and liver fat accumulation. Interestingly, the presence of preexisting obesity exaggerates the host response to LPS-induced liver injury. Compared to lean littermates, obesity prone zucker (fa/fa) rats developed significant steatohepatitis and hepatic injury after *i.p.* administration of LPS. Although $TNF-\alpha$ production by Kupffer cells was similar, the phagocytic activity of Kupffer cells was significantly increased in obese animals. This data suggests that the liver in metabolic endotoxemia likely primes the Kupffer cells to LPS making them more sensitive to toxic effects of $TNF-\alpha$ [56].

Additional data confirming the importance of intestinal microbiome in NAFLD came from studies investigating probiotics in NAFLD. In animal studies, treatments with probiotics lead to significant improvement in serum endotoxemia, intestinal barrier function, IR, and liver fat content [57].

These observations were confirmed in human studies where treatment with VSL#3, a mix of probiotic strains, lead to significant improvement in serum $TNF-\alpha$ levels and hepatic inflammation [58]. More recently in a cross-sectional cohort, relative deficiency in intestinal microbial species of *Bacteroides* and *Prevotella* was associated with steatohepatitis compared to healthy subjects and those with simple hepatic steatosis [59]. Additionally, compared to those with simple hepatic steatosis, those with steatohepatitis had higher fecal content of *Clostridium coccoides*. This association was independent of dietary fat intake and BMI, suggesting a role of intestinal microbiome in the development of steatohepatitis [59]. In another cross-sectional study comparing NAFLD with healthy controls, there was overrepresentation of Firmicutes (Lactobacillaceae, Veillonellaceae, and Lachnospiraceae families) and Proteobacteria (Kiloniellaceae and Pasteurellaceae families) while a relative decrease in *Bacteroides* (Porphyromonadaceae) [60]. Volatile organic compounds (VOC) are microbial-derived compounds whose effects are unknown in the human gut. Interestingly, ester VOCs were identified more frequently in fecal samples of those with NAFLD, although the clinical implication of these findings is unclear at this point [60].

Furthermore, this chronic inflammatory state has been shown to promote hepatocarcinogenesis in mice [61]. Mice treated with constituently low levels of LPS had increased tumor size and number in carbon tetrachloride ($CCl_4$)-induced hepatocarcinogenesis [61]. This increase in tumor burden is likely related to TLR-4-dependent pathways, as TLR-4-deficient mice had an 80–90% reduction in tumor size and number [61]. Additionally, reduced tumor burden was noted in germfree mice and in mice that underwent gut sterilization, implicating the intestinal microbiome as a key mediator of hepatocellular carcinoma progression [61].

However, there is significant variability and even contradictory findings in human studies attempting to better characterize intestinal microbiome in NAFLD [59, 60, 62, 63]. These discrepant findings could potentially be due to differences in demographics (i.e., geographic locations, ethnicities, age, etc.), methodology, small sample size, and nonhistological characterization of NAFLD.

### Choline deficiency and hepatic steatosis

Choline is an integral component of biological membranes and necessary for triglyceride secretion into very low-density lipoprotein (VLDL) from the liver [64–66]. Choline deficiency results in decreased hepatic triglyceride clearance and hepatic steatosis, which can be reversed with choline supplementation [65, 67]. Relative reduction in intestinal concentrations of Gammaproteobacteria and Erysipelotrichi is associated with choline deficiency and hepatic steatosis in humans [63]. Intestinal microbiome-mediated choline deficiency is likely multifactorial. Enzymes produced by the gut microbiota catalyze the first step in the conversion of dietary choline to methylamines, dimethylamine, and trimethylamine [68]. Methylamines are subsequently absorbed through the microvilli and reach the liver via portal vein where they activate inflammatory pathways leading to hepatic injury. Furthermore, conversion of choline into methylamines reduces the bioavailability of choline for production of phosphatidylcholine [69]. The relative choline and phosphatidylcholine deficiency subsequently interferes with VLDL assembly and triglyceride secretion from the liver leading to hepatic steatosis [69] (Figure 10.3).

### Endogenous ethanol production in NAFLD

Some of the microbial species in the intestinal microbiome produce potentially hepatotoxic agents like ethanol even in the absence of exogenous alcohol consumption.

Endogenous ethanol is metabolized into acetate and acetaldehyde, which are subsequently transported to the liver via portal circulation [62]. In the liver, acetate can be used as a substrate for *de novo* lipogenesis, while acetaldehyde can activate Kupffer cells to produce reactive oxygen species (ROS) leading to hepatic injury. Compared to obese controls, the microbiome of patients with steatohepatitis was found to be enriched with Proteobacteria, a major source of endogenous ethanol production in humans [70]. The increase in relative concentration of Proteobacteria was associated with a parallel increase in blood ethanol concentration.

### Conclusion

The role of intestinal microbiome in pathogenesis of NALFD is being continually defined. Although some of these mechanisms are likely linked to the development of other metabolic disorders like IR and obesity, other mechanisms are more specific to the liver like Kupffer cell activation, increase in *de novo* lipogenesis, and endogenous ethanol production.

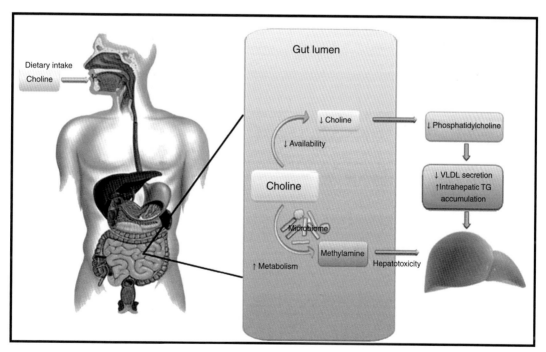

**FIG 10.3** The gut microbiota catalyzes the conversion of dietary choline into methylamines, which enter the portal circulation and promote hepatocellular injury. The conversion of choline to methylamines also reduces the bioavailability of choline, leading to phosphatidylcholine deficiency, which impairs VLDL secretion and promotes steatosis. (*See insert for color representation of the figure.*)

## References

1. Browning JD, Szczepaniak LS, Dobbins R, Nuremberg P, Horton JD, Cohen JC, Grundy SM, et al. Prevalence of hepatic steatosis in an urban population in the united states: Impact of ethnicity. Hepatology 2004; 40(6): 1387–1395.

2. Bhala N, Angulo P, van der Poorten D, Lee E, Hui JM, Saracco G, Adams LA, et al. The natural history of nonalcoholic fatty liver disease with advanced fibrosis or cirrhosis: An international collaborative study. Hepatology 2011; 54(4): 1208–1216.

3. Bellentani S, Tiribelli C, Saccoccio G, Sodde M, Fratti N, De Martin C, Cristianini G. Prevalence of chronic liver disease in the general population of northern Italy: The dionysos study. Hepatology 1994; 20(6): 1442–1449.

4. Kallwitz ER, Kumar M, Aggarwal R, Berger R, Layden-Almer J, Gupta N, Cotler SJ. Ethnicity and nonalcoholic fatty liver disease in an obesity clinic: The impact of triglycerides. Dig Dis Sci 2008; 53(5): 1358–1363.

5. Adams LA, Lymp JF, St Sauver J, Sanderson SO, Lindor KD, Feldstein A, Angulo P. The natural history of nonalcoholic fatty liver disease: A population-based cohort study. Gastroenterology 2005; 129(1): 113–121.

6. Vernon G, Baranova A, Younossi ZM. Systematic review: The epidemiology and natural history of non-alcoholic fatty liver disease and non-alcoholic steatohepatitis in adults. Hepatology 2011; 34(3): 274–285.

7. Söderberg C, Stål P, Askling J, Glaumann H, Lindberg G, Marmur J, Hultcrantz R. Decreased survival of subjects with elevated liver function tests during a 28-year follow-up. Hepatology 2009; 51: 595–602.

8. Ekstedt M, Franzen LE, Mathiesen UL, Thorelius L, Holmqvist M, Bodemar G, Kechagias S. Long-term follow-up of patients with NAFLD and elevated liver enzymes. Hepatology 2006; 44(4): 865–873.

9. Charlton MR, Burns JM, Pedersen RA, Watt KD, Heimbach JK, Dierkhsing RA. Frequency and outcomes of liver transplantation for nonalcoholic steatohepatitis in the united states. Gastroenterology 2011; 141: 1249–1253.

10. Ludwig J, Viggiano TR, McGill DB, Oh BJ. Nonalcoholic steatohepatitis: Mayo clinic experiences with a hitherto unnamed disease. Mayo Clin Proc 1980; 55(7): 434–438.

11. Chalasani N, Younossi Z, Lavine JE, Diehl AM, Brunt EM, Cusi K, Charlton M, et al. The diagnosis and management of non-alcoholic fatty liver disease: Practice guideline by the American association for the study of liver diseases, American college of gastroenterology, and the American gastroenterological association. Hepatology 2012; 55(6): 2005–2023.

12. Bacon BR, Farahvash MJ, Janney CG, Neuschwander-Tetri BA. Nonalcoholic steatohepatitis: An expanded clinical entity. Gastroenterology 1994; 107(4): 1103–1109.

13. Matteoni CA, Younossi ZM, Gramlich T, Boparai N, Liu YC, McCullough AJ. Nonalcoholic fatty liver disease: A spectrum of clinical and pathological severity. Gastroenterology 1999; 116(6): 1413–1419.

14. Kleiner DE, Brunt EM, Van Natta M, Behling C, Contos MJ, Cummings OW, Ferrell LD, et al. Design and validation of a histological scoring system for nonalcoholic fatty liver disease. Hepatology 2005; 41(6): 1313–1321.

15. Brunt EM, Janney CG, Di Bisceglie AM, Neuschwander-Tetri BA, Bacon BR. Nonalcoholic steatohepatitis: A proposal for grading and staging the histological lesions. Am J Gastroenterol 1999; 94(9): 2467–2474.

16. Pagano G, Pacini G, Musso G, Gambino R, Mecca F, Depetris N, Cassader M, et al. Nonalcoholic steatohepatitis, insulin resistance, and metabolic syndrome: Further evidence for an etiologic association. Hepatology 2002; 35(2): 367–372.

17. Sanyal AJ, Campbell-Sargent C, Mirshahi F, Rizzo WB, Contos MJ, Sterling RK, Luketic VA, et al. Nonalcoholic steatohepatitis: Association of insulin resistance and mitochondrial abnormalities. Gastroenterology 2001; 120(5): 1183–1192.

18. Fracanzani AL, Valenti L, Bugianesi E, Andreoletti M, Colli A, Vanni E, Bertelli C, et al. Risk of severe liver disease in nonalcoholic fatty liver disease with normal aminotransferase levels: A role for insulin resistance and diabetes. Hepatology 2008; 48(3): 792–798.

19. Savage DC. Microbial ecology of the gastrointestinal tract. Annu Rev Microbiol 1977; 31: 107–133.

20. Backhed F, Ding H, Wang T, Hooper LV, Koh GY, Nagy A, Semenkovich CF, et al. The gut microbiota as an environmental factor that regulates fat storage. Proc Natl Acad Sci U S A 2004; 101(44): 15718–15723.

21. Backhed F, Ley RE, Sonnenburg JL, Peterson DA, Gordon JI. Host-bacterial mutualism in the human intestine. Science 2005; 307(5717): 1915–1920.

22. Xu J, Bjursell MK, Himrod J, Deng S, Carmichael LK, Chiang HC, Hooper LV, et al. A genomic view of the human-bacteroides thetaiotaomicron symbiosis. Science 2003; 299(5615): 2074–2076.

23. Tilg H, Moschen AR, Kaser A. Obesity and the microbiota. Gastroenterology 2009; 136(5): 1476–1483.

24. Tilg H, Kaser A. Gut microbiome, obesity, and metabolic dysfunction. J Clin Invest 2011; 121(6): 2126–2132.

25. Tilg H. Obesity, metabolic syndrome, and microbiota: Multiple interactions. J Clin Gastroenterol 2010; 44(Suppl 1): S16–S18.

26. Amar J, Burcelin R, Ruidavets JB, Cani PD, Fauvel J, Alessi MC, Chamontin B, et al. Energy intake is associated with endotoxemia in apparently healthy men. Am J Clin Nutr 2008; 87(5): 1219–1223.

27. Brun P, Castagliuolo I, Di Leo V, Buda A, Pinzani M, Palu G, Martines D. Increased intestinal permeability in obese mice: New evidence in the pathogenesis of nonalcoholic steatohepatitis. Am J Physiol Gastrointest Liver Physiol 2007; 292(2): G518–G525.

28. Cani PD, Amar J, Iglesias MA, Poggi M, Knauf C, Bastelica D, Neyrinck AM, et al. Metabolic endotoxemia initiates obesity and insulin resistance. Diabetes 2007; 56(7): 1761–1772.

29. Backhed F, Manchester JK, Semenkovich CF, Gordon JI. Mechanisms underlying the resistance to diet-induced obesity in germ-free mice. Proc Natl Acad Sci U S A 2007; 104(3): 979–984.

30. Turnbaugh PJ, Ley RE, Mahowald MA, Magrini V, Mardis ER, Gordon JI. An obesity-associated gut microbiome with increased capacity for energy harvest. Nature 2006; 444(7122): 1027–1031.

31. Turnbaugh PJ, Backhed F, Fulton L, Gordon JI. Diet-induced obesity is linked to marked but reversible alterations in the mouse distal gut microbiome. Cell Host Microbe 2008; 3(4): 213–223.

32. Ley RE, Turnbaugh PJ, Klein S, Gordon JI. Microbial ecology: Human gut microbes associated with obesity. Nature 2006; 444(7122): 1022–1023.

33. Le Chatelier E, Nielsen T, Qin J, Prifti E, Hildebrand F, Falony G, Almeida M, et al. Richness of human gut microbiome correlates with metabolic markers. Nature 2013; 500(7464): 541–546.

34. Cotillard A, Kennedy SP, Kong LC, Prifti E, Pons N, Le Chatelier E, Almeida M, et al. Dietary intervention impact on gut microbial gene richness. Nature 2013; 500(7464): 585–588.

35. Sonnenburg JL, Xu J, Leip DD, Chen CH, Westover BP, Weatherford J, Buhler JD, et al. Glycan foraging in vivo by an intestine-adapted bacterial symbiont. Science 2005; 307(5717): 1955–1959.

36. Samuel BS, Shaito A, Motoike T, Rey FE, Backhed F, Manchester JK, Hammer RE, et al. Effects of the gut microbiota on host adiposity are modulated by the short-chain fatty-acid binding G protein-coupled receptor, Gpr41. Proc Natl Acad Sci U S A 2008; 105(43): 16767–16772.

37. Chawla A, Nguyen KD, Goh YP. Macrophage-mediated inflammation in metabolic disease. Nat Rev Immunol 2011; 11(11): 738–749.

38. Lolmede K, Durand de Saint Front V, Galitzky J, Lafontan M, Bouloumie A. Effects of hypoxia on the expression of proangiogenic factors in differentiated 3T3-F442A adipocytes. Int J Obes Relat Metab Disord 2003; 27(10): 1187–1195.

39. Weisberg SP, McCann D, Desai M, Rosenbaum M, Leibel RL, Ferrante AW, Jr. Obesity is associated with macrophage accumulation in adipose tissue. J Clin Invest 2003; 112(12): 1796–1808.

40. Xu H, Barnes GT, Yang Q, Tan G, Yang D, Chou CJ, Sole J, et al. Chronic inflammation in fat plays a crucial role in the development of obesity-related insulin resistance. J Clin Invest 2003; 112(12): 1821–1830.

41. Sabate JM, Jouet P, Harnois F, Mechler C, Msika S, Grossin M, Coffin B. High prevalence of small intestinal bacterial overgrowth in patients with morbid obesity: A contributor to severe hepatic steatosis. Obes Surg 2008; 18(4): 371–377.

42. Miele L, Valenza V, La Torre G, Montalto M, Cammarota G, Ricci R, Masciana R, et al. Increased intestinal permeability and tight junction alterations in nonalcoholic fatty liver disease. Hepatology 2009; 49(6): 1877–1887.

43. Anderson JM, Van Itallie CM. Tight junctions and the molecular basis for regulation of paracellular permeability. Am J Physiol 1995; 269(4 Pt 1): G467–G475.

44. Furuse M, Hirase T, Itoh M, Nagafuchi A, Yonemura S, Tsukita S, Tsukita S. Occludin: A novel integral membrane protein localizing at tight junctions. J Cell Biol 1993; 123(6 Pt 2): 1777–1788.

45. Furuse M, Fujita K, Hiiragi T, Fujimoto K, Tsukita S. Claudin-1 and -2: Novel integral membrane proteins localizing at tight junctions with no sequence similarity to occludin. J Cell Biol 1998; 141(7): 1539–1550.

46. Kakiyama G, Pandak WM, Gillevet PM, Hylemon PB, Heuman DM, Daita K, Takei H, et al. Modulation of the fecal bile acid profile by gut microbiota in cirrhosis. J Hepatol 2013; 58(5): 949–955.

47. Inagaki T, Moschetta A, Lee YK, Peng L, Zhao G, Downes M, Yu RT, et al. Regulation of antibacterial defense in the small intestine by the nuclear bile acid receptor. Proc Natl Acad Sci U S A 2006; 103(10): 3920–3925.

48. Tanaka N, Matsubara T, Krausz KW, Patterson AD, Gonzalez FJ. Disruption of phospholipid and bile acid homeostasis in mice with nonalcoholic steatohepatitis. Hepatology 2012; 56(1): 118–129.

49. Mudaliar S, Henry RR, Sanyal AJ, Morrow L, Marschall HU, Kipnes M, Adorini L, et al. Efficacy and safety of the farnesoid X receptor agonist obeticholic acid in patients with type 2 diabetes and nonalcoholic fatty liver disease. Gastroenterology 2013; 145(3): 574–582.e1.

50. Mydel P, Takahashi Y, Yumoto H, Sztukowska M, Kubica M, Gibson FC, III, Kurtz DM, Jr, et al. Roles of the host oxidative immune response and bacterial antioxidant rubrerythrin during porphyromonas gingivalis infection. PLoS Pathog 2006; 2(7): e76.

51. Roncon-Albuquerque R, Jr, Moreira-Rodrigues M, Faria B, Ferreira AP, Cerqueira C, Lourenco AP, Pestana M, et al. Attenuation of the cardiovascular and metabolic complications of obesity in CD14 knockout mice. Life Sci 2008; 83(13–14): 502–510.

52. Shi H, Kokoeva MV, Inouye K, Tzameli I, Yin H, Flier JS. TLR4 links innate immunity and fatty acid-induced insulin resistance. J Clin Invest 2006; 116(11): 3015–3025.

53. Laugerette F, Vors C, Peretti N, Michalski MC. Complex links between dietary lipids, endogenous endotoxins and metabolic inflammation. Biochimie 2011; 93: 39–45.

54. Ruiz AG, Casafont F, Crespo J, Cayon A, Mayorga M, Estebanez A, Fernadez-Escalante JC, et al. Lipopolysaccharide-binding protein plasma levels and liver TNF-alpha gene expression in obese patients: Evidence for the potential role of endotoxin in the pathogenesis of non-alcoholic steatohepatitis. Obes Surg 2007; 17(10): 1374–1380.

55. Nolan JP. The role of intestinal endotoxin in liver injury: A long and evolving history. Hepatology 2010; 52(5): 1829–1835.

56. Yang SQ, Lin HZ, Lane MD, Clemens M, Diehl AM. Obesity increases sensitivity to endotoxin liver injury: Implications for the pathogenesis of steatohepatitis. Proc Natl Acad Sci U S A 1997; 94(6): 2557–2562.

57. Li Z, Yang S, Lin H, Huang J, Watkins PA, Moser AB, Desimone C, et al. Probiotics and antibodies to TNF inhibit inflammatory activity and improve nonalcoholic fatty liver disease. Hepatology 2003; 37(2): 343–350.

58. Loguercio C, Federico A, Tuccillo C, Terracciano F, D'Auria MV, De Simone C, Del Vecchio Blanco C. Beneficial effects of a probiotic VSL#3 on parameters of liver dysfunction in chronic liver diseases. J Clin Gastroenterol 2005; 39(6): 540–543.

59. Mouzaki M, Comelli EM, Arendt BM, Bonengel J, Fung SK, Fischer SE, McGilvray ID, et al. Intestinal microbiota in patients with nonalcoholic fatty liver disease. Hepatology 2013; 58(1): 120–127.

60. Raman M, Ahmed I, Gillevet PM, Probert CS, Ratcliffe NM, Smith S, Greenwood R, et al. Fecal microbiome and volatile organic compound metabolome in obese humans with non-alcoholic fatty liver disease. Clin Gastroenterol Hepatol 2013; 11(7): 868–875.e1-3.

61. Dapito DH, Mencin A, Gwak GY, Pradere JP, Jang MK, Mederacke I, Caviglia JM, et al. Promotion of hepatocellular carcinoma by the intestinal microbiota and TLR4. Cancer Cell 2012; 21(4): 504–516.

62. Zhu L, Baker SS, Gill C, Liu W, Alkhouri R, Baker RD, Gill SR. Characterization of the gut microbiome in non-alcoholic steatohepatitis (NASH) patients: A connection between endogenous alcohol and NASH. Hepatology 2013; 57(2): 609–609.

63. Spencer MD, Hamp TJ, Reid RW, Fischer LM, Zeisel SH, Fodor AA. Association between composition of the human gastrointestinal microbiome and development of fatty liver with choline deficiency. Gastroenterology 2011; 140(3): 976–986.

64. Zeisel SH, da Costa KA. Choline: An essential nutrient for public health. Nutr Rev 2009; 67(11): 615–623.

65. Rinella ME, Elias MS, Smolak RR, Fu T, Borensztajn J, Green RM. Mechanisms of hepatic steatosis in mice fed a lipogenic methionine choline-deficient diet. J Lipid Res 2008; 49(5): 1068–1076.

66. Yao ZM, Vance DE. The active synthesis of phosphatidylcholine is required for very low density lipoprotein secretion from rat hepatocytes. J Biol Chem 1988; 263(6): 2998–3004.

67. Buchman AL, Dubin MD, Moukarzel AA, Jenden DJ, Roch M, Rice KM, Gornbein J, et al. Choline deficiency: A cause of hepatic steatosis during parenteral nutrition that can be reversed with intravenous choline supplementation. Hepatology 1995; 22(5): 1399–1403.

68. Zeisel SH, Wishnok JS, Blusztajn JK. Formation of methylamines from ingested choline and lecithin. J Pharmacol Exp Ther 1983; 225(2): 320–324.

69. Dumas ME, Barton RH, Toye A, Cloarec O, Blancher C, Rothwell A, Fearnside J, et al. Metabolic profiling reveals a contribution of gut microbiota to fatty liver phenotype in insulin-resistant mice. Proc Natl Acad Sci U S A 2006; 103(33): 12511–12516.

70. Clark DP. The fermentation pathways of *Escherichia coli*. FEMS Microbiol Rev 1989; 5(3): 223–234.

## 11 Can genetic influence in non-alcoholic fatty liver disease be ignored?

**Yang-Lin Liu[1], Christopher P. Day[1,2], and Quentin M. Anstee[1,2]**
[1] Institute of Cellular Medicine, Newcastle University, Newcastle upon Tyne, UK
[2] Liver Unit, Freeman Hospital, Newcastle upon Tyne, UK

### LEARNING POINTS

- NAFLD is a multifactorial complex disease trait determined by the integration of genetic and environmental factors.

- Although several genetic variants have been identified based on a priori hypotheses, some of the best validated gene variants have been identified through GWAS.

- PNPLA3 has been associated with steatosis, steatohepatitis, fibrosis and hepatocellular carcinoma risk.

- More recently, a variant in the TM6SF2 gene has been linked with both risk of progressive NAFLD and also cardiovascular disease risk.

- A key challenge is to understand the mechanisms and pathophysiological processes through which these genetic variants influence disease progression.

## Introduction

As has already been discussed, non-alcoholic fatty liver disease (NAFLD) represents a broad disease spectrum occurring in the absence of excessive alcohol consumption and ranging from steatosis (hepatocellular triglyceride accumulation >5%) [1], through steatohepatitis (NASH), to fibrosis/cirrhosis and in some cases, hepatocellular carcinoma (HCC). NAFLD is closely linked to central obesity, insulin resistance/type 2 diabetes mellitus (T2DM) and dyslipidaemia and thus with cardiovascular disease [1]. Due to sedentary lifestyles and the increasing consumption of diets enriched in fats and carbohydrates, these 'metabolic syndrome' risk factors have become endemic and so the

incidence of NAFLD has risen rapidly to become a leading cause of chronic liver disease worldwide [1].

Estimates of NAFLD prevalence vary somewhat according to population studied (different ethnicities, genders and comorbidities) and the sensitivity of the modality used employed such as radiology or histology [2, 3]. Studies in an unselected North American population determined that 35% of those studied exhibited NAFLD defined as [1]H-MRS measured hepatic triglyceride content (HTGC) >5.5%. Estimates increase further when populations with known risk factors are selected. For example, 91% of obese patients (BMI ≥ 30 kg/m$^2$), 67% of overweight (BMI 25–30) and 25% in normal weight individuals in the Italian Dionysos study had NAFLD, and 40–70% of T2DM patients have NAFLD [1]. An important paradox exists however: because the majority of patients with the metabolic syndrome develop steatosis, NAFLD is now extremely common, but only a minority of those with NAFLD will develop advanced liver disease characterised by NASH and hepatic fibrosis or experience any liver-related morbidity [1]. It is the recognition of this substantial inter-patient variability that prompted researchers to seek out those factors that drive pathogenesis and modify disease outcome.

## What evidence suggests a heritable component to NAFLD?

NAFLD is best considered a complex disease trait [4]. As with many common diseases, it is now appreciated that individual risk of NAFLD, development of NASH, fibrosis

*Clinical Dilemmas in Non-Alcoholic Fatty Liver Disease*, First Edition. Edited by Roger Williams and Simon D. Taylor-Robinson.
© 2016 John Wiley & Sons, Ltd. Published 2016 by John Wiley & Sons, Ltd.

progression and clinical outcome are the product of multi-directional interactions between *intrinsic factors* (genetic, epigenetic and age related) and a range of *extrinsic (environmental) influences* (including dietary/nutritional factors, intestinal flora/microbiome, xenobiotics as well as activity/behavioural factors). Together, these affect carbohydrate and lipid metabolism, modify endocrine function (in particular insulin sensitivity at both the cellular and tissue level), promote hepatocellular lipotoxicity and oxidative stress, influence inflammatory response and drive liver disease (from fibrosis to cirrhosis and onwards to primary liver cancer [HCC]) and cardiovascular disease. Unlike Mendelian disorders (e.g. cystic fibrosis) that are attributable to rare, highly penetrant single-gene mutations that are necessary and sufficient to cause disease, complex disease traits are attributable to multiple genetic modifiers (each of which alone is insufficient to cause disease) interacting with acquired exposures [4]. Thus, the contribution of each individual genetic variant is relatively modest but when taken together, in the presence of a permissive environment, these combine to produce a disease phenotype. In the case of NAFLD, the degree of heritability (fraction of the variation in the disease attributable to genetic causes) is estimated to be 26–27% for radiologically measured HTGC [5]. That there is a heritable component to NAFLD is further supported by observed interethnic variations in disease prevalence and familial disease clustering:

• *Interethnic differences in susceptibility* to NAFLD and NAFLD-related 'cryptogenic cirrhosis' have been reported in several studies [6, 7]. A large US study in an unselected multi-ethnic population found that NAFLD was present in 45% of Hispanics, 33% of whites and 24% of blacks, independent of BMI, insulin resistance or alcohol consumption [6]. Although some metabolic risk factors and socioeconomic characteristics associated with NAFLD differed between the ethnic groups, making precise interpretation of these data difficult, as discussed in the following, differences in population prevalence of patatin-like phospholipase domain-containing 3 (*PNPLA3*) genetic variants including the rs738409 polymorphism contributed to this variability and accounted for up to 72% of ethnic differences in the Dallas Heart Study cohort [8].

• *Familial aggregation* of NAFLD at levels greater than would be expected by chance has been described [4]. A study comparing HTGC in parents and sibs of children

with NAFLD to those of children with a similar degree of obesity but without NAFLD found that, even after adjusting for potential confounding factors, steatosis was significantly more common in the siblings and parents of the children with NAFLD than those without (59 and 78% vs. 17 and 37%, respectively) [9]. Importantly, MRI-determined hepatic fat fraction correlated more closely with body mass index in the families of index children with NAFLD than in those without [9]. Further support comes from a study comparing serum ALT and fasting serum insulin levels in twins where intra-pair correlations of were significantly higher in monozygotic than dizygotic twins [10].

## What genetic factors have been identified?

Candidate gene case–control association studies and genome-wide association studies (GWAS) have contributed greatly to our understanding of the genetic contribution to NAFLD pathogenesis and variability of prognosis (reviewed in Ref [4]). Until recently, candidate gene studies were the main method used by researchers to identify modifier genes of complex disease traits such as NAFLD. These studies assess correlations between specific genetic variants within large unrelated patient cohorts and phenotypes (disease) on a population scale and so have greater power to detect an effect. However, the selection of candidate genes for study is dependent upon there being an *a priori* hypothesis or knowledge of a biologically plausible physiological role to suggest that the gene may be relevant. The completion of the human genome sequence, and subsequent cataloguing of patterns of common sequence variation across the genome, revolutionised the study of complex diseases and paved the way for the development of GWAS technologies [4]. These allow investigators to simultaneously survey common variability (e.g., at a minor allele frequency >5%) across the entire human genome using single-nucleotide polymorphism (SNP) genotyping arrays and thus identify new genes that influence NAFLD pathogenesis where no *a priori* biological evidence for a role existed. Table 11.1 summarises the GWAS studies that have been published to date for NAFLD.

Several genes that influence susceptibility to NAFLD have been identified by GWAS, and their suggested effects have been independently confirmed in subsequent GWAS or candidate gene association studies (Table 11.2). Two

**TABLE 11.1** GWAS relevant to NAFLD

| | Population | Modality | N | Number of SNPs | Modifier genes identified |
|---|---|---|---|---|---|
| Romeo et al. [8] | United States (mixed ethnicity) | 1H-MRS steatosis | 2051 (B: 1,032; W: 636; H: 383) | 9229 | Chr 22: PNPLA3 (rs738409) |
| Yuan et al. [11] | European (mixed ethnicity) | Clinical biochemistry (ALT) | 12,419 (3 discovery and 3 replication groups) | — | Chr 22: PNPLA3 (rs738409) CPN1-ERLIN1-CHUK (rs11597390, rs11591741, rs11597086) |
| Chalasani et al. [12] | United States (all female, European Caucasian) | Histology | 236 | 324,623 | FDFT1 (rs2645424) COL13A1 (rs1227756) EFCAB4B (rs887304) PZP (rs6487679) Chromosome 7 (rs343062) |
| Speliotes et al. [5] | United States and Europe (meta-analysis of previous studies) | CT steatosis (with histological 'candidate gene' validation set) | 7176 | Range 329–618 k before imputation | Chr 22: PNPLA3 (rs738409) Chr 19: NCAN (rs2228603); GCKR (rs780094), LYPLAL1 (rs12137855), PPP1R3B (rs4240624) |
| Chambers et al. [13] | European (mixed ethnicity) | Clinical biochemistry (ALT) | 61,089 | ~2.6 million | Chr 22: PNPLA3 (rs738409) TRIB1 (rs2954021) Loci near HSD17B13 and MAPK10 (rs6834314) CPN1 (rs10883437) |
| Kawaguchi et al. [14] | Japan | Histology Japanese | 529 | 484,751 | Chr 22: PNPLA3 (rs738409) |
| Kitamoto et al. [15] | Histologically characterised NAFLD | | 392 | 261,540 | Chr 22: PNPLA3 (rs738409) |
| Feitosa et al. [16] | CT-measured steatosis | United States | 2705 | ~2.4 million | Chr 22: PNPLA3 (rs738409) PPP1R3B (rs2126259) ERLIN1–CHUK–CWF19L1 gene cluster (9 SNPs in two haplotype blocks) |
| Kozlitina et al. [17] | United States (mixed ethnicity) | 1H-MRS steatosis | 2736 (B: 1,324; W; 882; H:467; O: 63) | 138,374 (Exome) | Chr 22: PNPLA3 (rs738409) Chr 19: TM6SF2 |

Source: Modified and updated from Ref. [4] with permission.

**TABLE 11.2**  Additional genetic modifiers of NAFLD identified in candidate gene studies

| Gene | Protein | Comments |
|---|---|---|
| **Glucose metabolism and insulin resistance** | | |
| ENPP1, IRS1 | Ectonucleotide pyrophosphatase/ phosphodiesterase family member 1; insulin receptor substrate 1 | Functional variants in ENPP1/PC-1 and IRS1 impair insulin receptor signalling and promote insulin resistance<br>In 702 biopsy-proven NAFLD cases, carriage of non-synonymous SNPs in ENPP1 (rs1044498, encoding Lys121Gln) and IRS1 (rs1801278, encoding Gln972Arg) reduced AKT activation, promoted insulin resistance and were independently associated with greater fibrosis<br>A second smaller (underpowered) study on ENPP1 did not find a significant effect |
| GCKR | Glucokinase regulatory protein | GCKR SNP rs780094 is in strong LD with a functional non-synonymous SNP (rs1260326, encoding Pro446Leu) and has been associated with hepatic TAG accumulation in several studies |
| SLC2A1 | Solute carrier family 2, facilitated glucose transporter member 1 | A study examining 3072 SNPs across 92 candidate genes identified variants in SLC2A1 associated with NAFLD, independent of insulin resistance or T2DM[S8]<br>Down-regulation of SLC2A1 in vitro promoted lipid accumulation and increased oxidative stress, potentially linking the key pathogenic features of NAFLD: oxidative injury and increased lipid storage |
| TCF7L2 | Transcription factor 7-like 2 | A role for TCF7L2, which has a key role in Wnt signalling and has been implicated in T2DM, has been reported in NAFLD |
| PPARG | Peroxisome proliferator-activated receptor γ | A loss-of-function SNP (rs1805192, encoding Pro12Ala) impairs transcriptional activation and affects insulin sensitivity<br>Carriage of haplotypes including the Pro12Ala allele was associated with progressive NAFLD, but two studies found no association[S12,S13] |
| **Steatosis** | | |
| *Hepatic lipid import or synthesis* | | |
| SLC27A5 | Very long-chain acyl-CoA synthetase | Two principal isoforms of FATPs are expressed in the liver, SLC27A2 (also known as FATP2) and SLC27A5 (also known as FATP5)<br>Silencing Slc27a5 reverses diet-induced NAFLD and improves hyperglycaemia in mice<br>Carriage of the SLC27A5 rs56225452 promoter region polymorphism has been associated with higher ALT levels, and greater postprandial insulin and triglyceride levels<br>In patients with histologically proven NAFLD, the effect of BMI on degree of steatosis differed with SLC27A5 genotype |
| LPIN1 | Phosphatidate phosphatase LPIN1 | LPIN1 is required for adipogenesis and the normal metabolic flux between adipose tissue and liver, where it also acts as an inducible transcriptional co-activator to regulate fatty acid metabolism<br>Variants have been associated with multiple components of the metabolic syndrome<br>Although a large case–control study found no association with T2DM, obesity or related traits in 17,538 individuals, a meta-analysis in 8,504 individuals found that the LPIN1 rs13412852 [T] allele was associated with lower BMI and insulin levels<br>This same polymorphism was under-represented in paediatric (but not adult) NAFLD with a suggestion of less severe liver damage |

| Gene | Protein | Comments |
|---|---|---|
| *Hepatic lipid export or oxidation in steatosis* | | |
| PNPLA3 | Patatin-like phospholipase domain-containing 3 | The non-synonymous 617C >G nucleotide transversion mutation SNP (rs738409, encoding Ile148Met) has been consistently associated with steatosis, steatohepatitis and hepatic fibrosis; however, function remains incompletely understood |
| NR1I2 | Nuclear receptor subfamily 1 group I member 2 (also known as pregnane X receptor) | NR1I2 encodes a transcription factor that regulates hepatic detoxification and acts through CD36 (fatty acid translocase) and various lipogenic enzymes to control lipid metabolism<br>Nr1i2-deficient mice develop steatosis<br>Two SNPs (rs7643645 and rs2461823) were associated with NAFLD and were also a predictor of disease severity |
| PPARA | Peroxisome proliferator-activated receptor α | PPAR-α is a molecular sensor for long-chain fatty acids, eicosanoids and fibrates; activated by increased hepatocyte fatty acid load, it limits TAG accumulation by increasing fatty acid oxidation<br>Carriage of a non-synonymous SNP (rs1800234, encoding Val227Ala) increases activity and was associated with NAFLD despite reduced BMI |
| PEMT | Phosphatidylethanolamine N-methyltransferase | A loss-of-function polymorphism (rs1800206, encoding Leu162Val) was not associated with NAFLD<br>Two studies have reported an association between NAFLD and a non-synonymous PEMT exon 8 590G>A transversion (rs7946, encoding Val175Met) |
| MTTP | Microsome triglyceride transfer protein large subunit | MTTP mediates hepatic synthesis and secretion of VLDL<br>Abetalipoproteinaemia (OMIM#200100) results from a loss-of-function frameshift mutation in MTTP; however, whereas this mutation causes severe hepatic TAG accumulation, steatohepatitis and fibrosis are infrequent<br>A promoter region transversion (−493G >T; rs1800591), predisposed to steatosis and NASH in a small cohort, but a larger study in 131 patients found no association |
| APOC3 | Apolipoprotein C-III | Two promoter region SNPs −455T >C; rs2854116 and −482C >T; rs2854117) that increased steatosis were reported in small (n=95 and 163) cohorts of Asian Indian and non-Asian ethnicity<br>To date, studies together examining >4000 individuals have been unable to replicate these findings |
| ApoE | Apolipoprotein E | ApoE is a plasma protein involved in lipid transport and metabolism<br>Three alleles (ε2, ε3 and ε4) determine three isoforms (ApoE2, ApoE3 and ApoE4) resulting in six ApoE genotypes (E2/2, E3/3, E4/4, E2/3, E2/4, E3/4)<br>Overall homozygosity for the ε2 allele in one study was associated with dyslipidaemia but not NAFLD<br>In a subgroup of nonobese individuals, the ε2 allele and the E2/3 genotype were more prevalent in controls, suggesting this allele might be protective<br>Consistent with this result, the ApoE3/3 genotype was associated with NASH in a Turkish cohort, whereas ApoE3/4 was protective |

(continued)

TABLE 11.2 (continued)

| Gene | Protein | Comments |
|------|---------|----------|
| **Steatohepatitis** | | |
| *Oxidative stress* | | |
| HFE | Hereditary hemochromatosis protein | Hepatic iron accumulation promotes oxidative stress. Two studies, examining 177 patients, reported carriage of an *HFE* polymorphism (rs1800562, encoding Cys282Tyr) that was associated with more severe steatohepatitis and advanced fibrosis |
| | | However, three other studies have not shown increased carriage of either the Cys282Tyr or His63Asp (rs1799945) mutations |
| | | Meta-analyses have also provided conflicting results, with the latest finding no evidence of an effect |
| GCLC; GCLM | Glutamate–cysteine ligase catalytic unit; glutamate–cysteine ligase regulatory unit | Glutamate–cysteine ligase (γ-glutamyl cysteine synthetase) is the rate-limiting step in glutathione synthesis; absence of GCLC causes steatosis and liver failure in mice |
| | | A study of 131 patients with NAFLD found the *GCLC* promoter region polymorphism (−129C >T, rs17883901) was associated with steatohepatitis compared with simple steatosis |
| ABCC2 | ATP-binding cassette, subfamily C (CFTR/MRP), member 2 | Association studies support a role for *ABCC2* (also known as *MRP2*), which facilitates terminal excretion and detoxification of endogenous and xenobiotic organic anions, including lipid peroxidation products |
| SOD2 | Superoxide dismutase [Mn], mitochondrial | Carriage of the non-synonymous SNP (rs4880, encoding Ala16Val) has been associated with advanced hepatic fibrosis in NAFLD in both Japanese and European cohorts |
| *Endotoxin response* | | |
| TLR4 | Toll-like receptor 4 | Study of a spontaneous *TLR4* null mutation in C3H/J mice has established the contribution of TLR4/endotoxin to NAFLD pathogenesis in the laboratory |
| | | *TLR4* polymorphisms (rs4986791 and rs4986790) influence hepatitis C-related fibrosis, but no association with NAFLD and either *TLR4* or *NOD2* (bacterial cell wall peptidoglycan receptor) variants has been found |
| CD14 | Monocyte differentiation antigen CD14 | CD14 is a lipopolysaccharide receptor expressed on monocytes, macrophages and neutrophils that enhances TLR4 endotoxin signalling |
| | | An association with a promoter region polymorphism (−159C >T, rs2569190) that increases *CD14* expression has been reported |
| *Cytokines* | | |
| TNF | Tumour necrosis factor | A *TNF* (−238G >A, rs361525) promoter polymorphism has been associated with NASH, suggesting a primary role in the transition from steatosis to steatohepatitis; a separate study found that two other promoter region polymorphisms (−1031 T >C, rs1799964 and −863C >A, rs1800630) were more common in NASH than steatosis but were no more common in NAFLD than a control population |
| IL6 | Interleukin 6 | An *IL6* promoter region polymorphism (−174G >C, rs1800795) has been associated with NASH |
| **Fibrosis** | | |
| AGTR1 | Type 1 angiotensin II receptor | Two studies have linked the *ATGR1* rs3772622 SNP with grade of steatohepatitis and stage of fibrosis, with the most recent study also suggesting an interaction with *PNPLA3* genotype |
| KLF6 | Kruppel-like factor 6 | The *KLF6*-IVS1 −27G >A (rs3750861) SNP has been associated with milder NAFLD-related hepatic fibrosis in three separate European cohorts |

*Source:* Reproduced from Ref. [4] with permission.

ALT, alanine aminotransferase; FATP, fatty acid transport protein; LD, linkage disequilibrium; SNP, single-nucleotide polymorphism; TAG, triacylglycerol; T2DM, type 2 diabetes mellitus; VLDL, very low-density lipoprotein.

loci, on chromosome 22 and chromosome 19, which contain the *PNPLA3* and transmembrane 6 superfamily member 2 (*TM6SF2*) genes, respectively, deserve particular attention and so will be discussed in detail. Other than these, only a few loci associated with NAFLD have been independently validated and can be considered of proven importance. These include *glucokinase regulator* (*GCKR*), a key regulator of glucokinase activity that controls glucose metabolism [5]; mitochondrial *superoxide dismutase 2* (*SOD2*), which affects intracellular resistance to oxidative stress [18]; *phosphatidylethanolamine N-methyltransferase* (*PEMT*), which catalyses the conversion of phosphatidylethanolamine to phosphatidylcholine and so is needed for normal hepatic VLDL secretion [19]; and *Kruppel-like factor 6* (*KLF6*), a transcription factor that is highly expressed by activated stellate cells soon after injury [20].

## The chromosome 22 locus: *PNPLA3*

The first gene variant to be identified by GWAS in NAFLD was a non-synonymous SNP in *PNPLA3* (rs738409 c.444 C>G, p.I148M) [8]. This association has since been validated across multiple patient cohorts. As will be discussed in the following, carriage of this SNP has been robustly associated not only with steatosis but also with clinically relevant factors including severity of hepatic fibrosis/cirrhosis and development of NAFLD-related HCC [21–23].

*PNPLA3 and radiologically measured Steatosis (HTGC)*
The initial GWAS that highlighted the role of *PNPLA3* in NAFLD pathogenesis examined 9229 non-synonymous SNPs in a multi-ethnic population comprising 2051 patients (Hispanic, African American and European ancestry) from the Dallas Heart Study that had undergone HTGC measurement by MRI [24]. Carriage of the *PNPLA3* rs738409 variant that causes an amino acid substitution from an isoleucine to methionine (I148M) was significantly associated with steatosis ($P = 5.9 \times 10^{-10}$). The minor allele frequency (MAF) of this polymorphism was highest in Hispanics (0.49), the group with higher prevalence of aggressive NAFLD and increased levels of ALT and AST ($P = 3.7 \times 10^{-4}$). Whereas MAF was lower in European ancestry (0.23) and African Americans (0.17), partially explaining the ethnic differences in NAFLD that were described earlier. Subsequently, a number of other GWAS examining relevant phenotypes have validated the association of *PNPLA3* with NAFLD. These include a two-stage GWAS meta-analysis that independently confirmed the association between *PNPLA3* and HTGC [5]; studies

examining variation in routine clinical chemistry phenotypes (raised alanine transaminase); and several smaller studies that also report associations between histological steatosis and SNPs flanking *PNPLA3* (summarised in Table 11.1).

*PNPLA3 and histologically assessed steatohepatitis/fibrosis*
The link between *PNPLA3* and NAFLD was established in radiologically phenotyped cohorts; however such studies are unable to assess the presence of features such as NASH or stage of liver fibrosis that can only be detected histologically. This deficiency reflects the difficulty in assembling sufficiently large patient cohorts that have undergone invasive testing by liver biopsy to provide a well-powered fully phenotyped cohort and means that the majority of GWAS studies are radiologically based and so 'phenotype limited' to detecting variations in HTGC. Candidate gene disease association studies in histologically characterised patient cohorts have therefore been necessary to establish whether genetic variants identified by GWAS, such as *PNPLA3*, do indeed influence disease progression towards the more clinically relevant phenotypes. The *PNPLA3* rs738409 variant has been shown to increase the risk of NASH and advanced liver fibrosis, independent of potential confounding factors such as age, BMI or T2DM [4, 21].

*PNPLA3 and NAFLD-HCC*
The rise in the population prevalence of NAFLD coincides with a marked increase in the incidence of HCC in many countries. Whilst HCC remains an infrequent complication of NAFLD, its high prevalence means that NAFLD-related HCC contributes significantly to the disease burden. The *PNPLA3* rs738409 variant has been associated with increased HCC risk in alcohol-related liver disease, obesity and less consistently in chronic viral hepatitis. The largest study to test this association in NAFLD examined a well-characterised cohort of 100 European Caucasians with NAFLD-related HCC and 275 controls with histologically characterised NAFLD and so was able to control for any confounding effect of advanced fibrosis/cirrhosis on HCC risk. In a multivariate analysis adjusted for age, gender, diabetes, BMI and presence of cirrhosis, this demonstrated a strong association between *PNPLA3* rs738409 minor (G) allele carriage and NAFLD-HCC risk. Carriage of each copy of the minor (G) allele conferred an additive risk for HCC (adjusted OR 2.26 [95%CI 1.23–4.14], $p = 0.0082$), with GG homozygotes exhibiting a fivefold [1.47–17.29], $p = 0.01$ increased risk over CC. When compared to the UK

general population (1958 British Birth Cohort, $n = 1476$), the risk effect was more pronounced (GC vs. CC: unadjusted OR 2.52 [1.55–4.10], $p = 0.0002$; GG vs. CC: OR 12.19 [6.89–21.58], $p < 0.0001$) [23]. This equates to a Population Attributable Risk (PAR) of *PNPLA3* rs738409 for NAFLD-HCC of 55% and an AUROC of 0.68 attributable to this variant [23]. Given the mounting evidence of an association between *PNPLA3* and HCC [22], it is timely to consider the clinical utility of *PNPLA3* genotyping to assist in patient risk stratification. Although use of *PNPLA3* genotyping alone to *positively predict* the risk of HCC is unlikely to be tenable, the *negative predictive value* was substantially greater, suggesting that genetic testing may ultimately have a role in focussing surveillance or future risk-modifying treatments to those most likely to develop HCC. Clinical trials to assess the utility and health economic merits of a multifactorial risk stratification that incorporates *PNPLA3* rs738409 genotype along with other recognised risk factors for HCC may now be warranted.

### Biological function of *PNPLA3*: A strong modifier with an elusive function

The *PNPLA3* gene encodes a 481 amino acid protein (also referred to as adiponutrin) that belongs to a family of lipid hydrolases (patatin-like phospholipase domain-containing proteins, PNPLA1-9) [25]. Amongst the human PNPLA proteins, PNPLA3 is structurally related to *adipose triglyceride lipase* (*ATGL*, also known as *PNPLA2*), the major triglyceride hydrolase in adipose tissue [26, 27]. Hence, PNPLA3 was first thought to possess a similar function as ATGL. However, in contrast to the excessive TG accumulation that occurs following *ATGL* loss in mice, *PNPLA3* knockout mice do not show increased hepatic TG content [27]. Similarly, reduced TG content was not seen when the *PNPLA3* (I148) wild-type variant was overexpressed, whereas this did occur with *ATGL* overexpression [28]. These studies both suggest that the function of PNPLA3/adiponutrin differs substantially from ATGL.

Evidence established so far suggests that there are some differences in tissue distribution of PNPLA3 expression between humans and mice that have made study of PNPLA3 function more difficult. Amongst metabolically active organs, *PNPLA3* is mainly expressed in the liver of humans [29] whilst adipose tissue expression dominates in mice [30]. The expression of *PNPLA3* is controlled in a nutrition-dependent manner: on fasting, the expression is down-regulated whilst consumption of a high-carbohydrate diet up-regulates expression [31]. Apart from dietary intake and release from adipose tissue, *de novo* synthesis is also a source for free fatty acids/triglycerides uptake. *PNPLA3* is regulated by carbohydrate response element-binding protein (ChREBP) [32, 33], a key transcription factor that activates *de novo* synthesis under hyperglycemia promoting hepatic glycolysis and lipogenesis of what the excessive glucose is converted into free fatty acids. Insulin controls postprandial *PNPLA3* expression through liver X receptor–retinoid X receptor and the transcription factor sterol regulatory element-binding protein-1c (SREBP-1c) that also increases *de novo* hepatic lipogenesis [34, 35].

Despite the plethora of genetic evidence for an effect, the physiological role of *PNPLA3* and how it is perturbed by carriage of the rs738409 (I148M) variant has remained elusive. Although, some progress has been made, the data is at times conflicting and there remains some debate as to whether the variant is a true loss-of-function mutation or not. *In vitro* studies with both wild-type and mutant isoforms of recombinant adiponutrin indicate that PNPLA3 mediates hydrolyses of acylglycerols and that maximal hydrolytic activity is towards any of the three major glycerolipids (triacylglycerol, diacylglycerol and monoacylglycerol) as substrates, with a strong preference for oleic acid as the acyl moiety [28, 36]. Compared to the PNPLA3 wild-type protein, the I148M variant possesses substantially reduced enzymatic activity but there does not appear to be any change in substrate affinity [28, 36]. These findings are consistent with the results of stable isotope tracer studies in overweight or obese men and *in vitro* studies that show that carriage of the rs738409 (I148M) variant reduces VLDL secretion, an effect attributed to failure to mobilise TG from intracellular lipid droplets [37]. Arguing against a simple loss-of-function effect; however, *PNPLA3* knockout mice do not develop steatosis [38]. Indeed, others have suggested that the I148M substitution acts as a gain-of-function mutation with the variant form possessing some lysophosphatidic acid acetyltransferase activity, leading to an increase of TG synthesis [39]. Supporting this, murine overexpression of wild-type PNPLA3 does not induce steatosis but overexpression of the variant (I148M) form does [40]. Taken together, the currently available data would suggest that the PNPLA3 I148M variant alters TG remodelling in lipid droplets within hepatocytes [40, 41].

Beyond steatosis, the underlying mechanisms through which *PNPLA3* influences progression to NASH and hepatic fibrosis still remained uncertain. Recent data suggests that *PNPLA3* may have a role in retinol metabolism, acting as retinyl-palmitate hydrolase in human hepatic stellate cells (HSCs), which are dominant players in fibrogenesis [42]. Overexpressed wild-type PNPLA3 in HSCs resulted in a substantial reduction of lipid droplets, an effect that was lost with I148M. However, how this alters HSC activation and affects collagen deposition and fibrosis is not known; however it does suggest that PNPLA3 may have specific roles in different cell types and metabolic conditions, which each contribute to the progression of NAFLD from steatosis to fibrosis. Thus, challenges remain in which cell types to target and what kinds of experimental conditions should be applied in order to investigate the comprehensive role of *PNPLA3* in NAFLD.

## The chromosome 19 locus: *TM6SF2*

Evidence to support an association of NAFLD with part of chromosome 19 stems from the same GWAS meta-analysis that first validated the association of *PNPLA3* with HTGC [5]. This two-stage meta-analysis examined 2.4 million SNPs by imputation across combined cohorts totalling 7176 cases and initially identified 45 loci associating with CT-measured HTGC. Adopting a candidate gene approach, in a separate smaller cohort with histological confirmed NAFLD, these associations were then retested. Other than *PNPLA3*, a number of new associations were also reported by this study, including a region on chromosome 19 (19p13.11) that contains several genes including *neurocan* (*NCAN*) and *TM6SF2* as well as *CILP2* and *PBX4* [5]. This region had also been associated with variations in plasma cholesterol, triglyceride and low-density lipoprotein levels in previous studies [43, 44].

Initial research focussed on *NCAN* as the lead candidate gene for this association, which was replicated for steatosis, inflammation and fibrosis. However, *NCAN* lacked biologically plausible evidence of a functional role in NAFLD [4]. The use of a genome-wide exome chip genotyping approach in 2736 individuals, combined with detailed association analysis conditioning on previously published variants across the 19p13.11 region, determined that the causative non-synonymous variant affecting HTGC is in strong linkage disequilibrium ($D' = 0.926$, $r^2 = 0.798$) with the previously identified *NCAN* gene variants but actually lies within the neighbouring gene, *TM6SF2* (rs58542926, c.449 C > T, p.E167K) [17]. Carriage of the *TM6SF2* rs58542926 minor (T) allele was associated with increased HTGC.

Coincidentally, another group demonstrated that carriage of the common (C) allele was also associated with increased circulating cholesterol levels and greater cardiovascular disease (CVD) risk [45]. Independent studies in a large ($n = 1074$) histologically characterised European Caucasian NAFLD cohort confirmed the primacy of *TM6SF2* and showed that carriage of the *TM6SF2* minor (T) allele was associated not only with increased HTGC but also with NAFLD-associated advanced liver fibrosis/cirrhosis [46]. The odds ratio for advanced fibrosis with each copy of the minor (T) allele carried was 1.88 (1.4–2.5), independent of confounding factors including age, T2DM, obesity or *PNPLA3* rs738409 genotype [46]. These findings have been replicated in another European study, further confirming that minor (T) allele carriage is associated with progression to NASH and advanced fibrosis but is also protective against atherosclerosis and cardiovascular disease [47].

### Biological function of TM6SF2: A work in progress

Reflecting the recent nature of these discoveries, little is currently known about the biological function of the protein encoded by the *TM6SF2* gene; however expression within hepatocytes appears to be localised to the endoplasmic reticulum/ER-Golgi intermediate compartment [48]. Functional studies *in vivo* [17, 45] and *in vitro* [17, 45, 48] suggest that the gene controls hepatic lipid efflux, with its deletion resulting in a reduction of lipoprotein secretion (VLDL, TG and APOB) coincident with increased hepatocellular lipid droplet size and content. Consistent with the SNP being a loss-of-function allele, Kozlitina et al. showed that expression of *TM6SF2* variant form (E167K) protein was lower than the wild type [17]. They also found that knock-down of mouse *Tm6sf2* resulted in increased hepatic lipid accumulation, decreased hepatic VLDL secretion and decreased serum TG and LDL [17].

*TM6SF2* therefore provides new insights into not only the mechanistic basis of progressive NAFLD but also the association between NAFLD and CVD. Based on the available data, it appears that *TM6SF2* is an important determinant of clinical outcome across several facets of metabolic syndrome-related end-organ damage. Carriage of the *TM6SF2* rs58542926 minor (T) allele mediates hepatic retention of triglyceride and cholesterol, predisposing to steatohepatitis and NAFLD-associated fibrosis. In contrast, carriage of the common (C) allele promotes

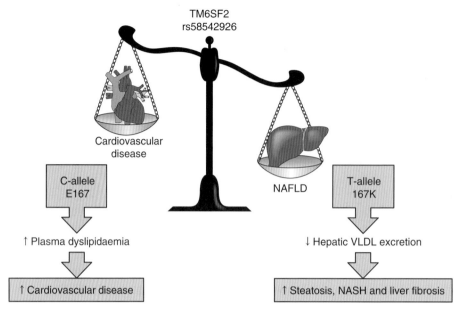

TM6SF2
rs58542926

Cardiovascular
disease

NAFLD

C-allele
E167

T-allele
167K

↑ Plasma dyslipidaemia

↓ Hepatic VLDL excretion

↑ Cardiovascular disease

↑ Steatosis, NASH and liver fibrosis

**FIG 11.1** Outcomes of the metabolic syndrome: *TM6SF2* dissociates NAFLD from cardiovascular disease.

hepatic VLDL excretion, protecting the liver but at the expense of an increased risk of atherosclerosis and ultimately cardiovascular disease (Figure 11.1). Thus, although the metabolic syndrome and NAFLD are in general associated with increased cardiovascular disease, individuals carrying the minor (T) allele of *TM6SF2* rs58542926 may be more prone to experience liver-related rather than cardiovascular morbidity and mortality. Further research is needed to establish the precise function of the TM6SF2 protein and to determine how this knowledge can be exploited clinically.

## Conclusions and clinical relevance

NAFLD is best considered a complex disease trait in which subtle inter-patient genetic variations and environmental factors interact to determine disease phenotype and progression. Recent technical advances have led to the identification of important genetic modifiers, in particular non-synonymous gene variants in *PNPLA3* (I148M) and *TM6SF2* (E167K) that are independently associated with degree of steatosis, grade of steatohepatitis and stage of fibrosis/cirrhosis also, for PNPLA3, HCC risk. These are important discoveries but it should be remembered that our genetic make-up has been stable for thousands of years

and so environmental (dietary/lifestyle) changes must largely be responsible for the observed recent rapid rise in NAFLD prevalence. To ignore the role of genetic factors in complex diseases such as NAFLD would however be unwise. Although this knowledge has not yet reached 'the bedside' or clinic, understanding how genetic variation exerts its effects is already informing our understanding of disease pathogenesis and may in the future guide a personalised medicine approach to risk stratification or the development of new pharmacological treatments that exploit this knowledge.

## References

1. Anstee QM, Targher G, Day CP. Progression of NAFLD to diabetes mellitus, cardiovascular disease or cirrhosis. Nat Rev Gastroenterol Hepatol. 2013;10(6):330–44.

2. Musso G, Gambino R, Cassader M, Pagano G. Meta-analysis: natural history of non-alcoholic fatty liver disease (NAFLD) and diagnostic accuracy of non-invasive tests for liver disease severity. Ann Med. 2011;43(8):617–49.

3. Argo CK, Caldwell SH. Epidemiology and natural history of non-alcoholic steatohepatitis. Clin Liver Dis. 2009;13(4): 511–31.

4. Anstee QM, Day CP. The genetics of NAFLD. Nat Rev Gastroenterol Hepatol. 2013;10(11):645–55.

5. Speliotes EK, Yerges-Armstrong LM, Wu J, Hernaez R, Kim LJ, Palmer CD, et al. Genome-wide association analysis identifies variants associated with nonalcoholic fatty liver disease that have distinct effects on metabolic traits. PLoS Genet. 2011;7(3):e1001324.

6. Browning JD, Szczepaniak LS, Dobbins R, Nuremberg P, Horton JD, Cohen JC, et al. Prevalence of hepatic steatosis in an urban population in the United States: impact of ethnicity. Hepatology. 2004;40(6):1387–95.

7. Bambha K, Belt P, Abraham M, Wilson LA, Pabst M, Ferrell L, et al. Ethnicity and nonalcoholic fatty liver disease. Hepatology. 2012;55(3):769–80.

8. Romeo S, Kozlitina J, Xing C, Pertsemlidis A, Cox D, Pennacchio LA, et al. Genetic variation in PNPLA3 confers susceptibility to nonalcoholic fatty liver disease. Nat Genet. 2008;40(12):1461–5.

9. Schwimmer JB, Celedon MA, Lavine JE, Salem R, Campbell N, Schork NJ, et al. Heritability of nonalcoholic fatty liver disease. Gastroenterology. 2009;136(5):1585–92.

10. Makkonen J, Pietilainen KH, Rissanen A, Kaprio J, Yki-Jarvinen H. Genetic factors contribute to variation in serum alanine aminotransferase activity independent of obesity and alcohol: a study in monozygotic and dizygotic twins. J Hepatol. 2009;50(5):1035–42.

11. Yuan X, Waterworth D, Perry JR, Lim N, Song K, Chambers JC, et al. Population-based genome-wide association studies reveal six loci influencing plasma levels of liver enzymes. Am J Hum Genet. 2008;83:520–8.

12. Chalasani N, Guo X, Loomba R, Goodarzi MO, Haritunians T, Kwon S, et al. Genome-wide association study identifies variants associated with histologic features of nonalcoholic Fatty liver disease. Gastroenterology. 2010;139:1567–76, 1576.e1561–6.

13. Chambers JC, Zhang W, Sehmi J, Li X, Wass MN, Van der Harst P, et al. Genome-wide association study identifies loci influencing concentrations of liver enzymes in plasma. Nat Genet. 2011;43:1131–8.

14. Kawaguchi T, Sumida Y, Umemura A, Matsuo K, Takahashi M, Takamura T, et al. Genetic polymorphisms of the human PNPLA3 gene are strongly associated with severity of non-alcoholic fatty liver disease in Japanese. PLoS One. 2012;7:e38322.

15. Kitamoto T, Kitamoto A, Yoneda M, Hyogo H, Ochi H, Nakamura T, et al. Genome-wide scan revealed that polymorphisms in the PNPLA3, SAMM50, and PARVB genes are associated with development and progression of nonalcoholic fatty liver disease in Japan. Hum Genet. 2013;132:783–92.

16. Feitosa MF, Wojczynski MK, North KE, Zhang Q, Province MA, Carr JJ, et al. The ERLIN1-CHUK-CWF19L1 gene cluster influences liver fat deposition and hepatic inflamma-tion in the NHLBI Family Heart Study. Atherosclerosis. 2013;228:175–80.

17. Kozlitina J, Smagris E, Stender S, Nordestgaard BG, Zhou HH, Tybjaerg-Hansen A, et al. Exome-wide association study identifies a TM6SF2 variant that confers susceptibility to nonalcoholic fatty liver disease. Nat Genet. 2014;46(4):352–6.

18. Al-Serri A, Anstee QM, Valenti L, Nobili V, Leathart JB, Dongiovanni P, et al. The SOD2 C47T polymorphism influences NAFLD fibrosis severity: evidence from case-control and intra-familial allele association studies. J Hepatol. 2012;56(2):448–54.

19. Dong H, Wang J, Li C, Hirose A, Nozaki Y, Takahashi M, et al. The phosphatidylethanolamine N-methyltransferase gene V175M single nucleotide polymorphism confers the susceptibility to NASH in Japanese population. J Hepatol. 2007;46(5):915–20.

20. Miele L, Beale G, Patman G, Nobili V, Leathart J, Grieco A, et al. The Kruppel-like factor 6 genotype is associated with fibrosis in nonalcoholic fatty liver disease. Gastroenterology. 2008;135(1):282–91.e1.

21. Valenti L, Al-Serri A, Daly AK, Galmozzi E, Rametta R, Dongiovanni P, et al. Homozygosity for the patatin-like phospholipase-3/adiponutrin I148M polymorphism influences liver fibrosis in patients with nonalcoholic fatty liver disease. Hepatology. 2010;51(4):1209–17.

22. Trepo E, Nahon P, Bontempi G, Valenti L, Falleti E, Nischalke HD, et al. Association between the PNPLA3 (rs738409 C > G) variant and hepatocellular carcinoma: evidence from a meta-analysis of individual participant data. Hepatology. 2013;59(6):2170–7.

23. Liu YL, Patman GL, Leathart JB, Piguet AC, Burt AD, Dufour JF, et al. Carriage of the PNPLA3 rs738409 C > G polymorphism confers an increased risk of non-alcoholic fatty liver disease associated hepatocellular carcinoma. J Hepatol. 2014;61(1):75–81.

24. Victor RG, Haley RW, Willett DL, Peshock RM, Vaeth PC, Leonard D, et al. The Dallas Heart Study: a population-based probability sample for the multidisciplinary study of ethnic differences in cardiovascular health. Am J Cardiol. 2004;93(12):1473–80.

25. Park WD, Blackwood C, Mignery GA, Hermodson MA, Lister RM. Analysis of the heterogeneity of the 40,000 molecular weight tuber glycoprotein of potatoes by immunological methods and by NH(2)-terminal sequence analysis. Plant Physiol. 1983;71(1):156–60.

26. Kienesberger PC, Lee D, Pulinilkunnil T, Brenner DS, Cai L, Magnes C, et al. Adipose triglyceride lipase deficiency causes tissue-specific changes in insulin signaling. J Biol Chem. 2009;284(44):30218–29.

27. Zimmermann R, Strauss JG, Haemmerle G, Schoiswohl G, Birner-Gruenberger R, Riederer M, et al. Fat mobilization in adipose tissue is promoted by adipose triglyceride lipase. Science. 2004;306(5700):1383–6.

28. He S, McPhaul C, Li JZ, Garuti R, Kinch L, Grishin NV, et al. A sequence variation (I148M) in PNPLA3 associated with nonalcoholic fatty liver disease disrupts triglyceride hydrolysis. J Biol Chem. 2010;285(9):6706–15.

29. Wilson PA, Gardner SD, Lambie NM, Commans SA, Crowther DJ. Characterization of the human patatin-like phospholipase family. J Lipid Res. 2006;47(9):1940–9.

30. Lake AC, Sun Y, Li JL, Kim JE, Johnson JW, Li D, et al. Expression, regulation, and triglyceride hydrolase activity of Adiponutrin family members. J Lipid Res. 2005;46(11): 2477–87.

31. Dubuquoy C, Robichon C, Lasnier F, Langlois C, Dugail I, Foufelle F, et al. Distinct regulation of adiponutrin/PNPLA3 gene expression by the transcription factors ChREBP and SREBP1c in mouse and human hepatocytes. J Hepatol. 2011;55(1):145–53.

32. Rae-Whitcombe SM, Kennedy D, Voyles M, Thompson MP. Regulation of the promoter region of the human adiponutrin/PNPLA3 gene by glucose and insulin. Biochem Biophys Res Commun. 2010;402(4):767–72.

33. Perttila J, Huaman-Samanez C, Caron S, Tanhuanpaa K, Staels B, Yki-Jarvinen H, et al. PNPLA3 is regulated by glucose in human hepatocytes, and its I148M mutant slows down triglyceride hydrolysis. Am J Physiol Endocrinol Metab. 2012;302(9):E1063–9.

34. Shimomura I, Bashmakov Y, Horton JD. Increased levels of nuclear SREBP-1c associated with fatty livers in two mouse models of diabetes mellitus. J Biol Chem. 1999;274(42): 30028–32.

35. Huang Y, He S, Li JZ, Seo YK, Osborne TF, Cohen JC, et al. A feed-forward loop amplifies nutritional regulation of PNPLA3. Proc Natl Acad Sci U S A. 2010;107(17):7892–7.

36. Huang Y, Cohen JC, Hobbs HH. Expression and characterization of a PNPLA3 protein isoform (I148M) associated with nonalcoholic fatty liver disease. J Biol Chem. 2011;286(43): 37085–93.

37. Pirazzi C, Adiels M, Burza MA, Mancina RM, Levin M, Stahlman M, et al. Patatin-like phospholipase domain-containing 3 (PNPLA3) I148M (rs738409) affects hepatic VLDL secretion in humans and in vitro. J Hepatol. 2012;57(6): 1276–82.

38. Basantani MK, Sitnick MT, Cai L, Brenner DS, Gardner NP, Li JZ, et al. Pnpla3/Adiponutrin deficiency in mice does not contribute to fatty liver disease or metabolic syndrome. J Lipid Res. 2011;52:318–29.

39. Kumari M, Schoiswohl G, Chitraju C, Paar M, Cornaciu I, Rangrez AY, et al. Adiponutrin functions as a nutritionally regulated lysophosphatidic acid acyltransferase. Cell Metab. 2012;15(5):691–702.

40. Li JZ, Huang Y, Karaman R, Ivanova PT, Brown HA, Roddy T, et al. Chronic overexpression of PNPLA3I148M in mouse liver causes hepatic steatosis. J Clin Invest. 2012;122: 4130–44.

41. Ruhanen H, Perttila J, Holtta-Vuori M, Zhou Y, Yki-Jarvinen H, Ikonen E, et al. PNPLA3 mediates hepatocyte triacylglycerol remodeling. J Lipid Res. 2014;55(4):739–46.

42. Pirazzi C, Valenti L, Motta BM, Pingitore P, Hedfalk K, Mancina RM, et al. PNPLA3 has retinyl-palmitate lipase activity in human hepatic stellate cells. Hum Mol Genet. 2014;23(15):4077–85.

43. Kathiresan S, Melander O, Guiducci C, Surti A, Burtt NP, Rieder MJ, et al. Six new loci associated with blood low-density lipoprotein cholesterol, high-density lipoprotein cholesterol or triglycerides in humans. Nat Genet. 2008;40(2):189–97.

44. Teslovich TM, Musunuru K, Smith AV, Edmondson AC, Stylianou IM, Koseki M, et al. Biological, clinical and population relevance of 95 loci for blood lipids. Nature. 2010;466(7307):707–13.

45. Holmen OL, Zhang H, Fan Y, Hovelson DH, Schmidt EM, Zhou W, et al. Systematic evaluation of coding variation identifies a candidate causal variant in TM6SF2 influencing total cholesterol and myocardial infarction risk. Nat Genet. 2014;46(4):345–51.

46. Liu YL, Reeves HL, Burt AD, Tiniakos D, McPherson S, Leathart JB, et al. TM6SF2 rs58542926 influences hepatic fibrosis progression in patients with non-alcoholic fatty liver disease. Nat Commun. 2014;5:4309.

47. Dongiovanni P, Petta S, Maglio C, Fracanzani AL, Pipitone R, Mozzi E, et al. TM6SF2 gene variant disentangles nonalcoholic steatohepatitis from cardiovascular disease. Hepatology. 2015;61:506–14.

48. Mahdessian H, Taxiarchis A, Popov S, Silveira A, Franco-Cereceda A, Hamsten A, et al. TM6SF2 is a regulator of liver fat metabolism influencing triglyceride secretion and hepatic lipid droplet content. Proc Natl Acad Sci U S A. 2014;111(24):8913–8.

## 12 Is there a mechanistic link between hepatic steatosis and cardiac rather than liver events?

**Soo Lim**

Department of Internal Medicine, Seoul National University College of Medicine, Seoul National University Bundang Hospital, Seoul, Korea

### LEARNING POINTS

- The mechanistic link exists between NAFLD and cardiometabolic disorders.

- Insulin resistance, oxidative stress, and endoplasmic reticulum (ER) stress are involved in this link.

- Inflammation, dyslipidemia, biomarkers, and genetic predisposition also play roles.

- NAFLD is a candidate for careful monitoring as a cardiovascular risk factor.

### Introduction

Non-alcoholic fatty liver disease (NAFLD) precedes non-alcoholic steatohepatitis (NASH), leading to liver cirrhosis [1, 2]. NAFLD is also a risk factor for liver cancer [3]. For decades, the two-hit theory has been accepted as the concept to explain this process [4]. Insulin resistance associated with visceral adipose tissue and oxidative stress induced by reactive oxygen species (ROS) represents these two hits.

The prevalence of NAFLD in the general population varies according to the diagnostic tools used to diagnose the condition. In the United States, liver biopsies performed on potential liver donors revealed that 20% of donors were ineligible for organ donation based on the degree of steatosis (>30%) [5]. A Korean study in which liver biopsies were performed on 589 consecutive potential liver transplant donors reported a NAFLD prevalence of 51% [6]. Although liver biopsy is the gold standard for NASH diagnosis and staging, it is invasive and cannot be used in population-based studies.

Autopsy series also showed a broad spectrum in the prevalence of NAFLD. The prevalence of NASH was 3% in an autopsy series of lean individuals from Canada reported in 1990 [7]. A study from India reported that 195 among 1230 adult autopsies (16%) had fatty liver [8]. Another study performed in Greece reported a NAFLD and NASH prevalence of 31 and 40%, respectively, in autopsied cases after exclusion of established liver disease [9].

Noninvasive imaging techniques, such as magnetic resonance imaging (MRI) and ultrasonography, have been used to assess fat accumulation in the liver. In the United States, a study based on MRI identified a NAFLD prevalence of 31% among a multiethnic population [10]. In a study performed in Spain, the prevalence of NAFLD on ultrasonography was 33% in men and 20% in women [11]. In an Italian study that used ultrasonography, the prevalence of NAFLD was 20% in subjects without suspected liver disease [12]. The prevalence of NAFLD identified via ultrasonography in a cohort of 35,519 Japanese individuals increased from 13 to 30% over 12 years [13].

Taken together, these results show that the prevalence of NAFLD in the general population is estimated to be 20–30% in Western countries and 5–20% in Asian countries and that it is increasing over time. However, these

*Clinical Dilemmas in Non-Alcoholic Fatty Liver Disease*, First Edition. Edited by Roger Williams and Simon D. Taylor-Robinson.
© 2016 John Wiley & Sons, Ltd. Published 2016 by John Wiley & Sons, Ltd.

rates vary according to the study population and the modality used to establish the diagnosis.

## Evidence supporting the association between NAFLD and CVD

Several studies have investigated the relationship between NAFLD and the incidence of cardiovascular (CV) events. In the Framingham Heart Study, fatty liver was associated with a clustering of CV risk after adjustment for other fat depots, including abdominal visceral fat [14]. Another study reported that intrahepatic lipid depots were more closely linked to CV complications than to abdominal visceral fat [15]. Rafiq et al. reported that patients with NAFLD had a significantly higher risk of developing cardiovascular disease (CVD) events than did the matched control population [16]. Several studies have demonstrated a high CVD mortality among patients with NAFLD. Of note, a 14-year follow-up study reported that patients with NAFLD died from CVD more than from liver-related death [17]. Another clinical trial indicated that mortality rates from CVD were the second most common cause of death in patients with NAFLD followed for 18 years and were similar to those of liver-related deaths [1]. Taken together, these findings show that CHD is the second most common cause of death in patients with NAFLD and that all-cause mortality is higher in these patients than it is in individuals without NAFLD [3]. More directly, NAFLD has been found to be an independent predictor of incident CV events in patients with type 2 diabetes mellitus (T2DM), as well as in normal subjects [18, 19].

## Mechanistic link between NAFLD and CVD

Several mechanisms have been proposed to explain the association between NAFLD/NASH and CV risk [14]. The hallmark features of atherosclerosis, such as atherogenic dyslipidemia, insulin resistance, inflammation, and oxidative and endoplasmic reticulum (ER) stress, are all associated with an increased risk of CVD in NAFLD/NASH.

## Disturbance of lipid metabolism in NAFLD/NASH

The progression of simple steatosis to steatohepatitis has been proposed to occur via the two-hit hypothesis, with the accumulation of lipids in the form of triglycerides

(TGs) as the first hit and oxidative stress leading to lipid peroxidation as the second hit, which is needed for the development of NASH [4]. However, emerging evidence from *in vivo* and *in vitro* studies suggests that fatty acid metabolites induce the hepatocellular injury in NASH [1]. Increased levels of FFAs released from adipose tissue to the liver play a key role in the onset and progression of lipotoxic liver injury. Ectopic fat accumulation in the liver and the subsequent activation of the inflammation pathway cause cellular dysfunction. The cross talk between dysfunctional adipocytes and the liver recruits multiple cell populations, including macrophages and other immune cells, which contribute to the development of CVD.

The liver plays an important role in lipid synthesis, storage, and release and is an important site for insulin clearance [20] and production of inflammatory cytokines [21, 22]. A large body of clinical and experimental data shows that increased flux of FFAs from increased visceral adipose tissue can lead to hepatic steatosis and insulin resistance [23]. However, the association between adiposity and abnormal liver function remains controversial. Some researchers have demonstrated prospectively a relationship between increased alanine aminotransferase (ALT) activity and T2DM, independent of obesity [24]. Others have demonstrated that fat accumulation in the liver in normal individuals is associated with insulin resistance, independent of total adiposity [25]. In a different context, the concept of hypertriglyceridemic waist was used as an indicator of visceral adiposity [26], and additive effects of waist circumference (WC) and TG concentration on ALT activity were observed in individuals who consumed alcohol and in nondrinkers.

In addition to their critical role in TG synthesis and storage, hepatocytes contain lipid droplets in the lumen of the ER, where VLDL particles are assembled [27]. Thus, the liver secretes TG into the blood in apolipoprotein B (apoB)-containing VLDL particles. NAFLD leads to hepatic insulin resistance, which induces hepatic VLDL production via changes in the rate of apoB synthesis and degradation or *de novo* lipogenesis [28].

FFAs also appear to induce c-Jun N-terminal kinase (JNK) activation, which also leads to insulin resistance via insulin receptor substrate 1 (IRS1) and IRS2 serine phosphorylation. Several lines of evidence have shown the critical role of visceral obesity as a source of FFAs that feed into the portal circulation and cause NAFLD, which results in metabolic disorders and, finally, atherosclerosis and CVD [26, 29].

## Role of insulin resistance in the development of NAFLD and CVD

Insulin resistance is the main pathophysiological feature of NAFLD. Recently, enzymes associated with liver function, (which are associated with insulin resistance), have much attraction, as hepatic dysfunction resulting from intrahepatic lipid deposition may contribute to the development of T2DM. Levels of ALT, aspartate aminotransferase (AST), and γ-glutamyltranspeptidase (GGT) are known indicators of hepatocellular health, and abnormal hepatocellular function is associated with the onset of diabetes. ALT is the most specific marker of this hepatic pathology. Many prospective studies have shown that elevated liver enzymes, including ALT, AST, and GGT, may be a predictor of the development of insulin resistance, metabolic syndrome, and T2DM [21, 30]. Most of these studies were performed in Western countries. In middle-aged Japanese men, serum GGT was an important predictor of the development of metabolic syndrome and T2DM [31]. In a prospective community-based study performed in Korea, we also found that increased activity of liver enzymes, notably of ALT, was associated with a twofold increase in the risk of T2DM, independent of conventional risk factors [32].

In a study of nonobese NAFLD subjects and control subjects closely matched for age and body composition, the pattern of metabolic defects observed in NAFLD subjects was consistent with insulin resistance involving the liver and peripheral tissues, including adipose tissue and skeletal muscle [33]. Thus, NAFLD is emerging as a component of metabolic syndrome based on insulin resistance [34].

Taken together, these findings suggest that fat accumulation in the liver is a critical determinant of metabolic fluxes and inflammatory processes, thereby representing an important therapeutic target in insulin resistance and T2DM.

## NAFLD/NASH and CVD share an inflammatory process

Fat accumulation in the liver stimulates the production of inflammatory cytokines [35]. In particular, NASH may instigate the pathogenesis of CVD through the systemic release of several inflammatory, prothrombotic, and oxidative stress mediators [36]. Nuclear factor-κB (NF-κB) and JNK are known as the main intracellular signaling pathways involved in the mechanistic link between NAFLD and inflammation. The activation of the NF-κB pathway in the liver of patients with NAFLD leads to steatosis or NASH, which in turn enhances the transcription

of several genes, such as the intercellular adhesion molecule-1 and monocyte chemoattractant protein-1, which are associated with the development or progression of atherosclerosis [37]. In a different context, JNK aggravates insulin resistance via the phosphorylation and degradation of IRS1 and contributes to the inhibition of the intracellular signaling pathway downstream of the insulin receptor [38].

Elevated liver enzyme activity may reflect inflammation, which impairs insulin signaling both locally and systemically [22]. Furthermore, increased inflammatory cytokines, such as the high-sensitivity C-reactive protein (hsCRP), were observed in patients with NAFLD [39, 40]. In a Japanese study, elevated ALT activity was an independent marker of the activation of systemic inflammation and increased oxidative stress [41]. We also showed that individuals in the top ALT quartile had the highest levels of hsCRP, which was also an independent predictor of T2DM [42].

Recent reports showed a novel role for inflammatory mediators of the link between fatty liver and inflammation. In the Multi-Ethnic Study of Atherosclerosis, which is a longitudinal, population-based study of four ethnic groups free of CV disease at the baseline, the levels of hsCRP and interleukin-6 (IL-6) were significantly associated with liver fat assessed via CT after adjusting for other risk factors for atherosclerosis [43].

The activation of pro-inflammatory pathways is mediated by Toll-like receptors (TLRs), which are fundamental to the innate immune system [44]. TLRs are well-characterized immune receptors that enhance inflammation [45]. Among TLRs, TLR2 and TLR4 induce insulin resistance, which is pivotal in the pathogenesis of NAFLD, obesity, and metabolic syndrome. TLR4 is activated by fatty acids and endotoxinemia, resulting in the activation of NF-κB and increased release of inflammatory cytokines, such as IL-6, IL-1β, TNFα, and the monocyte chemotactic protein-1, which play a critical role in the pathophysiology of atherosclerosis and CVD.

## Oxidative stress is a critical factor in NAFLD and CVD

Oxidative stress plays an important role in the progression from simple steatosis to steatohepatitis (Figure 12.1) [46, 47]. Oxidative stress induces the hepatic production of adhesion molecules and interleukins, which can perpetuate the vicious cycle of inflammation [48]. Based on this concept, a systematic review and meta-analysis have

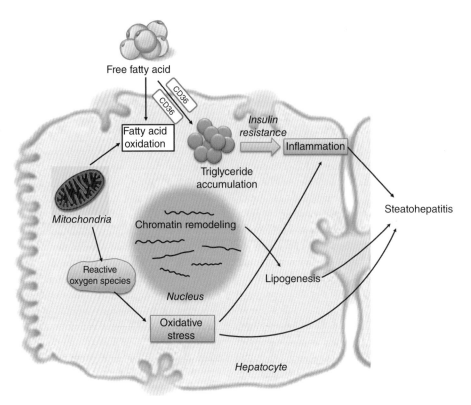

**FIG 12.1** Role of oxidative stress in the pathogenesis of steatohepatitis. Under conditions of insulin resistance, an increased amount of free fatty acids (FFAs) is released from the adipose tissue and is taken up by the liver. This overflow of FFAs increases reactive oxygen species (ROS) production and decreases the activity of antioxidant systems, thereby inducing oxidative stress.

shown that oxidative stress may be the key link between NAFLD and CVD [49].

The association between oxidative stress and NAFLD in humans has been demonstrated by the immunohistochemical detection of lipid peroxidation products and 8-hydroxy-deoxyguanosine in the plasma and in liver biopsies from patients with NAFLD [50]. In addition to insulin resistance and inflammation, elevated ALT activity may result from increased oxidative stress caused by increased delivery of FFAs to the portal circulation [51]. There is also evidence in support of the activation of oxidative stress and increased levels of homocysteine in NAFLD [52]. These data suggest that some component of oxidative stress, perhaps induced by the disease process in NAFLD, is involved in the pathogenesis of CVD. Thus, NAFLD may amplify oxidative stress and systemic inflammation, thus turning on the switch for the initiation of atherosclerosis and CVD.

## ER stress: Another factor associated with NAFLD and CVD

ER stress is also associated with the development of NAFLD or NASH [53]. ER stress is defined as a condition in which the protein-processing capacity of the ER is exceeded by nascent proteins, resulting in the accumulation of unfolded or misfolded proteins. The unfolded protein response (UPR) is a cellular self-defense mechanism that alleviates ER stress by limiting *de novo* protein synthesis, enhancing protein-folding capacity via the upregulation of specific ER chaperones, and increasing the degradation of irreversibly misfolded proteins [54].

Accumulating evidence supports a causative role for ER stress in the development or progression of atherosclerosis. Several independent CV risk factors, including obesity, cigarette smoking, hyperglycemia, and hyperhomocysteinemia, have been associated with the activation of the UPR [55, 56]. Elevated levels of diagnostic markers of ER stress and increased glycogen synthase kinase-3β (GSK3β) activity were also found in the livers and atherosclerotic lesions of three different animal models: hyperglycemic, hyperhomocysteinemic, and high-fat-fed mice [53]. These data support a role for ER stress-induced GSK3β activity in the accelerated development of hepatic steatosis and atherosclerosis.

There is robust evidence of the fundamental roles of the adaptive and proapoptotic pathways of the UPR in the development and progression of CVD, including atherosclerosis, coronary heart diseases, and heart failure [57]. ER stress can also activate caspases and promote the apoptosis of endothelial cells, macrophages, and other cell types, which are associated with the development of atherosclerosis [58].

### Other factors related with NAFLD and CVD

Patients with NAFLD exhibit low levels of adiponectin, which are associated with endothelial dysfunction, atherosclerosis, and CVD [59]. The reduced production

of adiponectin associated with insulin resistance and obesity may in turn contribute to the progression of NAFLD [60].

Factors that are related with fibrinolysis and hemostasis (e.g., fibrinogen, tissue plasminogen activator, and plasminogen activator inhibitor-1 (PAI-1)) are strongly associated with NAFLD [61]. Plasma PAI-1 levels are more closely associated with fat accumulation in the liver than in the adipose tissue, suggesting that fat deposition in the liver is an important source of PAI-1 production [62].

### Genetic association between fatty liver and cardiometabolic risk

Theoretically, genetic variation in candidate genes related to insulin resistance may contribute to the pathogenesis of NAFLD. A genetic study reported that 21 candidate genes were involved in NAFLD and insulin resistance among a

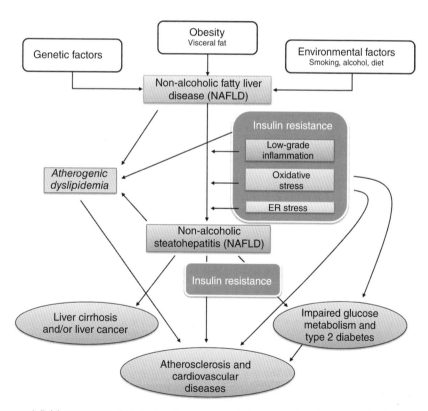

**FIG 12.2** Pathogenetic link between non-alcoholic fatty liver disease and atherosclerosis and cardiovascular diseases. ER, endoplasmic reticulum.

pool of thousands of genes, as assessed by a significance analysis of a microarray method [63].

Several genetic factors, such as patatin-like phospholipase 3 or apolipoprotein C3, have been characterized in NAFLD [64]. An allele of patatin-like phospholipase 3, which encodes a protein of unknown function with homology to lipid acyl hydrolases, is associated with fat accumulation in the liver. Apolipoprotein C3 gene variants are associated with insulin resistance and NAFLD. A more comprehensive investigation aimed at finding genes that are potentially pathogenic in the development of NAFLD related with insulin resistance or CVD is warranted.

## Conclusion

NAFLD is a chronic liver condition that is characterized by hepatic fat accumulation and/or hepatic inflammation. Individuals with obesity, insulin resistance, and dyslipidemia are at the greatest risk of developing NAFLD. NAFLD is considered as one of the phenotypes of metabolic syndrome or insulin resistance. In conclusion, NAFLD and NASH are likely to play a part in the pathogenesis of CVD via the systemic release of several inflammatory, prothrombotic, and oxidative stress mediators or via the contribution of NAFLD to insulin resistance and atherogenic dyslipidemia (Figure 12.2).

Future studies focusing on the molecular mechanism and signal transduction of the common denominators of NAFLD and CVD may allow the development of new therapeutic agents for NAFLD and related CVD.

## References

1. Matteoni CA, Younossi ZM, Gramlich T et al. Nonalcoholic fatty liver disease: a spectrum of clinical and pathological severity. Gastroenterology 1999; 116: 1413–1419.
2. Masarone M, Federico A, Abenavoli L, Loguercio C, Persico M. Non alcoholic Fatty liver: epidemiology and natural history. Rev Recent Clin Trials 2014; 9: 126–133.
3. Adams LA, Lymp JF, St Sauver J et al. The natural history of nonalcoholic fatty liver disease: a population-based cohort study. Gastroenterology 2005; 129: 113–121.
4. Mehta K, Van Thiel DH, Shah N, Mobarhan S. Nonalcoholic fatty liver disease: pathogenesis and the role of antioxidants. Nutr Rev 2002; 60: 289–293.
5. Marcos A, Fisher RA, Ham JM et al. Selection and outcome of living donors for adult to adult right lobe transplantation. Transplantation 2000; 69: 2410–2415.
6. Lee JY, Kim KM, Lee SG et al. Prevalence and risk factors of non-alcoholic fatty liver disease in potential living liver donors in Korea: a review of 589 consecutive liver biopsies in a single center. J Hepatol 2007; 47: 239–244.
7. Wanless IR, Lentz JS. Fatty liver hepatitis (steatohepatitis) and obesity: an autopsy study with analysis of risk factors. Hepatology 1990; 12: 1106–1110.
8. Amarapurkar A, Ghansar T. Fatty liver: experience from western India. Ann Hepatol 2007; 6: 37–40.
9. Zois CD, Baltayiannis GH, Bekiari A et al. Steatosis and steatohepatitis in postmortem material from Northwestern Greece. World J Gastroenterol 2010; 16: 3944–3949.
10. Williams CD, Stengel J, Asike MI et al. Prevalence of nonalcoholic fatty liver disease and nonalcoholic steatohepatitis among a largely middle-aged population utilizing ultrasound and liver biopsy: a prospective study. Gastroenterology 2011; 140: 124–131.
11. Caballeria L, Pera G, Auladell MA et al. Prevalence and factors associated with the presence of nonalcoholic fatty liver disease in an adult population in Spain. Eur J Gastroenterol Hepatol 2010; 22: 24–32.
12. Bedogni G, Miglioli L, Masutti F et al. Prevalence of and risk factors for nonalcoholic fatty liver disease: the Dionysos nutrition and liver study. Hepatology 2005; 42: 44–52.
13. Kojima S, Watanabe N, Numata M, Ogawa T, Matsuzaki S. Increase in the prevalence of fatty liver in Japan over the past 12 years: analysis of clinical background. J Gastroenterol 2003; 38: 954–961.
14. Speliotes EK, Massaro JM, Hoffmann U et al. Fatty liver is associated with dyslipidemia and dysglycemia independent of visceral fat: the Framingham Heart Study. Hepatology 2010; 51: 1979–1987.
15. Fabbrini E, Magkos F, Mohammed BS et al. Intrahepatic fat, not visceral fat, is linked with metabolic complications of obesity. Proc Natl Acad Sci U S A 2009; 106: 15430–15435.
16. Rafiq N, Bai C, Fang Y et al. Long-term follow-up of patients with nonalcoholic fatty liver. Clin Gastroenterol Hepatol 2009; 7: 234–238.
17. Ekstedt M, Franzen LE, Mathiesen UL et al. Long-term follow-up of patients with NAFLD and elevated liver enzymes. Hepatology 2006; 44: 865–873.
18. Targher G, Bertolini L, Rodella S et al. Nonalcoholic fatty liver disease is independently associated with an increased incidence of cardiovascular events in type 2 diabetic patients. Diabetes Care 2007; 30: 2119–2121.
19. Hamaguchi M, Kojima T, Takeda N et al. Nonalcoholic fatty liver disease is a novel predictor of cardiovascular disease. World J Gastroenterol 2007; 13: 1579–1584.
20. Michael MD, Kulkarni RN, Postic C et al. Loss of insulin signaling in hepatocytes leads to severe insulin resistance and progressive hepatic dysfunction. Mol Cell 2000; 6: 87–97.

21. Hanley AJ, Williams K, Festa A et al. Liver markers and development of the metabolic syndrome: the insulin resistance atherosclerosis study. Diabetes 2005; 54: 3140–3147.

22. Vozarova B, Stefan N, Lindsay RS et al. High alanine aminotransferase is associated with decreased hepatic insulin sensitivity and predicts the development of type 2 diabetes. Diabetes 2002; 51: 1889–1895.

23. Perry IJ, Wannamethee SG, Shaper AG. Prospective study of serum gamma-glutamyltransferase and risk of NIDDM. Diabetes Care 1998; 21: 732–737.

24. Ohlson LO, Larsson B, Bjorntorp P et al. Risk factors for type 2 (non-insulin-dependent) diabetes mellitus. Thirteen and one-half years of follow-up of the participants in a study of Swedish men born in 1913. Diabetologia 1988; 31: 798–805.

25. Seppala-Lindroos A, Vehkavaara S, Hakkinen AM et al. Fat accumulation in the liver is associated with defects in insulin suppression of glucose production and serum free fatty acids independent of obesity in normal men. J Clin Endocrinol Metab 2002; 87: 3023–3028.

26. Despres JP. Intra-abdominal obesity: an untreated risk factor for Type 2 diabetes and cardiovascular disease. J Endocrinol Invest 2006; 29: 77–82.

27. Wang H, Quiroga AD, Lehner R. Analysis of lipid droplets in hepatocytes. Methods Cell Biol 2013; 116: 107–127.

28. Meshkani R, Adeli K. Hepatic insulin resistance, metabolic syndrome and cardiovascular disease. Clin Biochem 2009; 42: 1331–1346.

29. Liu KH, Chan YL, Chan WB, Chan JC, Chu CW. Mesenteric fat thickness is an independent determinant of metabolic syndrome and identifies subjects with increased carotid intima-media thickness. Diabetes Care 2006; 29: 379–384.

30. Sattar N, Scherbakova O, Ford I et al. Elevated alanine aminotransferase predicts new-onset type 2 diabetes independently of classical risk factors, metabolic syndrome, and C-reactive protein in the west of Scotland coronary prevention study. Diabetes 2004; 53: 2855–2860.

31. Nakanishi N, Suzuki K, Tatara K. Serum gamma-glutamyltransferase and risk of metabolic syndrome and type 2 diabetes in middle-aged Japanese men. Diabetes Care 2004; 27: 1427–1432.

32. Cho NH, Jang HC, Choi SH et al. Abnormal liver function test predicts type 2 diabetes: a community-based prospective study. Diabetes Care 2007; 30: 2566–2568.

33. Kotronen A, Juurinen L, Tiikkainen M, Vehkavaara S, Yki-Jarvinen H. Increased liver fat, impaired insulin clearance, and hepatic and adipose tissue insulin resistance in type 2 diabetes. Gastroenterology 2008; 135: 122–130.

34. Marchesini G, Brizi M, Bianchi G et al. Nonalcoholic fatty liver disease: a feature of the metabolic syndrome. Diabetes 2001; 50: 1844–1850.

35. Lo L, McLennan SV, Williams PF et al. Diabetes is a progression factor for hepatic fibrosis in a high fat fed mouse obesity model of non-alcoholic steatohepatitis. J Hepatol 2011; 55: 435–444.

36. Targher G, Day CP, Bonora E. Risk of cardiovascular disease in patients with nonalcoholic fatty liver disease. N Engl J Med 2010; 363: 1341–1350.

37. Stefan N, Kantartzis K, Haring HU. Causes and metabolic consequences of Fatty liver. Endocr Rev 2008; 29: 939–960.

38. Shoelson SE, Lee J, Goldfine AB. Inflammation and insulin resistance. J Clin Invest 2006; 116: 1793–1801.

39. Lavie CJ, Milani RV, Verma A, O'Keefe JH. C-reactive protein and cardiovascular diseases—is it ready for primetime? Am J Med Sci 2009; 338: 486–492.

40. Dowman JK, Tomlinson JW, Newsome PN. Pathogenesis of non-alcoholic fatty liver disease. QJM 2010; 103: 71–83.

41. Yamada J, Tomiyama H, Yambe M et al. Elevated serum levels of alanine aminotransferase and gamma glutamyltransferase are markers of inflammation and oxidative stress independent of the metabolic syndrome. Atherosclerosis 2006; 189(1): 198–205.

42. Herder C, Peltonen M, Koenig W et al. Systemic immune mediators and lifestyle changes in the prevention of type 2 diabetes: results from the Finnish Diabetes Prevention Study. Diabetes 2006; 55: 2340–2346.

43. Hamirani YS, Katz R, Nasir K et al. Association between inflammatory markers and liver fat: the multi-ethnic study of atherosclerosis. J Clin Exp Cardiolog 2014; 5: 344.

44. Kiechl S, Lorenz E, Reindl M et al. Toll-like receptor 4 polymorphisms and atherogenesis. N Engl J Med 2002; 347: 185–192.

45. Jialal I, Kaur H, Devaraj S. Toll-like receptor status in obesity and metabolic syndrome: a translational perspective. J Clin Endocrinol Metab 2014; 99: 39–48.

46. Colak Y, Senates E, Yesil A et al. Assessment of endothelial function in patients with nonalcoholic fatty liver disease. Endocrine 2013; 43: 100–107.

47. Lim S and Barter P. Antioxidant effects of statins in the management of cardiometabolic disorders. J Atheroscler Thromb 2014; 21: 997–1010.

48. Hotamisligil GS. Inflammatory pathways and insulin action. Int J Obes Relat Metab Disord 2003; 27(Suppl 3): S53–S55.

49. Cakir E, Ozbek M, Colak N, Cakal E, Delibasi T. Is NAFLD an independent risk factor for increased IMT in T2DM? Minerva Endocrinol 2012; 37: 187–193.

50. Bhatia LS, Curzen NP, Byrne CD. Nonalcoholic fatty liver disease and vascular risk. Curr Opin Cardiol 2012; 27: 420–428.

51. Cassader M, Gambino R, Musso G et al. Postprandial triglyceride-rich lipoprotein metabolism and insulin sensitivity in nonalcoholic steatohepatitis patients. Lipids 2001; 36: 1117–1124.

52. Leach NV, Dronca E, Vesa SC et al. Serum homocysteine levels, oxidative stress and cardiovascular risk in non-alcoholic steatohepatitis. Eur J Intern Med 2014; 25: 762–767.

53. McAlpine CS, Bowes AJ, Khan MI, Shi Y, Werstuck GH. Endoplasmic reticulum stress and glycogen synthase kinase-3beta activation in apolipoprotein E-deficient mouse models of accelerated atherosclerosis. Arterioscler Thromb Vasc Biol 2012; 32: 82–91.

54. Pahl HL. Signal transduction from the endoplasmic reticulum to the cell nucleus. Physiol Rev 1999; 79: 683–701.

55. Ozcan U, Cao Q, Yilmaz E et al. Endoplasmic reticulum stress links obesity, insulin action, and type 2 diabetes. Science 2004; 306: 457–461.

56. Khan MI, Pichna BA, Shi Y, Bowes AJ, Werstuck GH. Evidence supporting a role for endoplasmic reticulum stress in the development of atherosclerosis in a hyperglycaemic mouse model. Antioxid Redox Signal 2009; 11: 2289–2298.

57. Minamino T, Komuro I, Kitakaze M. Endoplasmic reticulum stress as a therapeutic target in cardiovascular disease. Circ Res 2010; 107: 1071–1082.

58. Zinszner H, Kuroda M, Wang X et al. CHOP is implicated in programmed cell death in response to impaired function of the endoplasmic reticulum. Genes Dev 1998; 12: 982–995.

59. Lim S, Koo BK, Cho SW et al. Association of adiponectin and resistin with cardiovascular events in Korean patients with type 2 diabetes: the Korean atherosclerosis study (KAS): a 42-month prospective study. Atherosclerosis 2008; 196: 398–404.

60. Pagano C, Soardo G, Esposito W et al. Plasma adiponectin is decreased in nonalcoholic fatty liver disease. Eur J Endocrinol 2005; 152: 113–118.

61. Tuyama AC, Chang CY. Non-alcoholic fatty liver disease. J Diabetes 2012; 4: 266–280.

62. Alessi MC, Bastelica D, Mavri A et al. Plasma PAI-1 levels are more strongly related to liver steatosis than to adipose tissue accumulation. Arterioscler Thromb Vasc Biol 2003; 23: 1262–1268.

63. Wang XC, Zhan XR, Li XY, Yu JJ, Liu XM. Identification and validation co-differentially expressed genes with NAFLD and insulin resistance. Endocrine 2015; 48(1): 143–151.

64. Tilg H, Moschen A. Update on nonalcoholic fatty liver disease: genes involved in nonalcoholic fatty liver disease and associated inflammation. Curr Opin Clin Nutr Metab Care 2010; 13: 391–396.

**PART III**
# Diagnosis and Scoring

# 13 How to best diagnose NAFLD/NASH?

## Vlad Ratziu

Service d'hépatogastroentérologie, Hôpital Pitié salpêtrière, Institute for Cardiometabolism and Nutrition, Université Pierre et Marie Curie, Paris, France

### LEARNING POINTS

- In an exceedingly large number of cases, NAFLD is of primary origin and is associated with one or several metabolic risk factors. However, rare secondary causes should not be overlooked. NAFLD can coexist with other chronic liver diseases and documenting past or present exposure to metabolic risk factors is then key to the diagnosis.

- The distinction between NASH and non-NASH NAFLD (also called NAFL) is useful for the overall prognosis. It can currently be done only by liver biopsy. While some noninvasive panels of biomarkers perform well for diagnosing steatosis, there is no well-validated biomarker of steatohepatitis.

- Fibrosis has a major prognostic value and should be assessed, initially, noninvasively. Both serum markers and transient elastometry have been well studied, and both are especially performant for their negative predictive value. Ideally they should be tested in combination. Low values for both are strongly indicative of no/mild fibrosis, which should reduce the need for liver biopsy. Persistently discordant results should be adjudicated through liver biopsy.

- In clinical practice the decision to perform a liver biopsy should be done on a case by case basis taking into account associated comorbidities and treatments. The histological examination still provides major diagnostic and prognostic information. It should not be performed in a metabolically unstable patient and especially if recent weight loss with improvement of liver enzymes or of insulin resistance surrogates. The histological diagnosis of steatohepatitis does not rely on the NAS score.

Non-alcoholic fatty liver disease (NAFLD) is characterized by excessive hepatic fat accumulation [1–3]. The disease spectrum encompasses steatosis, varying degrees of inflammation, and fibrosis, which are features of the progressive form; non-alcoholic steatohepatitis (NASH); and ultimately cirrhosis and hepatocellular carcinoma [4]. NAFLD is associated with insulin resistance in patients that are overweight or obese but even lean NAFLD patients usually display insulin resistance, glycemic dysregulation, and visceral adiposity to a higher degree than non-NAFLD individuals with the same BMI [5]. Steatosis by itself can worsen insulin resistance and increases the incidence of comorbidities associated with the metabolic syndrome. Given the expanding epidemic of obesity and diabetes, NAFLD affects up to a third of the population worldwide and is becoming the leading cause of chronic liver disease and a major health concern owing to hepatic and extrahepatic complications, mainly related to NASH with fibrosis [6–8]. Moreover, the coexistence of NASH with other chronic liver diseases has been increasingly recognized in many cases with a higher risk of advanced liver injury [9, 10].

A key issue in the diagnosis and management of NAFLD is the distinction between simple steatosis and NASH, as the former is considered an indolent condition and the latter a progressive form with increased morbidity and mortality [11–14]. In addition a wide spectrum of extrahepatic comorbidities (cardiovascular and renal diseases, endocrinopathies, cancers, postsurgical complications, obstructive sleep apnea, psychological disorders) can occur in NAFLD patients. Some of these are triggered or worsened by NAFLD and affect quality of life and prognosis

---

*Clinical Dilemmas in Non-Alcoholic Fatty Liver Disease*, First Edition. Edited by Roger Williams and Simon D. Taylor-Robinson.
© 2016 John Wiley & Sons, Ltd. Published 2016 by John Wiley & Sons, Ltd.

while possibly interacting with liver disease progression [15–21]. Therefore, in addition to a hepatological workup, a complete metabolic and cardiovascular assessment is advisable in patients with NAFLD.

This chapter aims to give practical recommendations about the diagnostic workup of patients with suspicion of NAFLD. It will also summarize the performance and limitations of available methods for NAFLD diagnosis, NASH detection, and fibrosis staging. A more in-depth discussion of these topics is available in dedicated chapters of this book.

## Primary or secondary NAFLD?

A very large majority maybe between 90 and 99% of NAFLD cases are due to primary NAFLD, that is, NAFLD associated with insulin resistance, usually in a patient with metabolic risk factors (Table 13.1) [2]. Yet, it is important not to miss the diagnosis of secondary NAFLD mainly because specific interventions may be available. Table 13.2 lists a number of diseases that result in excessive fat accumulation in the liver. A detailed discussion of secondary causes of NAFLD is available elsewhere in this book.

A second important aspect is the recognition that NAFLD can coexist with other chronic liver diseases. Given the current high prevalence of overweight and

**TABLE 13.1** Metabolic risk factors

Body mass index >25 kg/m$^2$ and/or waist circumference >94 cm in men, 80 cm in women (Caucasians)
Arterial hypertension >135/85 mmHg
Fasting serum glucose >6.1 mmol/L
Serum triglycerides >1.7 mmol/L
HDL cholesterol <1 mmol/L (men); <1.3 mmol/L (women)
Serum ferritin >350 µg/L
First degree relatives of obesity and/or diabetes

**TABLE 13.2** Causes of secondary NAFLD

Drugs (amiodarone, corticosteroids, tamoxifen, methotrexate)
Chronic hepatitis C
Wilson's disease
Panhypopituitarism
Industrial toxins
A/hypobetalipoproteinemia
Lipodystrophies
Cholesteryl storage disease
Citrate deficiency

diabetes in the general population, some patients with chronic liver diseases other than NAFLD may have concurrent NAFLD. In some cases the association of NAFLD with another liver disease, such as chronic hepatitis C, alcoholic liver disease, or possibly hemochromatosis, can result in more severe liver damage [22–24]. Sorting out the respective contribution of each condition to the overall hepatic damage might not always be possible. But the recognition of lipotoxicity occurring in insulin resistance as the main pathogenic mechanism in NAFLD/NASH [25, 26] should help acknowledge that a positive definition of NAFLD/NASH is needed. This definition should be based on the presence of an underlying cause rather than the absence of an unrelated condition.

## Histological diagnosis

Liver biopsy is essential for the diagnosis of NASH and for prognostic risk stratification of NAFLD patients despite limitations due to sampling variability [27, 28]. Currently, liver biopsy is the only diagnostic procedure that can reliably differentiate steatohepatitis (i.e., NASH) from NAFL (non-alcoholic fatty liver).

### Steatohepatitis

The diagnosis of steatohepatitis is based on the association of liver fat (macrovacuolar or mixed steatosis of 5% or more), hepatocyte ballooning, and lobular inflammation [29–31]. Perisinusoidal fibrosis is a useful and frequent diagnostic feature but not included formally in the diagnostic criteria of steatohepatitis. In the early stages, the pattern of injury follows a centrilobular accentuation, although at later stages the zonular distribution is usually lost. Both the NASH CRN and the FLIP consortium contributed toward an accurate and homogenous histological definition of NASH [29, 30, 32]. The FLIP algorithm has been prospectively designed, and its use increases agreement for the overall diagnosis between observers. It also defines the grading for ballooning precisely, a cardinal feature of steatohepatitis that needs to be present for the diagnosis of NASH to be made [30]. Currently, no recommendation can be made for the use of any particular stain to identify ballooned hepatocytes reliably, although cytokeratin 18 might be useful in special cases [33]. In some, but not all, patients with cirrhosis, steatosis, inflammation, and ballooning may regress to show only "extinct" cirrhosis. Many of these patients have a history of exposure to metabolic risk factors, and a clinical phenotype quite distinct from that of truly cryptogenic cirrhosis [34, 35]; therefore, in these patients, this condition should be labeled "burned-out NASH." Rarely, some patients display bridging fibrosis and steatosis but no ballooning or inflammation. It is unclear whether hepatocyte ballooning or inflammation becomes extinct at an earlier precirrhotic stage, or whether they were missed because of sampling variability at biopsy. For clinical management purposes, these patients should be considered as having NASH, as usually steatohepatitis but not NAFL (see in the following) is associated with bridging fibrosis. Other histological features can be seen in steatohepatitis but are not necessary for the diagnosis of NASH: portal inflammation, perisinusoidal fibrosis, polymorphonuclear infiltrates, Mallory–Denk bodies, apoptotic bodies, clear vacuolated nuclei, microvacuolar steatosis, and megamitochondria. Portal inflammation is a frequent feature in pediatric NASH but can be seen in adults and could be associated with more severe disease [36]. Fibrosis has typically a pericellular distribution (perisinusoidal fibrosis) and is more abundant in acinar zone 3 but it can also be portal based. Thus neither portal inflammation nor portal fibrosis excludes the diagnosis of NASH. When polymorphonuclear cells and Mallory–Denk bodies are numerous and well delineated (satellitosis), the diagnosis of alcoholic liver disease (alone or in association) should instead be considered.

## NAFL

When steatosis is present but lobular inflammation or ballooning are absent, the minimal requirements for steatohepatitis are not met, and the diagnosis should be NAFL (non-alcoholic fatty liver, i.e., non-NASH NAFLD) [31]. The terms probable or possible NASH should be abandoned as they create confusion both for the practicing clinician and for clinical trials. Therefore, NAFL encompasses either (i) steatosis alone or (ii) steatosis with lobular or portal inflammation, without ballooning, or (iii) steatosis with ballooning but without inflammation [31]. Recent studies suggest a distinction between steatosis with and without inflammation: steatosis with inflammation could progress to steatohepatitis (sometimes with bridging fibrosis) while progression seems exceptional for steatosis alone [37, 38]. Earlier studies have suggested that inflammation is highly associated with fibrosis progression [39]. The diagnosis of NAFLD should therefore be divided into (i) steatohepatitis (NASH) and (ii) NAFL (non-NASH NAFLD). The latter

can be further subdivided into steatosis alone or steatosis with inflammation. Although this dichotomized diagnostic approach (NAFL vs. NASH) is clinically useful, it is an oversimplification that does not reflect the histological complexity of the disease such as cases of steatofibrosis as mentioned previously. Indeed, and as for any other chronic liver diseases, NAFLD might display a wide continuous spectrum of histological lesions so that splitting the disease into NAFL and NASH is artificial. Therefore, semiquantitative scoring system might better mirror the complexity of the histological pattern.

## Scoring systems

Several scoring systems have been described in adults [29, 30]. The NAFLD Activity Score (NAS) is the unweighted sum of steatosis (0–3), inflammation (0–3), and ballooning (0–2). It is not designed to be a surrogate for the diagnosis of steatohepatitis but rather a crude evaluation of the severity of the disease once the diagnosis of NASH has been established by the overall pathological assessment [29, 32]. Although the NAS is correlated with aminotransferase and HOMA values [32], unfortunately, to date there is no demonstration of any prognostic value of the NAS [40, 41]. While patients with a NAS <3 and a NAS more than 4 are, respectively, bona fide NAFL and NASH, there is a gray zone (NAS = 3 or 4) that includes both cases with NAFL and NASH. Consequently, its use as an histological outcome in therapeutic trials is of questionable clinical relevance. The SAF score has the advantage of separating scores of steatosis (from 0 to 3), activity (0–4) (lobular inflammation 0–2 plus ballooning 0–2), and fibrosis (0–4) [30]. It has good reproducibility both with expert pathologists and specialized liver pathologists but has not yet been tested within therapeutic trials. Staging of fibrosis of NAFLD rely on the Kleiner fibrosis stage [29] (which is also used in a simplified pattern in the SAF score) [30]. Unfortunately, this scoring system underscores perisinusoidal fibrosis within the lobule, which is a common pattern, especially in patients with diabetes; Morphometry that measures the amount of fibrous tissue on digitalized images might be a useful adjunct, and it is done in many clinical trials. None of these fibrosis staging systems, unfortunately, distinguishes between early and advanced bridging fibrosis. The FLIP staging system has better reproducibility mainly because of reduced granularity of stage 1 [30].

A key issue is which histological features of NAFLD predict liver disease progression and liver-related events or mortality as these could be acceptable surrogates for therapeutic trials. Studies with large cohorts defined histologically by a central pathologist and with long follow-up for clinical events are necessary to answer this question. Two such studies have shown that both the diagnosis of steatohepatitis [40] and the stage of fibrosis [40, 42] (bridging fibrosis or cirrhosis) predict liver-related mortality [40]. Recently, a large international study of 619 cases with index biopsy and a median follow-up of 12.6 years has shown that both the diagnosis of NASH and liver fibrosis are associated with overall mortality and liver-related mortality [43]. As steatohepatitis most likely drives fibrogenesis, the demonstration of an independent effect of steatohepatitis from that of fibrosis can be difficult to delineate statistically because of colinearity between the two variables.

## Noninvasive diagnostic procedures

The identification and validation of noninvasive markers in patients with suspected NAFLD should aim at (i) identifying in primary care settings the individuals exposed to metabolic risk factors that are at high risk of NAFLD-related liver disease; in secondary and tertiary care settings, identifying those with advanced/severe NASH, as this carries prognostic information and selects patients in need for specific therapy; (ii) monitoring disease progression; and (iii) predicting response to pharmacological or nonpharmacological interventions. If these objectives are fulfilled, noninvasive methods could reduce the need or even replace liver biopsy as a diagnostic tool.

### Steatosis

The demonstration of steatosis establishes the diagnosis of NAFLD and therefore it is recommended both as an initial diagnostic procedure in the workup of patients suspected of NAFLD or, more broadly, for any suspicion of liver disease as steatosis can be a chance finding. Emerging data suggest that steatosis predicts the occurrence of some of the comorbidities associated with overweight/insulin resistance such as diabetes, cardiovascular events, and arterial hypertension. In contrast, there are insufficient data that the quantification of steatosis is yet of clinical interest except, probably, as a surrogate of efficacy for nonpharmacological interventions (diet and lifestyle changes) [44, 45] and maybe for certain pharmacological interventions [46]. Therefore, in clinical practice, the diagnosis but not the quantification of steatosis is recommended.

At an individual patient level, especially in tertiary care centers, steatosis should be identified by imaging studies, preferably an ultrasound, a more widely available and cheaper technique than CT scan or MRI. All imaging techniques have limited sensitivity for mild steatosis and do not reliably detect steatosis when <20% [47, 48] or in individuals with high BMI (>40 kg/m$^2$) [49]. Despite observer dependency (the inter- and intraobserver variability for the presence of increased fat is 72 and 76%, respectively), ultrasound (or CT scan [50]) robustly diagnoses moderate and severe steatosis and provides additional information, critical for a comprehensive hepatobiliary workup, hence the recommendation for a first-line diagnostic procedure. However, for large cohort screening of patients with metabolic risk factors, the use of serum biomarkers of steatosis is preferred, as, on a larger scale, availability and cost of ultrasound could significantly impact feasibility. The best validated steatosis biomarkers are the fatty liver index (FLI) [51] followed by SteatoTest [52, 53] and the NAFLD liver fat score [54]. FLI had a particularly extensive external validation in Europe [55, 56], Asia [57], and North America [58], including in the general population and predicted metabolic [59–61] and cardiovascular [62] outcomes, as well as hepatic [63] and cardiovascular mortality [64]. SteatoTest has been externally validated in the general population [65] and in morbidly obese patients [66] undergoing bariatric surgery and is correlated with overall mortality [67]. Although most of these serum markers are associated with insulin resistance and reliably predict the presence of steatosis, they do not accurately quantify steatosis [68, 69] and therefore they cannot be recommended for this purpose [69]. An imaging technique, the controlled attenuation parameter (CAP) that measures ultrasonic attenuation in the liver using signals acquired by a transient elastography probe, has shown good discriminative value for the prediction of steatosis but a limited ability to discriminate between steatosis grades defined histologically. Besides, the use of the CAP technology implies having access to the FibroScan device and can be limited by high BMI values [70]. Future studies testing the quantitative ability of serum markers or imaging methods should be performed against 3HMRspectroscopy or at least a morphometric assessment of liver fat instead of the semiquantitative pathological score [71].

### Steatohepatitis

NASH is the progressive form of NAFLD. Therefore, in a patient with suspected NAFLD, the diagnosis of steatohepatitis provides important prognostic information and places the patient at higher risk of fibrosis progression, cirrhosis, and possibly hepatocellular carcinoma than does steatosis alone (non-NASH NAFLD). It may also prompt a closer follow-up and possibly a higher need for more aggressive therapeutic management including pharmacological therapy.

Simple clinical or biochemical measurements or widely available imaging methods (ultrasound, CT scan, or MRI) cannot distinguish NASH from steatosis. A myriad of noninvasive procedures have been tested (reviewed in Refs. [72, 73]) including adipocytokines, chemokines, inflammatory markers, breath tests, complex models based on panels of biomarkers, scintigraphy, or NMR spectroscopy. Most of these have been performed in cohorts of small sample size, with insufficient histological documentation or variable histological definitions, without external validation; some were developed in specific populations (e.g., morbidly obese patients); and some provided discrepant results. Importantly, virtually none had so far convincing external validation, and many are too complex to perform for everyday clinical practice. Cytokeratin-18 (CK-18) fragments that are generated during cell death (M65 fragment) or apoptosis (M30 fragment) are the most widely studied NASH biomarker, either alone [74] or in combination with different adipocytokines [75], apoptosis markers [76] or standard biochemical items [77]. A meta-analysis shows that CK-18 has modest accuracy overall for diagnosing NASH (66% sensitivity, 82% specificity) [73]; optimized cutoffs can improve the diagnostic performance but these are highly variable between publications and therefore not consensual for clinical practice. Importantly, a large series has confirmed the limited accuracy of CK-18 for diagnosing NASH [78], and interventional studies with antiapoptotic agents have shown inconsistent changes in CK-18 despite significant reduction in ALT [79]. CK-18 changes parallel histological improvement but do not perform better than ALT in identifying histological responders [80]. To date there is no reliable, well-validated noninvasive procedure for the diagnosis of NASH.

### Fibrosis

Fibrosis is the most important prognostic factor in NAFLD and it is correlated with liver-related outcomes and mortality [40, 42]. Hence, patients with no or very early fibrosis should be identified as their management should be centered on the metabolic comorbidities. Alternatively, advanced fibrosis identifies a subgroup of NASH patients

that deserve in-depth hepatological exploration (including, in a case by case basis, the confirmation of advanced fibrosis by liver biopsy) and, possibly, pharmacological therapies. Monitoring of fibrosis progression is also necessary in all NAFLD patients, although at variable time intervals according to the type of NAFLD and the activity steatohepatitis.

Many serum markers have been studied such as the NAFLD fibrosis score (NFS) [81], FIB-4 [82], BARD [83], and also commercially available panels such as FibroTest [84], FibroMeter [85], and ELF [86]. All have shown acceptable diagnostic accuracy as defined by an area under the ROC curve (AUROC) >0.8. Few of these, such as FIB-4 and NFS, have been externally validated more than once in ethnically different NAFLD populations and with consistent results. NFS, FIB-4, and FibroTest predict overall mortality and cardiovascular mortality [67, 87–89] and liver-related mortality [88]. NFS predicts incident diabetes [90] and some data suggest that changes in NFS are associated with mortality [89]. Importantly, the negative predictive value for excluding severe (F3 and F4) fibrosis is higher than the positive predictive value for ruling in severe fibrosis in some studies [86, 91]; if a negative predictive value >90% is confirmed, the best use of these tests would be to identify patients at low risk of severe fibrosis and could therefore serve as a first-line triage test for risk stratification. However, predictive values depend on the prevalence of severe fibrosis in a given patient population [82] and therefore are not readily comparable between studies. Moreover, most of these studies have been conducted in tertiary centers where the pretest probability of severe fibrosis is much higher than in the general population. These tests perform best at distinguishing severe versus not severe fibrosis but not advanced (F2, F3, F4) or any (F1–F4) fibrosis versus no fibrosis [86].

Transient elastography is now a well-accepted method for fibrosis evaluation. Several studies are available in NAFLD (reviewed in Ref. [73]). It has an acceptable accuracy in diagnosing bridging (severe) fibrosis (sensitivity and specificity >80% for a threshold >8–10.4 kPa), an excellent accuracy for the diagnosis of cirrhosis (sensitivity and specificity >90% for a threshold >10.3–17.5 kPa) but a moderate accuracy (sensitivity and specificity <80%) for the diagnosis of advanced fibrosis (≥F2). For the M probe a large series identified a 7 kPa threshold for excluding advanced (F2) fibrosis with 84% NPV, a 8.7 kPa threshold for excluding severe (bridging) fibrosis with a 95% NPV, and a 10.3 kPa threshold for excluding cirrhosis with a 99% NPV [92]. Overall, elastometry has a higher rate of false positive results than of false negative results and higher negative than positive predictive values [92]; hence the ability to rule in bridging fibrosis or cirrhosis is, in most studies, insufficient for clinical decision-making based on elastometry results alone.

The main shortcoming of transient elastography in NAFLD patients is the failure and unreliable results rate, which are highly dependent on BMI and the thoracic fold thickness. In a large, unselected, European series, up to 20% of FibroScan™ (Echosens, Lyon, France) examinations yielded unreliable results [93]; in NAFLD patients with a BMI >30 kg/m², the unreliable result rate could be as high as 25% [92]. Therefore, in these patients, the XL probe should be used, as it reduces the failure rate. Obese subjects still have a high (35%) failure rate even with the XL probe [94]. As the absolute elastometry values are in average 1.5 kPa lower with the XL probe than with the M probe, one study identified cutoffs for bridging fibrosis at 7.2 kPa (with a negative predictive value of 89%) and for cirrhosis at 7.9 kPa with a NPV of 98% [94]. However, there is no consensus on precise thresholds or strategies of use in clinical practice when trying to avoid the use of liver biopsy. Some data have suggested that the combination of elastometry and serum fibrosis markers performs better than either method alone [95]. Importantly, longitudinal data are necessary to understand whether changes in histological fibrotic severity are reflected by changes in elastometry or serum markers.

Several alternatives to elastometry such as real-time shear wave elastography (Aixplorer™) [96, 97] and acoustic radiation force imaging (ARFI) [98, 99] are currently evaluated in chronic hepatitis C and NAFLD. Both technologies provide a measurement of liver stiffness using a probe that can be integrated into a conventional ultrasound machine. There are few studies comparing head to head these new techniques versus FibroScan™. Preliminary data suggested similar diagnostic performance with the advantage over FibroScan™ that multiple measurements in distinct areas of interest can be performed, thus possibly minimizing sampling variability. A promising imaging method is the two-dimensional magnetic resonance elastography (2D-MRE) that provides mapping of the distribution of fibrosis in the whole liver. A recent prospective study has found an excellent overall diagnostic value with very high negative predictive value of 0.97 for advanced

fibrosis but only a modest positive predictive value of 0.68. This imaging method will become more attractive with increased availability and decreased cost.

## Recommendations for diagnosis in clinical practice

### How should noninvasive procedures be used?

The presence of metabolic risk factors or persistently abnormal liver functions tests should prompt the search for NAFLD by imaging methods (ultrasonography). The quantification of steatosis is not yet useful in clinical practice. It is important to remember that patients with suspected liver disease of any other origin could have concurrent NAFLD, and the latter needs to be diagnosed. Ultrasound is the preferred first-line diagnostic procedure for steatosis as it provides additional useful diagnostic information about the liver, biliary tree, pancreas, and abdomen in addition to the study of the liver echotexture. Since ultrasonography does not have excellent sensitivity and therefore can miss early steatosis, an alternative method could be the confirmation of the absence of steatosis using either serum markers or the CAP probe from a FibroScan™ machine. Once the diagnosis of steatosis has been made, the next practical step would be to assess noninvasively the amount of fibrosis. Fibrosis serum markers as well as elastometry are acceptable first-line procedures for the identification of patients at low risk of severe fibrosis/cirrhosis. However, the combination of a serum marker and of elastometry probably confers additional diagnostic accuracy and should be used. The identification of advanced/severe fibrosis is less accurate and may necessitate, according to the clinical context, histological confirmation. Histology is not necessary if cirrhosis is well documented by serum markers, elastometry, endoscopy, and standard biological tests.

The Figure 13.1 summarizes a diagnostic algorithm that can be proposed for the large number of patients that are exposed to metabolic risk factors and therefore are at risk of NAFLD. Most of these patients are seen in primary care or by endocrine, diabetes, or nutrition specialists. The objectives are twofold. The aim is first to identify patients at low risk of significant fibrosis that do not necessitate more in-depth hepatological workup and specific pharmacological interventions for NASH. These patients can be monitored at longer intervals. Second, to identify patients at risk of more advanced disease that should be referred to

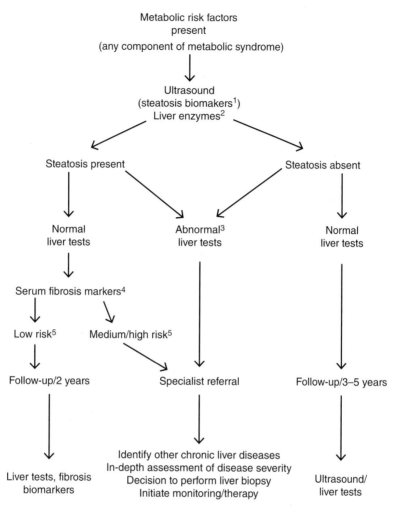

**FIG 13.1** Diagnostic workup to assess and monitor disease severity in patients with metabolic risk factors and suspected NAFLD. [1]Steatosis biomarkers: fatty liver index, SteatoTest, NAFLD fat score. [2]Liver tests: ALT AST, GGT. [3]Any increase in ALT, AST, or GGT. [4]Serum fibrosis markers: NAFLD fibrosis score, FIB-4, commercial tests (FibroTest, FibroMeter, ELF). [5]Low risk: indicative of no/mild fibrosis; Medium/high risk: indicative of significant fibrosis or cirrhosis.

a liver specialist. The consulting hepatologist will then undertake an in-depth assessment of liver injury, will decide upon the opportunity to perform a liver biopsy, and will initiate close monitoring or specific therapy, including inclusion in clinical trials, if appropriate.

## When should liver biopsy be performed in clinical practice?

The indications of liver biopsy are not consensual and cannot be generalized but only decided on an individual case basis. The decision to perform a liver biopsy in patients with suspected NAFLD or with NAFLD documented by imaging should take into account (i) the diagnostic and prognostic information provided by the biopsy such as the identification of a potentially progressive disease variety (i.e., steatohepatitis vs. NAFL), the severity of liver injury (i.e., grading of steatohepatitis as assessed by the NAS or the SAF score; presence of bridging fibrosis or of cirrhosis); (ii) the increased risk or increased complexity of the procedure in patients with concurrent antiaggregant or anticoagulant medication. Transjugular liver biopsy provides a safer alternative when these drugs cannot be discontinued; (iii) competing mortality due to comorbidities, and advanced age, and the possibility that successful management of NASH can be achieved within a timeline deemed compatible with life expectancy; this is particularly relevant in older individuals with numerous metabolic syndrome-related comorbidities.

The timing of liver biopsy should be guided by the metabolic condition: liver biopsy should be delayed in patients with unstable metabolic condition, for instance patients in the process of losing weight (patients with continuing weight loss) or patients with acute deterioration of diabetes. The decision to perform liver biopsy should be informed by results of noninvasive testing of fibrosis, preferably by two different methods such as elastometry and serum-based markers. If both methods unambiguously show that there is no or only mild fibrosis, liver biopsy could be delayed and fibrosis and metabolic monitoring initiated. If both methods are in favor of advanced (bridging) fibrosis, a biopsy can be recommended if the confirmation of advanced fibrosis is deemed necessary. In case of unexplained discordant results between the two methods, liver biopsy is necessary for fibrosis staging. If both methods are indicative of cirrhosis, liver biopsy may not be necessary for clinical practice and screening for the complications of cirrhosis should be initiated instead. As patients with normal aminotransferases can have significant liver disease [100, 101], liver biopsy should not be ruled out in these individuals.

## References

1. Loria P, Adinolfi LE, Bellentani S, et al. Practice guidelines for the diagnosis and management of nonalcoholic fatty liver disease. A decalogue from the Italian Association for the Study of the Liver (AISF) Expert Committee. Dig Liver Dis 2010;42(4):272–82.
2. Ratziu V, Bellentani S, Cortez-Pinto H, Day C, Marchesini G. A position statement on NAFLD/NASH based on the EASL 2009 special conference. J Hepatol 2010;53(2):372–84.
3. Chalasani N, Younossi Z, Lavine JE, et al. The diagnosis and management of non-alcoholic fatty liver disease: practice Guideline by the American Association for the Study of Liver Diseases, American College of Gastroenterology, and the American Gastroenterological Association. Hepatology 2012;55(6):2005–23.
4. Farrell GC, Larter CZ. Nonalcoholic fatty liver disease: from steatosis to cirrhosis. Hepatology 2006;43(2 Suppl 1):S99–112.
5. Younossi ZM, Stepanova M, Negro F, et al. Nonalcoholic fatty liver disease in lean individuals in the United States. Medicine (Baltimore) 2012;91(6):319–27.
6. Hui JM, Kench JG, Chitturi S, et al. Long-term outcomes of cirrhosis in nonalcoholic steatohepatitis compared with hepatitis C. Hepatology 2003;38(2):420–7.
7. Sanyal AJ, Banas C, Sargeant C, et al. Similarities and differences in outcomes of cirrhosis due to nonalcoholic steatohepatitis and hepatitis C. Hepatology 2006;43(4):682–9.
8. Bhala N, Angulo P, van der Poorten D, et al. The natural history of nonalcoholic fatty liver disease with advanced fibrosis or cirrhosis: an international collaborative study. Hepatology 2011;54(4):1208–16.
9. Clouston AD, Jonsson JR, Powell EE. Steatosis as a cofactor in other liver diseases: hepatitis C virus, alcohol, hemochromatosis, and others. Clin Liver Dis 2007;11(1):173–89, x.
10. Powell EE, Jonsson JR, Clouston AD. Metabolic factors and non-alcoholic fatty liver disease as co-factors in other liver diseases. Dig Dis 2010;28(1):186–91.
11. Teli MR, James OF, Burt AD, Bennett MK, Day CP. The natural history of nonalcoholic fatty liver: a follow-up study. Hepatology 1995;22(6):1714–19.
12. Matteoni CA, Younossi ZM, Gramlich T, Boparai N, Liu YC, McCullough AJ. Nonalcoholic fatty liver disease: a spectrum of clinical and pathological severity. Gastroenterology 1999;116(6):1413–19.
13. Soderberg C, Stal P, Askling J, et al. Decreased survival of subjects with elevated liver function tests during a 28-year follow-up. Hepatology 2010;51(2):595–602.
14. Musso G, Gambino R, Cassader M, Pagano G. Meta-analysis: natural history of non-alcoholic fatty liver disease (NAFLD) and diagnostic accuracy of non-invasive tests for liver disease severity. Ann Med 2011;43(8):617–49.
15. Adams LA, Lymp JF, St Sauver J, et al. The natural history of nonalcoholic fatty liver disease: a population-based cohort study. Gastroenterology 2005;129(1):113–21.
16. Wong VW, Wong GL, Tsang SW, et al. High prevalence of colorectal neoplasm in patients with non-alcoholic steatohepatitis. Gut 2011;60(6):829–36.
17. Aron-Wisnewsky J, Minville C, Tordjman J, et al. Chronic intermittent hypoxia is a major trigger for non-alcoholic fatty liver disease in morbid obese. J Hepatol 2012;56(1):225–33.
18. Reddy SK, Marsh JW, Varley PR, et al. Underlying steatohepatitis, but not simple hepatic steatosis, increases morbidity after liver resection: a case-control study. Hepatology 2012;56(6):2221–30.
19. Youssef NA, Abdelmalek MF, Binks M, et al. Associations of depression, anxiety and antidepressants with histological severity of nonalcoholic fatty liver disease. Liver Int 2013;33(7):1062–70.

20. Bonora E, Targher G. Increased risk of cardiovascular disease and chronic kidney disease in NAFLD. Nat Rev Gastroenterol Hepatol 2012;9(7):372–81.

21. Armstrong MJ, Adams LA, Canbay A, Syn WK. Extrahepatic complications of nonalcoholic fatty liver disease. Hepatology 2014;59:1174–97.

22. Bedossa P, Moucari R, Chelbi E, et al. Evidence for a role of nonalcoholic steatohepatitis in hepatitis C: a prospective study. Hepatology 2007;46(2):380–7.

23. Naveau S, Giraud V, Borotto E, Aubert A, Capron F, Chaput JC. Excess weight is a risk factor for alcoholic liver disease. Hepatology 1997;25:108–11.

24. Powell EE, Ali A, Clouston AD, et al. Steatosis is a cofactor in liver injury in hemochromatosis. Gastroenterology 2005; 129(6):1937–43.

25. Neuschwander-Tetri BA. Hepatic lipotoxicity and the pathogenesis of NASH: the central role of nontriglyceride fatty acid metabolites. Hepatology 2010;52:774–88.

26. Cusi K. Role of obesity and lipotoxicity in the development of nonalcoholic steatohepatitis: pathophysiology and clinical implications. Gastroenterology 2012;142(4):711–725.e6.

27. Ratziu V, Charlotte F, Heurtier A, et al. Sampling variability of liver biopsy in nonalcoholic fatty liver disease. Gastroenterology 2005;128(7):1898–906.

28. Merriman RB, Ferrell LD, Patti MG, et al. Correlation of paired liver biopsies in morbidly obese patients with suspected nonalcoholic fatty liver disease. Hepatology 2006;44(4):874–80.

29. Kleiner DE, Brunt EM, Van Natta M, et al. Design and validation of a histological scoring system for nonalcoholic fatty liver disease. Hepatology 2005;41(6):1313–21.

30. Bedossa P. Utility and appropriateness of the fatty liver inhibition of progression (FLIP) algorithm and steatosis, activity, and fibrosis (SAF) score in the evaluation of biopsies of nonalcoholic fatty liver disease. Hepatology 2014; 60(2):565–75.

31. Kleiner D, Brunt E. Nonalcoholic fatty liver disease: pathologic patterns and biopsy evaluation in clinical research. Semin Liver Dis 2012;32(1):3–13.

32. Brunt EM, Kleiner DE, Wilson LA, Belt P, Neuschwander-Tetri BA. Nonalcoholic fatty liver disease (NAFLD) activity score and the histopathologic diagnosis in NAFLD: distinct clinicopathologic meanings. Hepatology 2011;53(3):810–20.

33. Lackner C, Gogg-Kamerer M, Zatloukal K, Stumptner C, Brunt EM, Denk H. Ballooned hepatocytes in steatohepatitis: the value of keratin immunohistochemistry for diagnosis. J Hepatol 2008;48(5):821–8.

34. Caldwell SH, Oelsner DH, Iezzoni JC, Hespenheide EE, Battle EH, Driscoll CJ. Cryptogenic cirrhosis: clinical characterization and risk factors for underlying disease. Hepatology 1999;29:664–9.

35. Ratziu V, Bonyhay L, Di Martino V, et al. Survival, liver failure, and hepatocellular carcinoma in obesity-related cryptogenic cirrhosis. Hepatology 2002;35(6):1485–93.

36. Brunt EM, Kleiner DE, Wilson LA, et al. Portal chronic inflammation in nonalcoholic fatty liver disease (NAFLD): a histologic marker of advanced NAFLD-Clinicopathologic correlations from the nonalcoholic steatohepatitis clinical research network. Hepatology 2009;49(3):809–20.

37. Pais R, Charlotte F, Fedchuk L, et al. A systematic review of follow-up biopsies reveals disease progression in patients with non-alcoholic fatty liver. J Hepatol 2013;59:550–6.

38. Wong VWS, Wong GLH, Choi PCL, et al. Disease progression of non-alcoholic fatty liver disease: a prospective study with paired liver biopsies at 3 years. Gut 2010;59(7): 969–74.

39. Argo CK, Northup PG, Al-Osaimi AM, Caldwell SH. Systematic review of risk factors for fibrosis progression in non-alcoholic steatohepatitis. J Hepatol 2009;51(2):371–9.

40. Younossi ZM, Stepanova M, Rafiq N, et al. Pathologic criteria for nonalcoholic steatohepatitis: interprotocol agreement and ability to predict liver-related mortality. Hepatology 2011;53(6):1874–82.

41. Ekstedt M, Franzen LE, Mathiesen UL, Kechagias S. Low clinical relevance of the nonalcoholic fatty liver disease activity score (NAS) in predicting fibrosis progression. Scand J Gastroenterol 2012;47(1):108–15.

42. Ekstedt M, Hagstrom H, Nasr P, et al. Fibrosis stage is the strongest predictor for disease-specific mortality in NAFLD after up to 33 years of follow-up. Hepatology 2015; 61:1547–54.

43. Angulo P, Kleiner D, Dam-Larsen S, et al. Prognostic relevance of liver histology in NAFLD: the PREHLIN study. Hepatology 2014;60:226A.

44. Ryan MC, Itsiopoulos C, Thodis T, et al. The Mediterranean diet improves hepatic steatosis and insulin sensitivity in individuals with non-alcoholic fatty liver disease. J Hepatol 2013;59(1):138–43.

45. Kirk E, Reeds DN, Finck BN, Mayurranjan SM, Patterson BW, Klein S. Dietary fat and carbohydrates differentially alter insulin sensitivity during caloric restriction. Gastroenterology 2009;136(5):1552–60.

46. Safadi R, Konikoff FM, Mahamid M, et al. The fatty acid-bile acid conjugate aramchol reduces liver fat content in patients with nonalcoholic Fatty liver disease. Clin Gastroenterol Hepatol 2014;12(12):2085–91 e1.

47. Saadeh S, Younossi ZM, Remer EM, et al. The utility of radiological imaging in nonalcoholic fatty liver disease. Gastroenterology 2002;123(3):745–50.

48. Fishbein M, Castro F, Cheruku S, et al. Hepatic MRI for fat quantitation: its relationship to fat morphology, diagnosis, and ultrasound. J Clin Gastroenterol 2005;39(7):619–25.

49. Ryan CK, Johnson LA, Germin BI, Marcos A. One hundred consecutive hepatic biopsies in the workup of living donors for right lobe liver transplantation. Liver Transpl 2002; 8(12):1114–22.

50. Park SH, Kim PN, Kim KW, et al. Macrovesicular hepatic steatosis in living liver donors: use of CT for quantitative and qualitative assessment. Radiology 2006;239(1):105–12.

51. Bedogni G, Bellentani S, Miglioli L, et al. The Fatty Liver Index: a simple and accurate predictor of hepatic steatosis in the general population. BMC Gastroenterol 2006;6:33.

52. Poynard T, Lassailly G, Diaz E, et al. Performance of biomarkers FibroTest, ActiTest, SteatoTest, and NashTest in patients with severe obesity: meta analysis of individual patient data. PLoS One 2012;7(3):e30325.

53. Poynard T, Ratziu V, Naveau S, et al. The diagnostic value of biomarkers (SteatoTest) for the prediction of liver steatosis. Comp Hepatol 2005;4:10.

54. Kotronen A, Peltonen M, Hakkarainen A, et al. Prediction of non-alcoholic fatty liver disease and liver fat using metabolic and genetic factors. Gastroenterology 2009;137(3):865–72.

55. Cuthbertson DJ, Weickert MO, Lythgoe D, et al. External validation of the fatty liver index and lipid accumulation product indices, using 1H-magnetic resonance spectroscopy, to identify hepatic steatosis in healthy controls and obese, insulin-resistant individuals. Eur J Endocrinol 2014;171(5):561–9.

56. Zelber-Sagi S, Webb M, Assy N, et al. Comparison of fatty liver index with noninvasive methods for steatosis detection and quantification. World J Gastroenterol 2013;19(1): 57–64.

57. Jiang ZY, Xu CY, Chang XX, et al. Fatty liver index correlates with non-alcoholic fatty liver disease, but not with newly diagnosed coronary artery atherosclerotic disease in Chinese patients. BMC Gastroenterol 2013;13:110.

58. Ruhl CE, Everhart JE. Fatty liver indices in the multiethnic United States National Health and Nutrition Examination Survey. Aliment Pharmacol Ther 2015;41(1):65–76.

59. Bozkurt L, Gobl CS, Tura A, et al. Fatty liver index predicts further metabolic deteriorations in women with previous gestational diabetes. PLoS One 2012;7(2):e32710.

60. Ruckert IM, Heier M, Rathmann W, Baumeister SE, Doring A, Meisinger C. Association between markers of fatty liver disease and impaired glucose regulation in men and women from the general population: the KORA-F4-study. PLoS One 2011;6(8):e22932.

61. Balkau B, Lange C, Vol S, Fumeron F, Bonnet F. Nine-year incident diabetes is predicted by fatty liver indices: the French D.E.S.I.R. study. BMC Gastroenterol 2010;10:56.

62. Gastaldelli A, Kozakova M, Hojlund K, et al. Fatty liver is associated with insulin resistance, risk of coronary heart disease, and early atherosclerosis in a large European population. Hepatology 2009;49(5):1537–44.

63. Calori G, Lattuada G, Ragogna F, et al. Fatty liver index and mortality: the cremona study in the 15th year of follow-up. Hepatology 2011;54(1):145–52.

64. Lerchbaum E, Pilz S, Grammer TB, et al. The fatty liver index is associated with increased mortality in subjects referred to coronary angiography. Nutr Metab Cardiovasc Dis 2013;23(12):1231–8.

65. Zelber-Sagi S, Nitzan-Kaluski D, Goldsmith R, et al. Role of leisure-time physical activity in nonalcoholic fatty liver disease: a population-based study. Hepatology 2008;48(6): 1791–8.

66. Lassailly G, Caiazzo R, Hollebecque A, et al. Validation of non-invasive biomarkers (FibroTest, SteatoTest, and NashTest) for prediction of liver injury in patients with morbid obesity. Eur J Gastroenterol Hepatol 2011;23(6):499–506.

67. Perazzo H, Munteanu M, Ngo Y, et al. Prognostic value of liver fibrosis and steatosis biomarkers in type-2 diabetes and dyslipidaemia. Aliment Pharmacol Ther 2014;40(9): 1081–93.

68. Guiu B, Crevisy-Girod E, Binquet C, et al. Prediction for steatosis in type-2 diabetes: clinico-biological markers versus 1H-MR spectroscopy. Eur Radiol 2011;22(4):855–63.

69. Fedchuk L, Nascimbeni F, Pais R, Charlotte F, Housset C, Ratziu V. Performance and limitations of steatosis biomarkers in patients with nonalcoholic fatty liver disease. Aliment Pharmacol Ther 2014;40(10):1209–22.

70. de Ledinghen V, Vergniol J, Capdepont M, et al. Controlled attenuation parameter (CAP) for the diagnosis of steatosis: a prospective study of 5323 examinations. J Hepatol 2014;60(5):1026–31.

71. Boursier J, Cales P. Controlled attenuation parameter (CAP): a new device for fast evaluation of liver fat? Liver Int 2012;32(6):875–7.

72. Machado MV, Cortez-Pinto H. Non-invasive diagnosis of non-alcoholic fatty liver disease. A critical appraisal. J Hepatol 2013;58(5):1007–19.

73. Kwok R, Tse YK, Wong GL, et al. Systematic review with meta-analysis: non-invasive assessment of non-alcoholic fatty liver disease—the role of transient elastography and plasma cytokeratin-18 fragments. Aliment Pharmacol Ther 2014;39(3):254–69.

74. Feldstein AE, Wieckowska A, Lopez AR, Liu YC, Zein NN, McCullough AJ. Cytokeratin-18 fragment levels as noninvasive biomarkers for nonalcoholic steatohepatitis: a multicenter validation study. Hepatology 2009;50:1072–8.

75. Younossi ZM, Jarrar M, Nugent C, et al. A novel diagnostic biomarker panel for obesity-related nonalcoholic steatohepatitis. Obes Surg 2008;18(11):1430–7.

76. Tamimi TI, Elgouhari HM, Alkhouri N, et al. An apoptosis panel for nonalcoholic steatohepatitis diagnosis. J Hepatol 2011;54(6):1224–9.

77. Anty R, Iannelli A, Patouraux S, et al. A new composite model including metabolic syndrome, alanine aminotransferase and cytokeratin-18 for the diagnosis of non-alcoholic steatohepatitis in morbidly obese patients. Aliment Pharmacol Ther 2010;32(11–12):1315–22.

78. Cusi K, Chang Z, Harrison S, et al. Limited value of plasma cytokeratin-18 as a biomarker for NASH and fibrosis in patients with non-alcoholic fatty liver disease. J Hepatol 2014;60(1):167–74.

79. Ratziu V, Sheikh MY, Sanyal AJ, et al. A phase 2, randomized, double-blind, placebo-controlled study of GS-9450 in subjects with nonalcoholic steatohepatitis. Hepatology 2012;55(2):419–28.

80. Vuppalanchi R, Jain AK, Deppe R, et al. Relationship between changes in serum levels of keratin 18 and changes in liver histology in children and adults with nonalcoholic fatty liver disease. Clin Gastroenterol Hepatol 2014;12(12): 2121–2130.e2.

81. Angulo P, Hui JM, Marchesini G, et al. The NAFLD fibrosis score: a noninvasive system that identifies liver fibrosis in patients with NAFLD. Hepatology 2007;45(4):846–54.

82. Shah AG, Lydecker A, Murray K, Tetri BN, Contos MJ, Sanyal AJ. Comparison of noninvasive markers of fibrosis in patients with nonalcoholic fatty liver disease. Clin Gastroenterol Hepatol 2009;7(10):1104–12.

83. Harrison SA, Oliver D, Arnold HL, Gogia S, Neuschwander-Tetri BA. Development and validation of a simple NAFLD clinical scoring system for identifying patients without advanced disease. Gut 2008;57(10):1441–7.

84. Ratziu V, Massard J, Charlotte F, et al. Diagnostic value of biochemical markers (FibroTest-FibroSURE) for the prediction of liver fibrosis in patients with non-alcoholic fatty liver disease. BMC Gastroenterol 2006;6:6.

85. Cales P, Laine F, Boursier J, et al. Comparison of blood tests for liver fibrosis specific or not to NAFLD. J Hepatol 2009;50(1):165–73.

86. Guha IN, Parkes J, Roderick P, et al. Noninvasive markers of fibrosis in nonalcoholic fatty liver disease: validating the European Liver Fibrosis Panel and exploring simple markers. Hepatology 2008;47(2):455–60.

87. Kim D, Kim WR, Kim HJ, Therneau TM. Association between noninvasive fibrosis markers and mortality among adults with nonalcoholic fatty liver disease in the United States. Hepatology 2013;57(4):1357–65.

88. Angulo P, Bugianesi E, Bjornsson ES, et al. Simple noninvasive systems predict long-term outcomes of patients with nonalcoholic fatty liver disease. Gastroenterology 2013; 145(4):782–9 e4.

89. Treeprasertsuk S, Bjornsson E, Enders F, Suwanwalaikorn S, Lindor KD. NAFLD fibrosis score: a prognostic predictor for mortality and liver complications among NAFLD patients. World J Gastroenterol 2013;19(8):1219–29.

90. Chang Y, Jung HS, Yun KE, Cho J, Cho YK, Ryu S. Cohort study of non-alcoholic fatty liver disease, NAFLD fibrosis score, and the risk of incident diabetes in a Korean population. Am J Gastroenterol 2013;108(12):1861–8.

91. McPherson S, Anstee QM, Henderson E, Day CP, Burt AD. Are simple noninvasive scoring systems for fibrosis reliable in patients with NAFLD and normal ALT levels? Eur J Gastroenterol Hepatol 2013;25(6):652–8.

92. Wong VW, Vergniol J, Wong GL, et al. Diagnosis of fibrosis and cirrhosis using liver stiffness measurement in nonalcoholic fatty liver disease. Hepatology 2010;51(2):454–62.

93. Castera L, Foucher J, Bernard PH, et al. Pitfalls of liver stiffness measurement: a 5-year prospective study of 13,369 examinations. Hepatology 2010;51(3):828–35.

94. Wong VW, Vergniol J, Wong GL, et al. Liver stiffness measurement using XL probe in patients with nonalcoholic fatty liver disease. Am J Gastroenterol 2012;107(12): 1862–71.

95. Petta S, Vanni E, Bugianesi E, et al. The combination of liver stiffness measurement and NAFLD fibrosis score improves the noninvasive diagnostic accuracy for severe liver fibrosis in patients with nonalcoholic fatty liver disease. Liver Int 2015;35:1566–73.

96. Ferraioli G, Tinelli C, Dal Bello B, Zicchetti M, Filice G, Filice C. Accuracy of real-time shear wave elastography for assessing liver fibrosis in chronic hepatitis C: a pilot study. Hepatology 2012;56(6):2125–33.

97. Poynard T, Munteanu M, Luckina E, et al. Liver fibrosis evaluation using real-time shear wave elastography: applicability and diagnostic performance using methods without a gold standard. J Hepatol 2013;58(5):928–35.

98. Crespo G, Fernández-Varo G, Mariño Z, et al. ARFI, FibroScan®, ELF, and their combinations in the assessment of liver fibrosis: a prospective study. J Hepatol 2012;57(2): 281–7.

99. Cassinotto C, Lapuyade B, Mouries A, et al. Non-invasive assessment of liver fibrosis with impulse elastography: comparison of supersonic shear imaging with ARFI and FibroScan®. J Hepatol 2014;61(3):550–7.

100. Fracanzani AL, Valenti L, Bugianesi E, et al. Risk of severe liver disease in nonalcoholic fatty liver disease with normal aminotransferase levels: a role for insulin resistance and diabetes. Hepatology 2008;48(3):792–8.

101. Mofrad P, Contos MJ, Haque M, et al. Clinical and histologic spectrum of nonalcoholic fatty liver disease associated with normal ALT values. Hepatology 2003;37(6): 1286–92.

# 14

# The clinical utility of noninvasive blood tests and elastography

**Emmanuel A. Tsochatzis and Massimo Pinzani**

Institute for Liver and Digestive Health, University College London, Royal Free Hospital, London, UK

## LEARNING POINTS

- Risk stratification in patients with NAFLD is possible with simple noninvasive tests that consist of simple laboratory indices and clinical information.

- Although noninvasive methods require further validation, they are useful for selecting among NAFLD patients those who require secondary care referral or a liver biopsy.

- FIB4 and NAFLD fibrosis score can rule out advanced fibrosis with a negative predictive value of >95% and thus prevent unnecessary referrals in a significant number of patients.

- More refined noninvasive tests, such as elastography, FibroTest™, or ELF™, could be used as second tier tests to further characterize patients, although this sequential approach will need prospective validation.

## Introduction

NAFLD affects ~20% of the general population and encompasses a wide spectrum of liver disease, from simple steatosis to necroinflammation, fibrosis, and cirrhosis [1]. Non-alcoholic steatohepatitis (NASH) is the progressive form of NAFLD and affects 15–20% of patients with NAFLD [2]. Only patients with steatohepatitis have increased liver-related mortality [1].

Data on natural history of NAFLD are still scarce: in a meta-analysis of 10 studies comprising 221 patients, 37.6% had progressive fibrosis, 41.6% had no change, and 20.8% had improvement in fibrosis over a mean follow-up of 5.3 years [3]. Age and initial necroinflammation grade were the only factors associated with progression of fibrosis [3]. From a liver point of view and in the absence of specific treatment, the hallmarks in the progression of NAFLD are the development of NASH and the diagnosis of advanced fibrosis. The former is associated with potential progressive liver disease and the latter is the hallmark for targeted interventions and screening for complications of chronic liver disease, with a particular attention to the early development of hepatocellular carcinoma (HCC).

Therefore, NAFLD is a disease of high prevalence and relatively low severity in the majority of patients. Although liver biopsy is the gold standard for diagnosing steatohepatitis and assessing disease severity, it would be inappropriate to biopsy every patient diagnosed with NAFLD, as it is a costly and invasive procedure, which is associated with patient discomfort and potential side effects. In order to address this rising need, noninvasive tests and strategies have been developed that attempt to diagnose NASH and stage the disease.

In this chapter, we review the evidence on the use of noninvasive blood tests and imaging techniques based on elastography for diagnosing NASH and staging fibrosis.

## Use of noninvasive fibrosis tests in chronic liver diseases

During the last few years, there has been an explosive development and use of noninvasive fibrosis tests (NILTs) [4, 5]. The NILTs can be broadly divided into three categories: simple or indirect serum markers, direct serum markers, and imaging modalities [4].

*Clinical Dilemmas in Non-Alcoholic Fatty Liver Disease*, First Edition. Edited by Roger Williams and Simon D. Taylor-Robinson.
© 2016 John Wiley & Sons, Ltd. Published 2016 by John Wiley & Sons, Ltd.

Indirect serum markers or class II biomarkers consist of the combination of routine biochemical tests, such as transaminases, platelet count and albumin, and patient demographics that are associated with fibrosis, such as age or the presence of diabetes [4]. These tests usually have dual cutoffs: a high cutoff with high specificity and a low cutoff with high sensitivity. Depending on the clinical scenario and the disease prevalence, the low or high cutoff is used at the expense of increased false positives and false negatives, respectively. If these cutoffs are combined, then the numbers of false positives and false negatives are minimized. However, a number of patients will fall in the indeterminate range of fibrosis (i.e., their score will be between the low and the high cutoff) and will need either further noninvasive testing or liver biopsy.

Direct serum noninvasive tests (class I biomarkers) are supposed to detect extracellular matrix turnover and/or fibrogenic cell changes [4]. The most common markers used in current assays involve measuring products of extracellular matrix synthesis or degradation and the enzymes that regulate their production or modification, such as hyaluronic acid, serum collagenases and their inhibitors, and profibrogenic cytokines. It should be noted that these markers are not exclusively found in liver tissue; therefore, they reflect fibrogenic processes in various other organs and their diagnostic value become questionable in aging patients with comorbidities such as atherosclerosis and chronic lung disorders. Moreover, their sensitivity is low in the initial stages of fibrosis.

Various direct and indirect tests have been combined in patented commercial algorithms that improve the diagnostic accuracy of tests when used singly. In the case of NAFLD, these are FibroTest, ELF, and FibroMeters. Among them, FibroTest (FibroSure in the United States) is the most widely validated panel: it consists of five parameters and has been studied in viral hepatitis, NAFLD, and alcohol-related liver disease (ALD) [6]. FibroMeters are a family of 6 blood tests: one for staging and one for quantifying liver fibrosis in each of the 3 main causes of liver disease (chronic viral hepatitis, ALD, and NAFLD) [7]. The ELF biomarker is a panel of direct noninvasive markers that includes hyaluronic acid, type III collagen, and tissue inhibitor of metalloproteinase-1 (TIMP-1) [8].

New imaging modalities offer better sensitivity and specificity than conventional techniques, such as ultrasound, CT, and MRI. The latter can only identify cirrhosis, based on imaging findings of coarse echo-texture,

collaterals suggestive of portal hypertension and nodularity. These new modalities measure liver elasticity, or liver stiffness, based on MR or US techniques. The most widely used imaging modality is transient elastography or FibroScan™ (Echosens, Paris) [9]. Briefly, an ultrasound transducer, inducing an elastic shear wave that propagates within the liver, transmits vibrations of mild amplitude and low frequency. Pulse-echo ultrasonic acquisitions are performed to follow the shear wave and measure its speed, which is directly related to the tissue stiffness. Results are expressed in kilopascals (kPa) and correspond to the median value of ten validated measurements. The volume of liver tissue evaluated by TE is at least 100 times bigger than a liver biopsy. Moreover, TE is painless and rapid (<5 min) and thus highly acceptable for patients.

Other modalities include acoustic radiation force impulse (ARFI) [10], supersonic shear imaging (SSI) [11], and MR elastography (MRE) [12]. ARFI allows the evaluation of liver stiffness in a region of interest (ROI) involving mechanical excitation of tissue, by the use of short-duration acoustic pulses, while performing a real-time B-mode conventional hepatic U/S. Results are expressed in (m/s). Although the volume of liver explored is smaller than that for TE, a critical advantage is the possibility to choose the representative area of interest, therefore avoiding large vessels and ribs. An advantage over TE is that it can be easily incorporated into a modified US machine. It should be noted that quality criteria for ARFI have not yet been established.

SSI, also named shear wave elastography, is also built on an US device and does not require an external vibrator to produce the shear wave [11]. In contrast to FibroScan and ARFI where a single shear wave is emitted at a single frequency for each measurement, in SSI a plurality of pulse wave beams at increasing depths are emitted, using a very wide frequency band from 60 to 600 Hz, therefore allowing the synchronous evaluation of several shear wave fronts over a wide frequency range. By generating a real-time color mapping of the elasticity encoded pixel by pixel in an image superimposed on the standard B-mode, SSI allows a quantitative image of the tissue elasticity. By placing an ROI in the center of the color mapping, the calculated value is the mean of values with the ROI. MRE uses a modified phase-contrast method to evaluate the propagation of the shear waves within the liver. It is a very promising technique but is not yet widely available and cost might be an important limiting factor.

A major limitation of all the aforementioned NILTs is the absence of uniformly established and validated cutoffs for specific etiologies of liver disease and fibrosis stages and the poor methodological quality of many of the published studies. In a recent meta-analysis on transient elastography, only 6 of 41 included studies had both histological evaluation and FibroScan™ measurements optimally performed, while all studies had a high risk of bias, based on quality assessment by the QUADAS tool [13].

## Noninvasive diagnosis of NASH

NASH is the lynchpin between steatosis and cirrhosis in the spectrum of NAFLD and is characterized by necroinflammation, hepatocellular ballooning, and apoptosis that could lead to fibrosis and cirrhosis. Although there is a large clinical need for noninvasive assessment, the diagnosis of NASH is still largely based on liver biopsy, as there are no well-validated noninvasive tests.

The best-studied noninvasive marker for differentiating NASH is an apoptotic marker, namely, caspase generated cytokeratin 18 (CK-18) fragments in the serum. CK-18 is the major intermediate filament protein in the liver and is cleaved by effector caspases during the apoptotic process. Plasma CK-18 fragments have been evaluated in more than 10 cohort studies of patients with NAFLD, but the cutoffs for diagnosing NASH varied between studies and were not prospectively validated [14]. Feldstein evaluated CK-18 fragments in 139 patients with biopsy-proven NAFLD and 150 age-matched healthy controls and reported an AUROC of 0.83 with sensitivity and specificity of 0.75 and 0.81, respectively [15]. In the largest study to date, the initial enthusiasm on the use of CK-18 as a stand-alone test was tampered, as in a multiethnic cohort of 424 patients the sensitivity for NASH was low despite a high specificity, thus making this inadequate as a screening test [16].

All the other potential noninvasive tests for diagnosing NASH were evaluated in single studies and small cohorts of patients and therefore need further validation.

NashTest™ is a proprietary noninvasive algorithm for the diagnosis of NASH that combines 13 parameters [17]. This test categorizes patients into three groups: "not NASH," borderline NASH, and NASH with AUROCs that range between 0.69 and 0.83.

In a Japanese study with an estimation and validation cohort and 619 patients in total, serum ferritin ($\geq$200 ng/mL in females or $\geq$300 ng/mL in males), fasting insulin ($\geq$10 μU/mL), and type IV collagen 7S ($\geq$5.0 ng/mL) were combined in a weighted sum and formed a composite score for predicting NASH, called the NAFIC score [18]. This score had an AUROC of 0.78–0.85 for predicting NASH; however, it needs validation in Western populations as well.

In a single study, terminal peptide of procollagen III (PIIINP), which is involved in fibrogenesis, was identified as a potential biomarker of NASH using a derivation and validation cohort of 65 and 71 patients in respectively with an AUROC of 0.77–0.82 [19]. This will need validation in larger cohorts, as the sample size was low and the groups with simple steatosis/borderline NASH and NASH were disproportionate. All the aforementioned tests are summarized in Table 14.1.

Therefore, despite the huge clinical need, the tools for noninvasive diagnosis of NASH still remain inadequate. The fact that the diagnosis of NASH does not necessarily incorporate fibrosis and the considerable interobserver variability in the histological diagnosis of NASH further complicate this issue. A combination of biomarkers that evaluate apoptosis, necroinflammation, and fibrosis might be the most appropriate tool for diagnosing NASH and currently remains an unmet need.

**TABLE 14.1** Noninvasive tests for diagnosing NASH in patients with non-alcoholic fatty liver disease

| Test | Number of studies | Components | AUROC |
|---|---|---|---|
| CK-18 fragments | >5 | CK-18 | 0.83 |
| NashTest™ | 1 | Age, sex, height, weight, triglycerides, cholesterol, a2-macroglobulin, ALT, GGT, ALT, AST, bilirubin, haptoglobin, apolipoprotein a1 | 0.79 |
| NAFIC | 1 | Ferritin, fasting insulin, type IV collagen | 0.78–0.85 |
| PIIINP | 1 | PIIINP | 0.77–0.84 |

## Noninvasive fibrosis assessment

### Serum biomarkers

Various combinations and algorithms of potential serum biomarkers have been used in NAFLD as shown in Table 14.2. The combination of simple laboratory parameters with clinical variables has resulted in simple scores that can be used at the point of care and have an excellent negative predictive value of >95% for advanced fibrosis (≥F3) in unselected cohorts of NAFLD patients. The most commonly used scores are the NAFLD fibrosis score [20] and FIB4 [21]. NAFLD fibrosis score incorporates age, BMI, presence of diabetes, AST, ALT, platelet count, and albumin, whereas FIB4 consists of age, AST, ALT, and platelet count. They both have dual cutoffs, that is, a low cutoff with a high sensitivity and a high cutoff with a high specificity. Their main clinical utility derives from the low cutoff, which can be used to rule out patients from further investigations and/ or liver biopsy. Most importantly, they have been validated against clinical outcomes; in a retrospective cohort study of 320 patients with almost 10 years of follow-up, patients with intermediate and high risk of advanced fibrosis according to the NAFLD fibrosis score had a hazard ratio of 4.2 and 9.8 for death compared to the low-risk group [22].

APRI and the ratio of aspartate aminotransferase to alanine aminotransferase (AST/ALT) are other simple scores that diagnose cirrhosis rather than advanced fibrosis and have not been extensively validated in NAFLD [23]. The BARD score was created from the retrospective analysis of 827 patients with NAFLD and consists of body mass index (BMI), presence of diabetes, and AST/ALT ratio [24]. A cutoff point of 2 is used to predict advanced fibrosis; however, the diagnostic accuracy is lower than NAFLD fibrosis score and FIB4.

Serum ferritin has also been proposed as a marker of NASH; in the NASH CRN cohort of 628 patients, a serum ferritin >1.5 the upper limit of normal was an independent predictor of advanced fibrosis. In a cohort of 111 patients, serum ferritin was independently associated with both the presence of NASH and more severe fibrosis [25]. Clearly, these data need further validation and ideally ferritin should be incorporated in one of the algorithms of fibrosis assessment.

**TABLE 14.2** Noninvasive fibrosis tests in patients with non-alcoholic fatty liver disease

| Test | Components | Fibrosis stage assessed | Cutoff | AUROC/other measures |
|---|---|---|---|---|
| *Nonproprietary serum tests* | | | | |
| AST/ALT ratio | AST, ALT | F4 | 1 | NA |
| APRI | AST, platelet count | F2, F4 | F2: <0.5, >1.5 F4: <1, >2 | F4: 0.85 |
| FIB-4 | Age, AST, ALT, platelet count | F3 | <1.45, >3.25 | 0.85 |
| NAFLD fibrosis score | Age, BMI, diabetes. AST, ALT, platelet count, albumin | F3 | < −1.455, >0.676 | 0.88 |
| BARD | BMI, AST/ALT ratio, diabetes | F3 | ≥2 | NA |
| Hepascore | Age, sex, a2-macroglobulin, hyaluronic acid, bilirubin, GGT | F3 | 0.37 | 0.84 |
| *Proprietary serum tests* | | | | |
| FibroTest™ | Bilirubin, haptoglobin, GGT, a2-macroglobulin, apolipoprotein A | | <0.3, >0.7 | NPV:0.98 PPV: 0.60 |
| ELF™ | Hyaluronic acid, PIIINP, TIMP-1 | F2, F3, F4 | F3: 9.5 | 0.90 |
| FibroMeter™ | Age, weight, glucose, AST, ALT, platelet count, ferritin | F3 | <0.611, >0.715 | 0.94 |
| *Elastography modalities* | | | | |
| FibroScan™ | US based | All stages | F4: >10.5 | 0.92 |
| ARFI™ | US based | All stages | To be defined | >0.90 |
| Shear wave elastography | US based | All stages | No specific data on NAFLD | >0.90 |
| MR elastography | MR based | All stages | No specific data on NAFLD | >0.90 |

Finally, the Hepascore has been evaluated in a single study and showed an acceptable diagnostic accuracy ≥F3, although not significantly better than NAFLD fibrosis score and FIB4 [26].

## Proprietary panels

The FibroTest™, the FibroMeter NAFLD™, and the ELF™ score are the proprietary panels that have been used for fibrosis assessment in NAFLD (Table 14.2). The FibroTest™, which has been best validated in CHC, uses a dual cutoff to "rule in" or "rule out" patients with advanced fibrosis, but up to a third of patients will fall in the indeterminate range of values and thus will require further assessment and/or biopsy [27]. The FibroMeter NAFLD™ had an AUROC of 0.94 for predicting significant fibrosis in 235 patients with NAFLD and performs better than the NAFLD fibrosis score and APRI [28]. ELF™ was evaluated in 192 adults and had a sensitivity of 0.8 and a specificity of 0.93 for advanced fibrosis [29]. The diagnostic accuracy of ELF™ was even higher in pediatric patients with NASH, with an AUROC of 0.95. All the aforementioned proprietary panels need independent validation by groups not involved in their creation and also in non-Caucasian populations.

## Elastography

Transient elastography using FibroScan is the most widely evaluated imaging tool for fibrosis assessment in NAFLD. Although not as widely validated as in patients with CHC, FibroScan in patients with NAFLD has excellent diagnostic accuracy for the diagnosis of cirrhosis and acceptable but not ideal accuracy for the diagnosis of fibrosis stage, F2 [30]. Although not definitely proven, it appears that steatosis influences the liver stiffness measurements, thus resulting in slightly lower values than CHC. It should be noted that there are no validated cutoff values for specific fibrosis stages and this remains a weakness of FibroScan™ [13].

Using the conventional M probe, liver stiffness measurements are uninterpretable in 19% of the cases and this is mainly due to increased waist circumference and BMI, as is frequently the case in patients with NAFLD [31]. This drawback of FibroScan™ in patients with NAFLD was recently addressed by the development of a dedicated XL probe for patients with high BMI. The use of this probe in patients with high BMI reduces the rate of failures from 10 to 2% and also the rate of unreliable results from 33 to 25%, as shown in a cohort of 193 patients with NAFLD [32]. Pairwise examination showed that liver stiffness measurement by the XL was lower than by the M probe; thus, a separate set of diagnostic cutoff values need to be validated for the XL probe [32]. The controlled attenuation parameter (CAP) incorporated in the new FibroScan™ machines can also quantify steatosis, although this requires further validation [33]. As with other noninvasive fibrosis tests, FibroScan™ is reliable for diagnosing the extremes of the fibrosis spectrum (no fibrosis/cirrhosis) but of less value in intermediate fibrosis stages.

ARFI™ was compared with elastography in two small studies with <100 patients in NAFLD and was of similar diagnostic accuracy [23]. It resulted in less exam failures compared to FibroScan™ using the M probe, whereas there the success rates were similar when compared to the XL probe. Clearly, larger studies in NAFLD and the validation of specific cutoffs are needed.

There are no dedicated studies of SSI and MRE in patients with NAFLD to date. In a recent study comparing SSI with FibroScan and ARFI in 349 patients with chronic liver disease, SSI had a significantly higher accuracy than FibroScan for ≥F3 and a significantly higher accuracy than ARFI for ≥F2 [11]. MRE has shown AUROCs of >0.90 in cohorts of patients with various etiologies of liver disease; however, the inclusion of normal control might have resulted in the overestimation of diagnostic accuracy [12]. Both SSI and MRE need further validation in patients with NAFLD.

## Conclusions: Future directions

NAFLD is the most common cause of abnormal transaminases, and its prevalence will further increase given the current epidemic of obesity. Noninvasive strategies are urgently needed to diagnose NASH and stratify patients who will need secondary referral and specialist follow-up. Although the noninvasive diagnosis of NASH is still an unmet need, risk stratification is possible with simple noninvasive tests that consist of simple laboratory indices and clinical information. FIB4 and NAFLD fibrosis score can rule out advanced fibrosis with a negative predictive value of >95% and thus prevent unnecessary referrals in a significant number of patients. More refined noninvasive tests, such as elastography, FibroTest™, or ELF™, could be used as second tier tests to further characterize patients, although this sequential approach will need prospective validation. The development of such noninvasive algorithms, with the incorporation of efficacy and cost-effectiveness data, will likely limit the need for liver biopsy in a selected few in the future.

## References

1. Chalasani N, Younossi Z, Lavine JE, et al. The diagnosis and management of non-alcoholic fatty liver disease: practice guideline by the American Gastroenterological Association, American Association for the Study of Liver Diseases, and American College of Gastroenterology. Gastroenterology 2012;142:1592–609.
2. Qian MY, Yuwei JR, Angus P, et al. Efficacy and cost of a hepatocellular carcinoma screening program at an Australian teaching hospital. J Gastroenterol Hepatol 2010;25:951–6.
3. Argo CK, Northup PG, Al-Osaimi AM, et al. Systematic review of risk factors for fibrosis progression in non-alcoholic steatohepatitis. J Hepatol 2009;51:371–9.
4. Martinez SM, Crespo G, Navasa M, et al. Noninvasive assessment of liver fibrosis. Hepatology 2011;53:325–35.
5. Castera L. Noninvasive methods to assess liver disease in patients with hepatitis B or C. Gastroenterology 2012;142:1293–302.e4.
6. Imbert-Bismut F, Ratziu V, Pieroni L, et al. Biochemical markers of liver fibrosis in patients with hepatitis C virus infection: a prospective study. Lancet 2001;357:1069–75.
7. Cales P, Halfon P, Batisse D, et al. Comparison of liver fibrosis blood tests developed for HCV with new specific tests in HIV/HCV co-infection. J Hepatol 2010;52:S405.
8. Parkes J, Guha IN, Roderick P, et al. Enhanced Liver Fibrosis (ELF) test accurately identifies liver fibrosis in patients with chronic hepatitis C. J Viral Hepat 2011;18:23–31.
9. Castera L, Vergniol J, Foucher J, et al. Prospective comparison of transient elastography, FibroTest, APRI, and liver biopsy for the assessment of fibrosis in chronic hepatitis C. Gastroenterology 2005;128:343–50.
10. Lupsor M, Badea R, Stefanescu H, et al. Performance of a new elastographic method (ARFI technology) compared to unidimensional transient elastography in the noninvasive assessment of chronic hepatitis C. Preliminary results. J Gastrointestin Liver Dis 2009;18:303–10.
11. Cassinotto C, Lapuyade B, Mouries A, et al. Non-invasive assessment of liver fibrosis with impulse elastography: comparison of Supersonic Shear Imaging with ARFI and FibroScan(R). J Hepatol 2014;61:550–7.
12. Huwart L, Sempoux C, Vicaut E, et al. Magnetic resonance elastography for the noninvasive staging of liver fibrosis. Gastroenterology 2008;135:32–40.
13. Tsochatzis EA, Gurusamy KS, Ntaoula S, et al. Elastography for the diagnosis of severity of fibrosis in chronic liver disease: a meta-analysis of diagnostic accuracy. J Hepatol 2011;54:650–9.
14. Musso G, Gambino R, Cassader M, et al. Meta-analysis: natural history of non-alcoholic fatty liver disease (NAFLD) and diagnostic accuracy of non-invasive tests for liver disease severity. Ann Med 2011;43:617–49.
15. Feldstein AE, Wieckowska A, Lopez AR, et al. Cytokeratin-18 fragment levels as noninvasive biomarkers for nonalcoholic steatohepatitis: a multicenter validation study. Hepatology 2009;50:1072–8.
16. Cusi K, Chang Z, Harrison S, et al. Limited value of plasma cytokeratin-18 as a biomarker for NASH and fibrosis in patients with non-alcoholic fatty liver disease. J Hepatol 2014;60:167–74.
17. Poynard T, Ratziu V, Charlotte F, et al. Diagnostic value of biochemical markers (NashTest) for the prediction of non alcoholo steato hepatitis in patients with non-alcoholic fatty liver disease. BMC Gastroenterol 2006;6:34.
18. Sumida Y, Yoneda M, Hyogo H, et al. A simple clinical scoring system using ferritin, fasting insulin, and type IV collagen 7S for predicting steatohepatitis in nonalcoholic fatty liver disease. J Gastroenterol 2011;46:257–68.
19. Tanwar S, Trembling PM, Guha IN, et al. Validation of terminal peptide of procollagen III for the detection and assessment of nonalcoholic steatohepatitis in patients with nonalcoholic fatty liver disease. Hepatology 2013;57:103–11.
20. Angulo P, Hui JM, Marchesini G, et al. The NAFLD fibrosis score: a noninvasive system that identifies liver fibrosis in patients with NAFLD. Hepatology 2007;45:846–54.
21. Sumida Y, Yoneda M, Hyogo H, et al. Validation of the FIB4 index in a Japanese nonalcoholic fatty liver disease population. BMC Gastroenterol 2012;12.
22. Angulo P, Bugianesi E, Bjornsson ES, et al. Simple noninvasive systems predict long-term outcomes of patients with nonalcoholic fatty liver disease. Gastroenterology 2013;145:782–9.e4.
23. Castera L, Vilgrain V, Angulo P. Noninvasive evaluation of NAFLD. Nat Rev Gastroenterol Hepatol 2013;10:666–75.
24. Harrison SA, Oliver D, Arnold HL, et al. Development and validation of a simple NAFLD clinical scoring system for identifying patients without advanced disease. Gut 2008;57:1441–7.
25. Kowdley KV, Belt P, Wilson LA, et al. Serum ferritin is an independent predictor of histologic severity and advanced fibrosis in patients with nonalcoholic fatty liver disease. Hepatology 2012;55:77–85.
26. Adams LA, George J, Bugianesi E, et al. Complex noninvasive fibrosis models are more accurate than simple models in non-alcoholic fatty liver disease. J Gastroenterol Hepatol 2011;26:1536–43.
27. Ratziu V, Massard J, Charlotte F, et al. Diagnostic value of biochemical markers (FibroTest-FibroSure) for the prediction of liver fibrosis in patients with non-alcoholic fatty liver disease. BMC Gastroenterol 2006;6:6.
28. Cales P, Laine F, Boursier J, et al. Comparison of blood tests for liver fibrosis specific or not to NAFLD. J Hepatol 2009;50:165–73.

29. Guha IN, Parkes J, Roderick P, et al. Noninvasive markers of fibrosis in nonalcoholic fatty liver disease: validating the European liver fibrosis panel and exploring simple markers. Hepatology 2008;47:455–60.

30. Wong VWS, Vergniol J, Chan HLY, et al. Diagnostic power of FibroScan in predicting liver fibrosis in nonalcoholic fatty liver disease reply. Hepatology 2009;50:2049–50.

31. Castera L, Foucher J, Bernard PH, et al. Pitfalls of liver stiffness measurement: a 5-year prospective study of 13,369 examinations. Hepatology 2010;51:828–35.

32. Wong VW, Vergniol J, Wong GL, et al. Liver stiffness measurement using XL probe in patients with nonalcoholic fatty liver disease. Am J Gastroenterol 2012;107:1862–71.

33. Myers RP, Pollett A, Kirsch R, et al. Controlled Attenuation Parameter (CAP): a noninvasive method for the detection of hepatic steatosis based on transient elastography. Liver Int 2012;32:902–10.

# 15

# Are the guidelines—AASLD, IASL, EASL, and BSG—of help in the management of patients with NAFLD?

**Cristina Margini[1] and Jean-François Dufour[2]**

[1] Hepatology, Department of Clinical Research, University of Bern, Bern, Switzerland
[2] University Clinic for Visceral Surgery and Medicine, Inselspital University of Bern, Bern, Switzerland

---

## LEARNING POINTS

- An overview on the published guidelines with emphasis on the weak points and on the future research directions
- Guidelines position concerning screening policies
- A comparison of the diagnostic and therapeutic approach offered from the different guidelines
- Guidelines position concerning NAFLD in pediatric patients
- The increasing need of randomized controlled trial in order to establish evidence-based guidelines

---

What do we expect from a guideline? What should a guideline offer? In the context of constantly evolving scientific literature, guidelines should represent a reviewed and up-to-date source of information guiding physicians in their decisions and constitute the essential bridge connecting research to clinical practice. We expect guidelines to be helpful in patient management, to provide the stage for clinical research, and to be open to change and evolution. In the following pages, we will discuss the position of the European Association for the Study of the Liver (EASL) [1], the Italian Association for the Study of the Liver (IASL) [2], the American Association for the Study of Liver Diseases (AASLD) [3], the British Society of Gastroenterology (BSG), and the World Gastroenterology Organisation (WGO) [4].

## A definition problem

The published guidelines and position papers agree that the definition of NAFLD relies on two pillars: evidence of hepatic steatosis (by histology or imaging) and the absence of secondary causes of liver fat accumulation. On review of the same documents, it is clear that the second pillar is starting to creak because of two critical points. The diagnosis of suspected NAFLD includes the absence of *significant* alcohol consumption. As a recent review underlines, there are conflicting suggestions in the literature over this matter and what should be considered significant remains controversial [5]. Significant is defined as >21 drinks/week in men and >14 drinks/week in women by the AASLD, and >30 g/day in men and >20 g/day in women by the EASL and IASL, while a clear cutoff is not mentioned by the WGO. The problem of significant alcohol consumption is not just a definition but also an evaluation problem. As suggested by the IASL, this evaluation should not only consider the patients' interview but also specific biomarkers [6]; however, the limits of the available diagnostic methods [7] mean that the distinction in clinical practice between NAFLD and AFLD remains a challenge. This is actually more than a semantic problem since many patients have a combination of metabolic- and alcohol-induced steatosis.

The remaining reason accounting for the decline of the second pillar is the possible coexistence of NAFLD with other causes of liver disease. The EASL and IASL guidelines mention how NAFLD can coexist with hepatitis C

---

*Clinical Dilemmas in Non-Alcoholic Fatty Liver Disease*, First Edition. Edited by Roger Williams and Simon D. Taylor-Robinson.
© 2016 John Wiley & Sons, Ltd. Published 2016 by John Wiley & Sons, Ltd.

[8, 9] and hemochromatosis [10] and worsen their outcome. It is in this setting that the EASL position paper underlines the need for a change in nomenclature: from a substantially "negative" definition toward a more positive definition of NAFLD. A positive definition of NAFLD has to be considered the highest priority in this field. It will have deep implications way beyond the need to rename NAFLD.

## To screen or not to screen?

The suggestions for screening offered by the present guidelines refer to three main categories of subjects: general population, population at high risk for NAFLD, and the population with other causes of chronic liver disease. It is generally agreed that screening in the general population should not be suggested due to insufficient data on prevalence, impact of diagnosis [11], and treatment options. However, the recommendations relating to high-risk groups differ from those for the general population. The EASL position paper suggests that due to the established link between insulin resistance (IR) and NASH [12], patients with IR should be screened through liver function tests (LFTs) and ultrasound for advanced liver disease as the diagnosis could potentially change patient management. The WGO defines "triggers for considering a diagnosis of NASH and starting testing of liver enzymes" not only type 2 diabetes but also hypertension, sleep apnea, obesity, hyperlipidemia, and a sedentary lifestyle, extending the possible range of candidates for screening. The recommendations of the AASLD differ completely: they do not recommend any screening policy neither in the general population nor in obese and diabetic patients because of the uncertainty of diagnostic tests, treatment options, long-term benefit, and the cost-effectiveness of screening.

The EASL suggests that patients with other chronic liver diseases may be screened for metabolic risk factors, IR, and steatosis using ultrasound. This suggestion confirms the need for a change: NAFLD should not be considered an exclusion diagnosis but a possible concomitant cause of liver disease.

The varied positions on possible screening policies in NAFLD reflect the lack of extensive data concerning prevalence, incidence, impact of diagnosis, and availability of treatment options. Several reports suggest that NAFLD is associated with higher all-cause mortality [13], increased diabetes risk [14], and greater incidence of cardiovascular disease [15] compared with the general population. There is also general agreement on the great importance that NAFLD will play in the future due to aging of the population, better control of other causes of liver disease, and an ongoing epidemic of obesity and diabetes [16, 17]. Even though it is premature to establish clear screening policies for NAFLD, these elements are likely to improve our understanding of NAFLD in order to approach it on a global scale, as an increasingly relevant public health issue.

## The thin line between NAFL and NASH

The dichotomy concerning NAFLD is widely accepted: on one side there is NAFL, and on the other there is NASH [18, 19]. If uncomplicated fatty liver progresses to NASH in a minority of cases, NASH can lead to cirrhosis and hepatocellular carcinoma (HCC) [16], and it is associated with a reduced life expectancy and an increased frequency of cardiovascular disease [20]. All of the guidelines agree that distinguishing steatosis and steatohepatitis is a key aspect in patients' management, as it allows follow-up and therapeutic strategies to be tailored to the individual. However, in clinical practice this distinction remains a challenge. In fact, liver biopsy is considered the gold standard, both for diagnostic and prognostic purposes [21], but because of the heterogeneous distribution of pathologic changes [22, 23], ESPGHAN defines this same "gold standard" as "imperfect" [24]. Furthermore, the EASL highlights the lack of a widely accepted grading classification for NASH, and the presence of distinct histological pattern in particular categories, such as in children and in bariatric surgery patients. The SAF score, which was recently proposed by the FLIP consortium, is likely to become the standard [25]. Due to the biopsy-related morbidity, mortality, and costs, noninvasive methods and markers have been developed in order to select patients who might benefit from the procedure.

So, who should receive a liver biopsy? The answer is unanimous: patients at risk of steatohepatitis, those at risk of fibrosis, and patients in which a competing etiology cannot be otherwise ruled out. According to the AASLD, metabolic syndrome is a strong predictor of steatohepatitis [26] and could be a criterion for selecting patients for liver biopsy. CK-18 is defined as an "encouraging" (AASLD) and "promising" (EASL) marker of steatohepatitis, but as the AASLD reports, it is premature to recommend it in clinical practice since it may be confounded by the amount of fibrosis [27], and no cutoff value has been established. NAFLD fibrosis score is calculated through a published formula using six available variables (age, BMI, hyperglycemia, platelet count, albumin, and AST/ALT ratio) and according to the AASLD and IASL should be considered in selecting patients for liver biopsy [28]. Transient elastography [29–31] is a useful tool for measuring fibrosis, but the different guidelines agree concerning its limitations: the cutoff values are insufficiently defined; it is influenced by steatosis and inflammation; and it has a high failure rate in patients with higher BMI. Other tests, such as the ELF Panel [32], FibroMeter fatty liver [33], and FibroTest [34], are not yet recommended due to their limits and lack of extensive validation.

Equally important is timing: when should a liver biopsy be performed? The IASL and WGO recommend two slightly different algorithms. According to the WGO, only patients with signs of advanced disease should be directly evaluated for liver biopsy; meanwhile, the IASL suggests that the same diagnostic approach should also be used in subjects who present risk factors for steatohepatitis, such as IR or components of metabolic syndrome. Patients who do not agree to a liver biopsy should undergo a 6-month follow-up period aimed at lifestyle modification and appropriate control of metabolic syndrome, and only by persistently abnormal liver enzyme or unvaried steatosis on ultrasounds a liver biopsy should be considered. Also the EASL suggests a watching period of 4–6 months to enforce diet and lifestyle changes, but in cases where these measures do not result in weight loss, ALT normalization, and reduction of IR, the EASL recommends considering liver biopsy.

Liver biopsy, even though imperfect, still represents the gold standard for the diagnosis of NASH. The developed noninvasive markers of steatohepatitis and fibrosis lack extensive validation and cannot be conclusively combined in a diagnostic algorithm. Therefore, a personalized approach has been suggested in which time and first-line therapeutic options (lifestyle changes and treatment of metabolic syndrome) become part of the diagnostic process.

## Therapy: An open and evolving question

Therapy of NAFLD, as suggested by the EASL, can be divided into three main approaches: (i) correct IR and hyperinsulinemia and reduce fat mass; (ii) prevent and reverse hepatic damage induced by lipotoxicity; and (iii) treat and monitor metabolic and cardiovascular comorbidities.

All of the guidelines agree that the milestone of NAFLD treatment relies on lifestyle modifications through diet and physical exercise. A low-carbohydrate, low-saturated-fat diet is suggested by the IASL, while the AASLD recommends a more general hypocaloric diet; the WGO and EASL do not suggest a specific nutrition regimen but recommend a low consumption of soft drinks (high in fructose), industrial trans fat, and an increased consumption of omega-3 in order to increase the omega-3/omega-6 ratio. Physical activity should also be encouraged. The WGO suggests a moderate exercise program three to four times/week to achieve a heart rate of 65–70% of the age-based maximum, and the EASL suggests that patients with NAFLD have their physical activity targets derived from diabetes prevention trials applied: 150 min/week of moderate-intensity physical activity, 75 min/week of vigorous-intensity physical activity, and muscle-strengthening activities twice a week. Interestingly, the IASL describes how physical activity improves IR and LFT independent of weight loss, but as underlined by the AASLD, if exercise alone may improve steatosis, it is not known whether it could also reduce inflammation. It is not clear what the weight loss target should be in order to improve steatosis and inflammation; the recommendation varies from 3–5% according to the AASLD, to 7% (EASL), 5–10% (WGO), or 0.5 kg/week (IASL). The BSG guidelines underline that weight loss in cirrhotic patients with decompensated end-stage liver disease is not recommended, but in patients with compensated disease or HCC, it is appropriate to try to achieve some weight loss before transplant. Lifestyle interventions are a ready-available therapeutic option, but not equally simple to achieve; in fact, the IASL and EASL mention the need for cognitive behavioral therapy in order to ensure the long-term success of therapy. Once again, the approach should be multidisciplinary and personalized [35].

Concerning bariatric surgery, all of the guidelines share the same position: it should not be contraindicated in otherwise eligible obese patient, but it is premature to consider it as an established option to specifically treat NASH. Furthermore, the AASLD recommends that it should not be performed in cirrhotic patients. Posttransplant, the BSG recommends considering bariatric surgery in recipients with severe morbid obesity who failed treatment of obesity or in patients developing progressive NASH with fibrosis. At present, no medical treatment is specifically approved for NAFLD, and the general suggestion is to use pharmacological therapy to treat concomitant metabolic conditions. The EASL identifies the patients with steato-hepatitis and intermediate fibrosis (Kleiner stage 2) as target population for hepatic-specific pharmacological therapy.

All of the guidelines discuss the role of insulin sensitiz-ers such as metformin and glitazones. The IASL and WGO share the same position: insulin sensitizers should be used within randomized clinical trials in nonresponders to standard lifestyle changes. The EASL and AASLD agree that the available contrasting data on metformin do not allow its use as a specific treatment for NAFLD [36]. Glitazones have consistently shown some benefit in patients with NASH; the EASL therefore suggests a 1–2-year course with glitazone. As stated by the AASLD, pioglitazone can be used in patients with biopsy-proven NASH. The AASLD does however also highlight the following: that clinical trials with pioglitazone enrolled mainly nondiabetic patients; that the long-term safety and efficacy has not been established; and that side effects, such as weight gain, a correlation with heart failure, bladder cancer, and bone loss, have been reported.

Regarding agents such as vitamin E or ursodeoxycholic acid (UDCA), the position of the different associations varies. The WGO considers vitamin E experimental because of the limited number of double-blind controlled trials; the IASL underlines the positive preliminary data of vitamin E in association with UDCA [37]; the EASL sug-gests a 1–2-year course therapy with vitamin E based on the results of PIVENS trial [38]; and the AASLD suggests a daily dose of 800 IU of vitamin E in nondiabetic, noncir-rhotic adults with biopsy-proven NASH. The AASLD equally underlines the safety concerns related to vitamin E administration: the increased risk of prostate cancer [39] and the controversy of whether [40] or not [41] it increases all-cause mortality. While the EASL suggests high doses of UDCA may be given with glitazone or vitamin E, the IASL indicates there to be conflicting data on UDCA and, on that basis, offers no recommendation for UDCA treat-ment. The same position is shared by the AASLD, which does not recommend UDCA for NASH treatment [42].

Together with lifestyle modification, all patients should be evaluated for metabolic and cardiovascular risk factors and treated accordingly. In fact, several studies underline that cardiovascular disease is the most common cause of death in patients with NAFLD [15]. A key message of the EASL and AASLD is that statins, antihypertensive agents and antidiabetic drugs directed to correct the concurrent

metabolic disorders, should be given as needed, since NAFLD does not increase hepatotoxicity or other side effects of these drugs.

## Special population: Pediatric patients

Probably because of the limited data available, this popula-tion of NAFLD patients is somehow neglected by the pub-lished guidelines, and only the AASLD and BSG face the problem: although the incidence of NAFLD in pediatric patients is increasing, NAFLD remains underdiagnosed by healthcare providers. Some special features characterize this population. When considering the pediatric patient with suspected NAFLD, according to the AASLD, other etiologies should be ruled out first, including Wilson's disease, fatty acid oxidation defects, lysosomal storage dis-eases, peroxisomal disorders, and autoimmune hepatitis. A biopsy should be considered if the diagnosis is unclear or where multiple diagnoses are possible. Furthermore, pathologists interpreting biopsy in children should be aware of the unique pattern of NAFLD in these patients. If for adults there are only limited data available on treat-ment options, in pediatric patients this problem is further enhanced. In fact, only few clinical trials are available and the AASLD summarizes the results in its recommenda-tions: intensive lifestyle modifications are the first-line treatment in pediatric patients as it is in adults; metformin offers no benefits; and vitamin E 800 IU/day offers histo-logical benefits, but further studies are needed before its use can be recommended in clinical practice [43].

## Conclusions

Through a simple PubMed search using the key words "non-alcoholic fatty liver disease," a total of 4689 articles could be found (September 2014). Of those, 3527 were published in the last 4 years. An interesting point is that the number of articles fell drastically to 171 when the search was limited to article type of "clinical trial" (Figure 15.1). This great difference in the number of published articles and the number of clinical trials sug-gests an undeniable truth: we need more evidence to establish evidence-based clinical practice guidelines. Many points remain undiscovered, from diagnosis to therapy, from natural history to impact of medical interventions.

There is great need for approved therapeutic options in NASH and, in this context, it is crucial, as highlighted by the

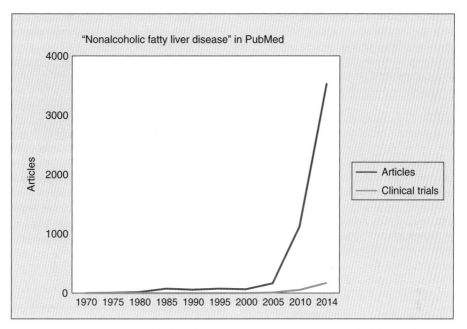

**FIG 15.1** Disproportionately low number of clinical trials in comparison with the large number of publications in the field of nonalcoholic fatty liver disease. Search in PubMed showing the number of publications over the time. Date of the search: September 26, 2014.

EASL, that registration clinical trials establish "relevant but also achievable endpoints," like improvement in NAS score, in steatohepatitis and necroinflammatory lesions, while harder endpoints (impact on fibrosis, reduction of incident cirrhosis) should be reserved to outcome trials. Considering the lack of an approved medical therapy for NASH, it could be argued what do all these efforts concerning diagnosis and follow-up aim for? This is not just to monitor complications and progression but also to get ready for "better times" when treatment options will be available in clinical practice. In this context, the development of reliable noninvasive markers of steatohepatitis and fibrosis is crucial, not only for diagnosis and staging but also as a fundamental instrument to monitor therapy success. We can see then how the improvement of diagnostic/staging knowledge should go hand in hand with the development of new therapeutic options.

## References

1. Ratziu V, Bellentani S, Cortez-Pinto H, Day C, Marchesini G. A position statement on NAFLD/NASH based on the EASL 2009 special conference. J Hepatol 2010;53:372–384.
2. Loria P, Adinolfi LE, Bellentani S, Bugianesi E, Grieco A, Fargion S, Gasbarrini A, et al. Practice guidelines for the diagnosis and management of nonalcoholic fatty liver disease. A decalogue from the Italian Association for the Study of the Liver (AISF) Expert Committee. Dig Liver Dis 2010;42:272–282.
3. Chalasani N, Younossi Z, Lavine JE, Diehl AM, Brunt EM, Cusi K, Charlton M, et al. The diagnosis and management of nonalcoholic fatty liver disease: practice guideline by the American Gastroenterological Association, American Association for the Study of Liver Diseases, and American College of Gastroenterology. Gastroenterology 2012;142:1592–1609.
4. LaBrecque DR, Abbas Z, Anania F, Ferenci P, Khan AG, Goh KL, Hamid SS, et al. World Gastroenterology Organisation global guidelines: nonalcoholic fatty liver disease and nonalcoholic steatohepatitis. J Clin Gastroenterol 2014;48:467–473.
5. Nascimbeni F, Pais R, Bellentani S, Day CP, Ratziu V, Loria P, Lonardo A. From NAFLD in clinical practice to answers from guidelines. J Hepatol 2013;59:859–871.
6. Niemela O. Biomarkers in alcoholism. Clin Chim Acta 2007;377:39–49.
7. Scaglioni F, Ciccia S, Marino M, Bedogni G, Bellentani S. ASH and NASH. Dig Dis 2011;29:202–210.
8. Moucari R, Asselah T, Cazals-Hatem D, Voitot H, Boyer N, Ripault MP, Sobesky R, et al. Insulin resistance in chronic hepatitis C: association with genotypes 1 and 4, serum HCV RNA level, and liver fibrosis. Gastroenterology 2008;134:416–423.
9. Leandro G, Mangia A, Hui J, Fabris P, Rubbia-Brandt L, Colloredo G, Adinolfi LE, et al. Relationship between steatosis, inflammation, and fibrosis in chronic hepatitis C: a meta-analysis of individual patient data. Gastroenterology 2006;130:1636–1642.

10. Powell EE, Ali A, Clouston AD, Dixon JL, Lincoln DJ, Purdie DM, Fletcher LM, et al. Steatosis is a cofactor in liver injury in hemochromatosis. Gastroenterology 2005;129:1937–1943.

11. Adams PC, Arthur MJ, Boyer TD, DeLeve LD, Di Bisceglie AM, Hall M, Levin TR, et al. Screening in liver disease: report of an AASLD clinical workshop. Hepatology 2004;39: 1204–1212.

12. Cusi K. Role of obesity and lipotoxicity in the development of nonalcoholic steatohepatitis: pathophysiology and clinical implications. Gastroenterology 2012;142:711–725.e716.

13. Musso G, Gambino R, Cassader M, Pagano G. Meta-analysis: natural history of non-alcoholic fatty liver disease (NAFLD) and diagnostic accuracy of non-invasive tests for liver disease severity. Ann Med 2011;43:617–649.

14. Ekstedt M, Franzen LE, Mathiesen UL, Thorelius L, Holmqvist M, Bodemar G, Kechagias S. Long-term follow-up of patients with NAFLD and elevated liver enzymes. Hepatology 2006;44:865–873.

15. Targher G, Day CP, Bonora E. Risk of cardiovascular disease in patients with nonalcoholic fatty liver disease. N Engl J Med 2010;363:1341–1350.

16. Farrell GC, Larter CZ. Nonalcoholic fatty liver disease: from steatosis to cirrhosis. Hepatology 2006;43:S99–S112.

17. Lazo M, Clark JM. The epidemiology of nonalcoholic fatty liver disease: a global perspective. Semin Liver Dis 2008;28: 339–350.

18. Day CP. Natural history of NAFLD: remarkably benign in the absence of cirrhosis. Gastroenterology 2005;129:375–378.

19. Bedogni G, Miglioli L, Masutti F, Tiribelli C, Marchesini G, Bellentani S. Prevalence of and risk factors for nonalcoholic fatty liver disease: the Dionysos nutrition and liver study. Hepatology 2005;42:44–52.

20. Gastaldelli A, Kozakova M, Hojlund K, Flyvbjerg A, Favuzzi A, Mitrakou A, Balkau B. Fatty liver is associated with insulin resistance, risk of coronary heart disease, and early atherosclerosis in a large European population. Hepatology 2009;49:1537–1544.

21. Farrell GC, Chitturi S, Lau GK, Sollano JD. Guidelines for the assessment and management of non-alcoholic fatty liver disease in the Asia-Pacific region: executive summary. J Gastroenterol Hepatol 2007;22:775–777.

22. Kleiner DE, Brunt EM, Van Natta M, Behling C, Contos MJ, Cummings OW, Ferrell LD, et al. Design and validation of a histological scoring system for nonalcoholic fatty liver disease. Hepatology 2005;41:1313–1321.

23. Ratziu V, Charlotte F, Heurtier A, Gombert S, Giral P, Bruckert E, Grimaldi A, et al. Sampling variability of liver biopsy in nonalcoholic fatty liver disease. Gastroenterology 2005;128:1898–1906.

24. Vajro P, Lenta S, Socha P, Dhawan A, McKiernan P, Baumann U, Durmaz O, et al. Diagnosis of nonalcoholic fatty liver disease in children and adolescents: position paper of the ESPGHAN Hepatology Committee. J Pediatr Gastroenterol Nutr 2012;54:700–713.

25. Bedossa P. Utility and appropriateness of the fatty liver inhibition of progression (FLIP) algorithm and steatosis, activity, and fibrosis (SAF) score in the evaluation of biopsies of non-alcoholic fatty liver disease. Hepatology 2014;60:565–575.

26. Vuppalanchi R, Chalasani N. Nonalcoholic fatty liver disease and nonalcoholic steatohepatitis: selected practical issues in their evaluation and management. Hepatology 2009;49:306–317.

27. Feldstein AE, Wieckowska A, Lopez AR, Liu YC, Zein NN, McCullough AJ. Cytokeratin-18 fragment levels as noninvasive biomarkers for nonalcoholic steatohepatitis: a multi-center validation study. Hepatology 2009;50:1072–1078.

28. Angulo P, Hui JM, Marchesini G, Bugianesi E, George J, Farrell GC, Enders F, et al. The NAFLD fibrosis score: a non-invasive system that identifies liver fibrosis in patients with NAFLD. Hepatology 2007;45:846–854.

29. Yoneda M, Yoneda M, Fujita K, Inamori M, Tamano M, Hiriishi H, Nakajima A. Transient elastography in patients with non-alcoholic fatty liver disease (NAFLD). Gut 2007;56: 1330–1331.

30. Yoneda M, Yoneda M, Mawatari H, Fujita K, Endo H, Iida H, Nozaki Y, et al. Noninvasive assessment of liver fibrosis by measurement of stiffness in patients with nonalcoholic fatty liver disease (NAFLD). Dig Liver Dis 2008;40:371–378.

31. Friedrich-Rust M, Ong MF, Martens S, Sarrazin C, Bojunga J, Zeuzem S, Herrmann E. Performance of transient elastography for the staging of liver fibrosis: a meta-analysis. Gastroenterology 2008;134:960–974.

32. Guha IN, Parkes J, Roderick P, Chattopadhyay D, Cross R, Harris S, Kaye P, et al. Noninvasive markers of fibrosis in nonalcoholic fatty liver disease: validating the European Liver Fibrosis Panel and exploring simple markers. Hepatology 2008;47:455–460.

33. Cales P, Laine F, Boursier J, Deugnier Y, Moal V, Oberti F, Hunault G, et al. Comparison of blood tests for liver fibrosis specific or not to NAFLD. J Hepatol 2009;50:165–173.

34. Ratziu V, Massard J, Charlotte F, Messous D, Imbert-Bismut F, Bonyhay L, Tahiri M, et al. Diagnostic value of biochemical markers (FibroTest-FibroSURE) for the prediction of liver fibrosis in patients with non-alcoholic fatty liver disease. BMC Gastroenterol 2006;6:6.

35. Bellentani S, Dalle Grave R, Suppini A, Marchesini G. Behavior therapy for nonalcoholic fatty liver disease: the need for a multidisciplinary approach. Hepatology 2008;47:746–754.

36. Vernon G, Baranova A, Younossi ZM. Systematic review: the epidemiology and natural history of non-alcoholic fatty liver disease and non-alcoholic steatohepatitis in adults. Aliment Pharmacol Ther 2011;34:274–285.

37. Dufour JF, Oneta CM, Gonvers JJ, Bihl F, Cerny A, Cereda JM, Zala JF, et al. Randomized placebo-controlled trial of ursodeoxycholic acid with vitamin E in nonalcoholic steatohepatitis. Clin Gastroenterol Hepatol 2006;4: 1537–1543.

38. Sanyal AJ, Chalasani N, Kowdley KV, McCullough A, Diehl AM, Bass NM, Neuschwander-Tetri BA, et al. Pioglitazone, vitamin E, or placebo for nonalcoholic steatohepatitis. N Engl J Med 2010;362:1675–1685.

39. Klein EA, Thompson IM, Jr., Tangen CM, Crowley JJ, Lucia MS, Goodman PJ, Minasian LM, et al. Vitamin E and the risk of prostate cancer: the Selenium and Vitamin E Cancer Prevention Trial (SELECT). JAMA 2011;306:1549–1556.

40. Miller ER, III, Pastor-Barriuso R, Dalal D, Riemersma RA, Appel LJ, Guallar E. Meta-analysis: high-dosage vitamin E supplementation may increase all-cause mortality. Ann Intern Med 2005;142:37–46.

41. Gerss J, Kopcke W. The questionable association of vitamin E supplementation and mortality—inconsistent results of different meta-analytic approaches. Cell Mol Biol 2009;55 Suppl:Ol1111-1120.

42. Lindor KD, Kowdley KV, Heathcote EJ, Harrison ME, Jorgensen R, Angulo P, Lymp JF, et al. Ursodeoxycholic acid for treatment of nonalcoholic steatohepatitis: results of a randomized trial. Hepatology 2004;39:770–778.

43. Lavine JE, Schwimmer JB, Van Natta ML, Molleston JP, Murray KF, Rosenthal P, Abrams SH, et al. Effect of vitamin E or metformin for treatment of nonalcoholic fatty liver disease in children and adolescents: the TONIC randomized controlled trial. JAMA 2011;305:1659–1668.

# 16 Imaging methods for screening of hepatic steatosis

**Hero K. Hussain**

Department of Radiology and MRI, University of Michigan Health System, Ann Arbor, MI, USA

## LEARNING POINTS

- To describe imaging modalities used for the assessment of hepatic steatosis

- To discuss advantages and limitations of each modality

- To review the reported accuracy of each modality for the detection and quantification of all degrees of hepatic steatosis and the distinction of simple steatosis from steatohepatitis and hepatic fibrosis

- To evaluate the practicality of each of these modalities for screening for hepatic steatosis and assessment of response to therapy

Hepatic steatosis is the abnormal and excessive accumulation of triglycerides in hepatocytes. For a long time, hepatic steatosis was considered inconsequential, but it is now known to be a causative or contributing factor in the development of end-stage liver disease, cancer, and other systemic disorders, such as diabetes and cardiovascular disease. It is also an independent risk factor for cardiovascular-related mortality [1–6]. In the liver, steatosis is the hallmark of non-alcoholic fatty liver disease (NAFLD), which can progress to cirrhosis [7]. Hepatic steatosis may reduce the efficacy of antiviral therapy in chronic hepatitis C infection [8] and has been shown to increase the risk of hepatocellular carcinoma even without cirrhosis [9]. Steatosis also compromises hepatic function and contributes to liver failure after resection or transplantation [10, 11]. Thus, hepatic steatosis is no longer considered inconsequential, and detection and accurate estimation of severity of hepatic steatosis, especially during therapeutic intervention, have become necessary.

Random percutaneous liver biopsy is considered the gold standard for the diagnosis of hepatic steatosis. This, however, is impractical for screening, because it is invasive, requires postprocedural recovery care, and is associated with risk of complications, such as bleeding and, rarely, death [7, 12]. Biopsy sample size is prone to sampling errors owing to undersampling of disease, which may be patchy in distribution [13].

Owing to the expeditious, noninvasive, and relatively risk-free nature of imaging, several imaging modalities have been used for the detection and quantification of hepatic steatosis. In the coming sections, these modalities will be discussed, with their advantages and limitations and suitability for screening.

## Ultrasound

Ultrasound (US) is the most commonly used modality for the assessment of fatty liver and often the first-line imaging test. The reported overall sensitivity and specificity of US for the detection of all grades of hepatic steatosis are 60–94% and 66–95%, respectively [14].

### Appearance of fatty liver on US

The normal liver parenchyma is homogeneous with echogenicity equal to or minimally higher than that of the adjacent kidney, and there is usually clear visualization of the intrahepatic vessels and diaphragm [15–17]. The fatty liver on US is characterized by increased echogenicity, relative to adjacent organs, not known to be affected by steatosis (such as the right kidney), and decreased echogenicity of the deep liver with poor visualization of the diaphragm and intrahepatic vessels [18, 19]. This increased echogenicity is due to increased beam scattering by fat droplets within hepatocytes. These fat droplets also reduce beam penetration through the liver resulting in a hypoechoic distant field [20]. In combination, these effects result in a hyperechoic featureless liver with decreased conspicuity of the diaphragm, intrahepatic portal venules, and gallbladder wall [20–22] and apparent dilatation of the hepatic veins and bile ducts [19].

## Advantages and limitations of US for screening

US is a widely available, noninvasive test that is affordable, is easy to perform, and lacks ionizing radiation. All these features make it highly attractive for screening patients with suspected fatty liver disease [19]. US screening has several advantages and limitations that are discussed in the following:

1.  Sensitivity of detection of hepatic steatosis: Using the sonographic features described earlier, US is highly sensitive for the detection of moderate and severe hepatic steatosis at histology (defined as ≥30% of hepatocytes affected by steatosis). In a recent meta-analysis, the pooled sensitivity for the detection of moderate and severe hepatic steatosis was reported at 84.8% (95% confidence interval: 79.5–88.9) [23] and as high as 96.4–100% in other individual studies [16, 24, 25]. However, US has low sensitivity for the detection of mild steatosis (<20–30% by histology) with reported sensitivities ranging from 47 to 55% [19, 24, 26]. The combination of increased liver echogenicity and portal vein blurring has been shown to be the best predictors of steatosis [24].

2.  Specificity of diagnosis of steatosis: The performance of US varies according to the exact definition of hepatic steatosis and the presence of coexisting chronic liver disease, such as fibrosis, which result in increased hepatic echogenicity [27, 28]. Coexistence of inflammation and fibrosis may result in increased hepatic echogenicity, thus reducing the US specificity for the diagnosis of steatosis [22, 26–28]. The specificity of US for detecting moderate to severe steatosis alone has been reported at 93.6% but is reduced to 79.2% with a lower positive predictive value in the presence of inflammation or fibrosis [23]. Other studies have suggested that this distinction is possible, as severe fibrosis does not result in posterior beam attenuation [27, 29].

3.  Patient-related factors: Sensitivity and specificity of US detection of hepatic steatosis have been reported to be reduced in morbidly obese patients to 49 and 75%, respectively [30]. This is secondary to beam attenuation by subcutaneous and visceral adipose tissue and can also be seen in patients with excessive intestinal gas [31].

4.  Operator dependency and technical factors: US is operator dependent and, therefore, nonreproducible. Technical factors, such as transducer frequency and equipment settings, may also affect perceived hepatic echogenicity [20].

5.  Quantification of hepatic fat: Assessment of the degree of steatosis on US is qualitative and determined by subjective visual assessment of liver echogenicity in comparison to the kidneys, conspicuity of intrahepatic vessel walls, and visualization of the diaphragm. It is graded into four grades (0–3) with 0 being normal. Grade 1 is mild steatosis and manifests diffuse mild increased liver echogenicity versus the kidney with normal visualization of the intrahepatic vessel walls and diaphragm. Grade 2 is moderate and manifests moderate increased liver echogenicity compared to the kidney with poor visualization of intrahepatic vessel walls. Grade 3 is severe and manifests marked diffuse increase in liver echogenicity with poor visualization of the deep liver and diaphragm [16, 19] (Figure 16.1).

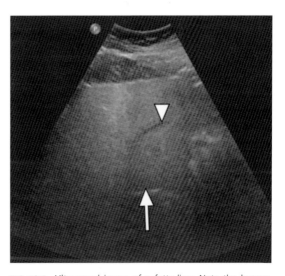

**FIG 16.1** Ultrasound image of a fatty liver. Note the hyperechoic featureless liver with poor visualization of the deep liver and diaphragm (arrow) and the intrahepatic vessel walls (arrowhead).

Owing to its qualitative nature, US assessment is subject to high intra- and interobserver variability [16, 23, 25, 32–34]. In a recent meta-analysis, the kappa values for intrarater agreement ranged from 0.54 to 0.92 and inter-rater agreement from 0.44 to 1 [23]. This variability makes US nonreproducible and limits its utility for the assessment of changes in the degree of hepatic steatosis. Also, categorizing steatosis into three major categories makes US unreliable for the assessment of small changes in liver fat content [34]. Quantitative methods for hepatic fat quantification on US using beam scattering and atten-uation have been proposed, but it is not used in routine clinical practice [35–37].

Thus, US is a well-established screening tool that has moderate sensitivity and specificity for the detection of hepatic steatosis. However, its operator dependency, quali-tative nature, and low accuracy in detecting mild steatosis and distinguishing steatosis from fibrosis preclude its usage for monitoring response to therapy. It is most useful for the diagnosis of moderate and severe steatosis in asymptomatic patients with elevated liver enzyme tests and suspected NAFLD. However, it does not help distin-guish steatosis from steatohepatitis.

## Computed tomography

Both unenhanced and contrast-enhanced computed tomography (CT) have been widely used for the evaluation of hepatic steatosis. Unlike US, CT is quantitative and utilizes tissue density measurements as a function of atten-uation measured in Hounsfield units (HU) [18, 20]. Tissue density is dependent on tissue composition. Unenhanced CT has a reported sensitivity of 74% and a specificity of 70% for the detection of all grades of hepatic steatosis and has been shown to be insensitive for mild steatosis (≤30% on histology) [38].

### Appearance of the steatotic liver on CT

Fat has very low attenuation on CT (−100 HU); therefore, fatty liver has reduced attenuation. Either absolute liver attenuation values (usually on unenhanced CT) or the dif-ference in the attenuation of the liver and spleen (liver minus spleen) (on unenhanced and enhanced CT) is used to assess for the presence of hepatic steatosis [18]. A ratio of liver to spleen attenuation has also been used. Unenhanced CT measures are generally preferred to enhanced CT in

order to minimize the effect of inhomogeneous liver perfu-sion on attenuation measurements.

On unenhanced CT, the normal liver is higher attenua-tion than the intrahepatic vasculature and spleen. As fatty liver becomes more severe, the attenuation of the liver decreases and the intrahepatic vessels appear brighter than the liver parenchyma, mimicking a contrast-enhanced study [20, 26] (Figure 16.2). A liver minus spleen (L-S) attenuation of −9 HU has been reported to have a sensitivity of 82% and a specificity of 100% of moderate and severe steatosis ≥30% at histology [39]. Park and colleagues [40] established the normal reference range of liver minus spleen attenuation at 1–18 HU and found that an absolute liver density of ≤48 HU and a difference of ≥ −2 HU between the attenuation of the liver and spleen have 100% specificity for the diagnosis of moderate and severe hepatic steatosis.

On contrast-enhanced CT, the attenuation of the liver is greatly influenced by perfusion effects related to the patient's circulation, injection rate, and phase of enhance-ment (early vs. late). The liver minus spleen attenuation on enhanced CT has a reported sensitivity of 0.54–0.71 for the detection of hepatic steatosis because of overlap in the attenuation values of normal and fatty livers [41]. In gen-eral, a liver–spleen difference in attenuation of more than −35 HU in the venous phase (>100 s after contrast) is con-sidered acceptable for the diagnosis of moderate to severe hepatic steatosis (Figure 16.3).

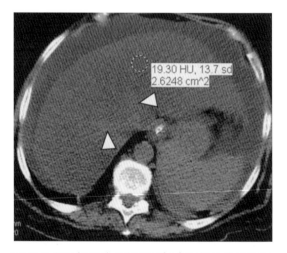

**FIG 16.2** Unenhanced CT image of a fatty liver. The intrahe-patic vessels (arrowheads) appear brighter than the low-atten-uation fatty liver parenchyma that measures 19 Hounsfield units (HU).

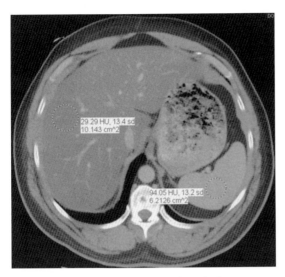

**FIG 16.3** Enhanced CT image of a fatty liver. The liver measures 29 HU and the spleen 94 HU. The liver spleen attenuation difference is −65 HU.

## Advantages and limitations of CT for screening

CT, especially unenhanced CT, is relatively available and fast; still, it is expensive and less available compared to US. Moreover, it utilizes ionizing radiation therefore not suitable for longitudinal studies and for children [20]. Other limitations of CT are discussed in the following:

1. Sensitivity of detection of hepatic steatosis: CT is not sensitive for the detection of mild steatosis, while it is more accurate for moderate to severe steatosis graded at ≥30% by histology [18, 32, 38, 42]. On unenhanced CT, the overall threshold values for CT indices vary according to the method used and study population [38, 39]. The absolute liver attenuation values may vary across scanners from different vendors; therefore, normalizing liver attenuation value with that of the spleen as the internal control is suggested [43–45].

2. Specificity of diagnosis of hepatic steatosis: Low attenuation of the hepatic parenchyma is not specific for steatosis. Other causes, such as fibrosis, inflammation, and edema, can reduce the attenuation value of the liver [41, 42]. Furthermore, steatosis can be masked by other causes of increased liver attenuation, such as glycogen, copper, and drugs, such as amiodarone [32].

Unenhanced CT therefore does not obviate liver biopsy in the majority of patients being considered for living donor liver transplantation [42].

3. Assessment of hepatic steatosis on enhanced CT is influenced by liver perfusion and underlying liver disease [32].

4. Quantification of hepatic fat on CT: Although HU are used to assess for the presence of hepatic steatosis, evaluation of the degree of steatosis is qualitative [39] and cannot be used to detect small changes in hepatic fat and, therefore, cannot be used to monitor response to therapy [39].

Although CT has the advantage of speed and relative availability, it has many shortcomings that prevent its utilization as a screening tool or for longitudinal follow-up of patients with steatosis. These include higher cost and limited availability compared to US and utilization of ionizing radiation. CT is also insensitive for the detection of mild steatosis or small changes in hepatic fat. Moreover, unenhanced liver CT attenuation values are influenced by the coexistence of other diffuse liver diseases or drug effects, and enhanced CT values by perfusion and timing of image acquisition.

## Magnetic resonance imaging

Unlike US and CT that utilize surrogate features of echogenicity and attenuation to determine the presence of hepatic fat, magnetic resonance imaging (MRI) techniques can be used to objectively measure the hepatic fat fraction (HFF) by measuring the signal that arises from fat protons.

MRI signal arises primarily from protons in water and fat molecules. The basic MR principle used to distinguish water from fat protons is the chemical shift of water and fat, which is the difference in the resonance frequency between water and fat protons. MR spectroscopy (MRS) is used to display signals at their respective resonance frequencies. Other quantitative MR techniques can be used to generate images that display the signal from fat and water protons.

MRI techniques are highly sensitive and specific for the detection and quantification of hepatic steatosis, but MRI has the disadvantage of limited availability and high cost. Several MRI techniques are used to display the HFF. Some of these techniques are used in daily clinical practice and are qualitatively examined for the presence of hepatic fat. Quantitative techniques have mostly been used in research studies because they require complex analysis. However, these quantification methods will soon be available for use on all commercial MR scanners. These techniques are discussed in details in the following.

## Qualitative estimation of hepatic fat on MRI

The presence of hepatic fat can be determined qualitatively or semiquantitatively in daily clinical practice by visual assessment and simple region-of-interest (ROI) analysis of following routinely used imaging techniques:

1.  Frequency-selected fat suppression (FS) techniques
2.  Opposed/in-phase (OIP) gradient recalled echo (GRE) imaging technique

### Frequency-selected FS technique

The presence of hepatic fat results in decreased signal intensity (SI) of the liver from nonfat-suppressed to fat-suppressed imaging on both $T_1$-weighted and $T_2$-weighted imaging. Conventional $T_2$-weighted fast spin-echo (FSE) imaging without and with frequency-selected FS has been shown to be reliable for detecting hepatic fat (Figure 16.4A and B). This signal decrease can be assessed visually or estimated semiquantitatively by placing matching ROI in the liver and spleen on the non-FS and FS images, normalizing the liver signal by that of the spleen (normalized SI), and applying the following formula [32, 46]:

$$\text{Normalized SI liver (non-FS)} - \text{normalized SI (FS)}/ \\ \text{normalized SI (non-FS)} \times 100$$

Two studies [32, 46] have shown moderate to good correlation between estimated signal loss on FS imaging and severity of steatosis on biopsy, sometimes exceeding that of OIP imaging [46] but with greater interobserver variability [32]. This technique suffers many limitations. For example, heterogeneous fat distribution in the liver can result in sampling errors when using ROI-based analysis. Also, estimation of signal loss on fat-suppressed images is confounded by technical factors related to inhomogeneous FS. Furthermore, no reference standard exists for correlating SI changes in the liver on fat-suppressed images with liver fat content at histology.

Since estimation of signal loss on fat-suppressed imaging is qualitative or semiquantitative, and subject to sampling error and technical limitation, this technique is not reliable or reproducible and, therefore, not widely used in daily clinical practice and cannot be utilized for longitudinal follow-up or estimation of small changes in hepatic fat content.

(A)

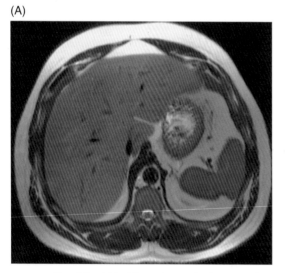

(B)

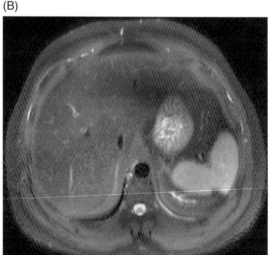

**FIG 16.4** $T_2$-weighted ($T_2$W) fast spin-echo (FSE) images of the liver without (A) and with (B) fat suppression. Note that the high signal intensity of the liver relative to the spleen on the nonfat-suppressed $T_2$W FSE image (A) decreases on the fat-suppressed $T_2$W FSE image (B).

## OIP imaging technique

This technique utilizes the difference in the resonance frequencies of the signal of protons in water and fat, which decreases with increasing field strength [7]. $T_1$-weighted dual-echo GRE images are acquired at specific echo times when water and fat signals are precessing in phase (IP) and out of phase such that their signals are added and subtracted, respectively. The echo times for OIP vary according to the field strength and are acquired at ~2.3 ms intervals at 1.5 T and 1.15 ms intervals at 3 T (i.e., standard opposed-phase (OP)/IP echo times are ~2.3 and 4.6 ms at 1.5 T and 1.15 and 2.3 ms at 3 T). The dual-echo GRE sequence is a part of all routine liver protocols.

In the nonfatty liver, no perceptible signal loss occurs between OP and IP imaging. In the presence of hepatic steatosis, signal loss is observed on OP images relative to IP (Figure 16.5A and B) due to signal cancellation related to the coexistence of water and fat in the same imaging voxel. This signal loss can be assessed qualitatively by visual estimation or semiquantitatively by measuring the SI of the liver on OP and IP using ROI and applying the following formula:

$$\text{SI liver (in phase)} - \text{SI liver (opposed phase)} / \text{SI liver (in phase)} \times 100$$

Although some authors suggest normalizing the liver signal by that of the spleen [32], this is unnecessary with current dual-echo acquisition techniques wherein the only difference between the images is the echo time [47].

Signal loss on OIP imaging has been shown in several studies to have good correlation with all grades of steatosis on biopsy in the absence of iron deposition and cirrhosis [32, 46, 48, 49]. There are limitations to this technique. For example, estimation of signal loss on routine dual-echo OIP images correlates with HFF but is not a true measure of HFF because the measured SI is confounded by the effect of relaxation times ($T_1$, $T_2^*$) and spectral complexity of hepatic fat. These confounding factors need to be addressed for accurate quantification of hepatic fat, as will be discussed later. Also, similar to any ROI-based analysis, heterogeneous fat distribution in the liver can result in sampling error and a single measure may not be reflective of the entire fat content of the liver. Furthermore, no reference standard exists for SI loss on OIP imaging in relationship with liver fat content at histology.

Since estimation of signal loss as a measure of hepatic steatosis on routine OIP imaging is qualitative or at best semiquantitative and is subject to errors related to sampling, relaxation parameters, and underestimation of the total hepatic fat, this technique is not reproducible and therefore not reliable for longitudinal follow-up and estimation of small changes in hepatic fat content. It is, however, the most reliable qualitative and semiquantitative for the detection of hepatic fat and therefore may be the most suitable for screening.

(A)  (B)

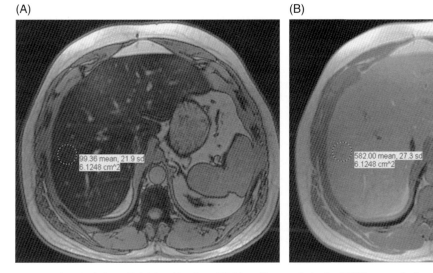

**FIG 16.5** Opposed-phase (OP) (A) and in-phase (IP) (B) gradient recalled echo (GRE) images of a fatty liver. There is signal loss in the liver on the OP image (A) relative to the IP image (B) due to hepatic steatosis.

## Quantitative estimation of hepatic fat on MRI

In addition to the simple qualitative and semiquantitative methods that can be used in daily clinical practice to determine if there is hepatic fat, MRI can be used to quantitatively estimate the hepatic fat and thus used to monitor patients and detect small changes in HFF. MRI techniques detect the abnormal triglycerides that accumulate within hepatocytes (fat vacuoles) [50]. Two methods are generally used for quantitative estimation of HFF, and both utilize the chemical shift between water and fat protons:

1. Magnitude-based techniques using standard OIP GRE images: These utilize the SI of the liver on standard 2-D GRE OIP images to calculate the HFF. Usually six OP and IP echoes are acquired for this calculation (Figure 16.6).
2. Complex-based techniques using standard water (W) and fat (F) separation GRE images: These utilize both the SI and phase information of the liver on 3-D GRE water and fat separation images (water only, fat only—Dixon, Iterative Decomposition of water and fat with Echo Asymmetry and Least-squares estimation (IDEAL)) to calculate the HFF (Figure 16.7). Usually 6 echoes are acquired at appropriate echo times to separate water and fat signal [50].

As a principle, HFF can be measured from the previously described images using the following formulas:

$$\text{HFF (OIP)} = \text{SI liver IP} - \text{SI liver OP}/ 2 \times \text{SI liver IP}$$
$$\text{HFF (W-F separation)} = \text{SI liver (F only)} / \text{SI liver}$$
$$\text{(F only)} + \text{SI liver (W only)}$$

However, estimation of signal loss and HFF on routine clinical uncorrected OIP or water-only and fat-only images is confounded by factors such as those related to relaxation times $(T_1, T_2^*)$ and spectral complexity of hepatic fat. For example, coexistence of iron in the liver leads to $T_2^*$ shortening, which results in decreased signal in the liver on all images leading to underestimation of HFF. Also, the OIP echo times are based on the chemical shift between water and only the dominant methylene peak of fat [7] without taking into consideration the other types of hepatic fat leading to underestimation of the total hepatic fat content.

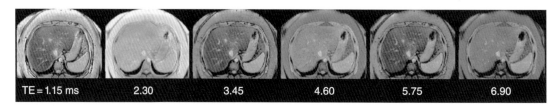

**FIG 16.6** Standard 6 echo opposed-phase/in-phase GRE sequence at 3T used for measuring the hepatic fat fraction (HFF). The measured signal needs to be corrected for $T_1$ and $T_2^*$ bias and spectral fat complexity.

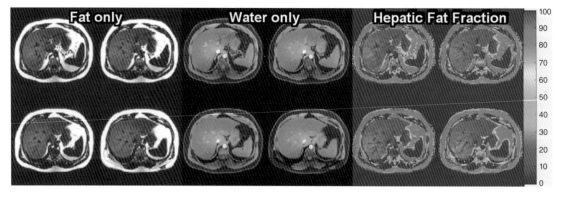

**FIG 16.7** The hepatic fat fraction (HFF) map calculated using water and fat separation GRE images. The color scale on the side indicates the percent HFF. (*See insert for color representation of the figure.*)

In order to accurately estimate the HFF from OIP and water-only/fat-only MR images, confounders related to relaxation times ($T_1$ and $T_2^*$), spectral fat complexity, and other factors should be minimized. These confounders are mitigated by changing acquisition parameters ($T_1$), calculating and correcting the signal ($T_2^*$), accounting for all types of fat in the liver (spectral fat modeling), and mitigating other biases as discussed in the following:

1. $T_1$ bias [47]: The repetition time (TR) and flip angle used for standard GRE imaging are optimized to provide $T_1$-weighted imaging, which results in overestimation of the HFF when these images are used. Reducing the flip angle minimizes the $T_1$ effect and provides proton density (PD)-weighted images that can be used to estimate the PD-HFF without $T_1$ bias.

2. $T_2^*$ bias: The $T_2^*$ shortening effect on the signal, often due to the coexistence of iron, can lead to severe errors in fat quantification, mostly underestimation of the PD-HFF. $T_2^*$ can be calculated from the images acquired and used to correct the signal [47, 51–55].

3. Spectral complexity of fat: Unlike water, hepatic fat is not a single, sharp spectral resonance; rather, it comprises at least six distinct spectral peaks of different resonant frequencies [7, 56]. Accurate fat quantification should therefore include signal from all the fat resonances and not only the dominant resonances. This can be achieved by incorporating spectral modeling of fat in the calculation of HFF [51, 52].

Additional confounders need to be addressed such as noise bias and phase errors that pertain mostly to water and fat separation methods [7, 51, 57–60]. Noise bias occurs because areas of low signal have positive noise on magnitude images and can lead to overestimation of the HFF at very low liver fat fractions. This can be addressed using magnitude discrimination and phase-constrained methods described by Liu et al. [57]. Noise bias can also affect magnitude-based technique at 50% fat content when the signal on OP images approaches 0%. Phase errors can degrade HFF estimation using water and fat separation techniques that incorporate phase information in their calculations. These errors result from the rapid switching of gradients between echoes that can lead to gradient delays and eddy currents and can be addressed using hybrid acquisition methods [58, 59].

One major difference between the multiecho OIP and water–fat separation techniques is that the latter allows estimation of the entire range of HFF from 0 to 100%, whereas the former allows calculation of the range of HFF between 0 and 50%, which is the clinically relevant range as hepatic fat signal rarely exceeds 50%. This limitation can be overcome using a dual-flip-angle technique [47]. Using either of these methods, a map of the PD-HFF of the entire liver can be generated on a pixel-by-pixel basis (Figure 16.8), thus eliminating the sampling error associated with biopsy.

PD-HFF calculations on MRI at 1.5 T and 3 T have been shown to be highly accurate for all grades of steatosis in comparison with MRS measurements and biopsy with reported accuracy of up to 96% [47, 61–65], but it may be affected by coexisting fibrosis [66]. The techniques are reproducible [67], are field strength independent [68], and can be used to detect as small as 1% changes in hepatic fat [67, 69]. Still, these techniques have several limitations as discussed in the following:

1. While both OIP and water–fat separation techniques are highly accurate for estimation of the PD-HFF of all degrees of severity, these are not yet commercially available for clinical use and are usually applied in a research context because of the complex analysis required. Therefore, these methods are currently not practical for screening.

2. Until recently, no reference standard was available to correlate the PD-HFF with severity of steatosis on histology. A PD-HFF of 5.56% or larger is considered abnormal [70]. A recent publication [64] suggested that in patients with NAFLD, PD-HFF of 8.9% corresponds to grade 1 histological steatosis, 16.3% to grade 2, and 25% to grade 3. It is important to remember that determination of steatosis on histology is semiquantitative and estimates the % hepatocytes with fat vacuoles.

3. High cost and limited availability of MRI remains to be an issue.

## MRS

Proton MRS is a technique that measures and displays the signal amplitude of protons as a function of their resonance frequency [18]. Within the liver, fat and water protons are the most abundant and contribute to most of the identifiable peaks. The water resonance is seen as a single peak at 4.7 parts per million (ppm) and fat as multiple peaks due to the coexistence of several types of fat protons in the liver that vary in their chemical bonds. The largest fat resonance

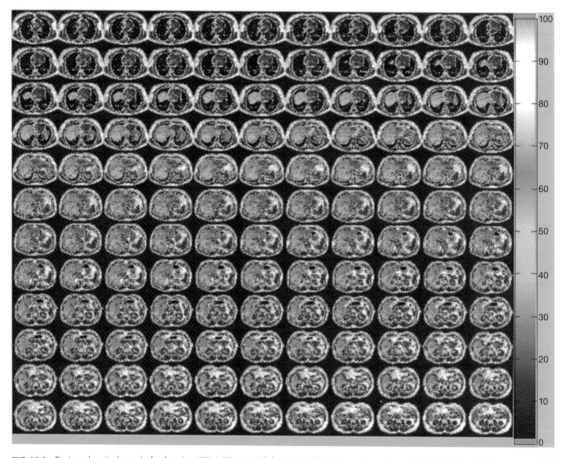

**FIG 16.8** Proton density hepatic fat fraction (PD-HFF) map of the entire liver. The color scale on the side indicates the percent HFF. (*See insert for color representation of the figure.*)

in the liver spectrum is the methylene peak at 1.3 ppm, and there are at least five other peaks with slightly different resonance frequencies, two of which are closely aligned to the water resonance [56] (Figure 16.9).

MRS techniques: Single-voxel MRS is the most commonly used technique. The voxel is typically $3 \times 3 \times 3$ cm in size and is manually placed in the liver parenchyma (Figure 16.10). Shimming (an old ploughing term, originally meaning to straighten furrows in an agricultural field) is necessary to achieve a homogeneous magnetic field across the voxel [18]. Either a stimulated echo acquisition mode (STEAM) or a point-resolved spectroscopy sequence (PRESS) is used to acquire the MR spectra. PRESS sequence is preferred because of higher signal-to-noise ratio and reduced susceptibility [71, 72]. MRS can be performed during free breathing or preferably

in a breath-hold to avoid motion-related issues [61, 62, 65, 73, 74].

Similar to other MRI methods, and in order to obtain accurate PD-HFF measurements, relaxation effects ($T_1$ and $T_2$) should be minimized when using MRS sequences. A long repetition time (TR) reduces $T_1$ bias. Multiecho MRS with multiple spectra acquired at different echo times (TE) best mitigate the $T_2$ relaxation effect that can lead to erroneous estimations of the HFF [61, 62, 65, 73–75].

Fat within the liver can be quantified by spectral tracing of each peak. The PD-HFF can be calculated as the sum of signal from all fat peaks divided by the sum of water and fat signal [6]. If only the area under the main fat peak is calculated without including the smaller fat peaks, the hepatic fat can be underestimated by up to 30% [56].

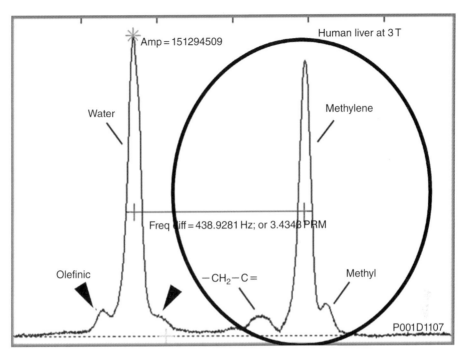

**FIG 16.9** Liver proton spectrum at 3 T. Hepatic fat and water protons are displayed as a function of their resonance frequency. There is a single water peak at 4.7 parts per million (ppm) and several fat peaks. The dominant fat peak is the methylene peak at 1.3 ppm with three smaller adjacent peaks encompassed by the black circle and two additional small peaks (arrowheads) in close proximity to the water peak.

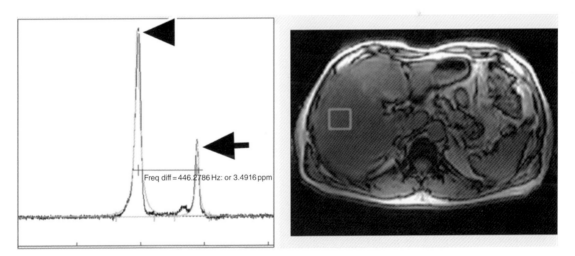

**FIG 16.10** Single-voxel proton MR spectroscopy of a fatty liver at 1.5 T. Note the small red voxel placed in the right lobe of the liver and the water (arrowhead) and dominant fat (methylene) (arrow) peaks in the sampled parenchyma. (*See insert for color representation of the figure.*)

MRS accuracy: Proton MRS is considered to be the gold standard MR method for hepatic fat quantification. Reported MRS sensitivities for the detection of hepatic fat ≥5% even without signal correction methods have been at 80–91% [25, 38]. MRS measurements are highly reproducible [62]. The main advantage of MRS over CT and US is that assessment of steatosis is objective and quantitative and highly reproducible [61, 62, 68, 70]. It can be used for diagnosis of all degrees of hepatic steatosis and for follow-up to assess for changes in hepatic steatosis in response to treatment or lifestyle changes.

Despite the safety and high accuracy of MRI for quantification of all degrees of hepatic steatosis, MRS is not widely available and expensive, and the acquisition and analysis of MRS data require expertise. Also, when using the single-voxel technique, the data are often collected from a small voxel of the liver and not the entire liver, therefore subject to sampling error.

Although histological estimation of degree of severity of hepatic steatosis is still considered the gold standard, several studies have shown that PD-HFF measured by MRI and MRS are better reference standards due to their high accuracy, reproducibility, and better correlation with biochemical lipid assays and computerized analysis of microscopic images of liver samples [76–78].

Assessment of PD-HFF on MRI and MRS is more quantitative than histology, which relies on the pathologist subjective visual estimation of the number of hepatocytes containing fat vacuoles [47]. Also, histological cutoffs of 30% between grades are too wide and are not sensitive for the detection of small changes in hepatic fat. However, MRI- and MRS-determined PD-HFF scale of severity of hepatic steatosis is different than that of histology. Moreover, biopsy suffers from sampling error, which is not an issue with MRI techniques that can be used to determine the PD-HFF throughout the liver on a pixel-by-pixel basis.

In summary, US should be used as the first-line screening test in patients with suspected hepatic steatosis. US is sensitive for moderate and severe hepatic steatosis, is readily available, and is affordable. When available, simple OIP MR imaging is a potential alternative and a complimentary test for those patients with negative US, as it is a more sensitive for the detection of milder degrees of hepatic steatosis. MRS is another option for these patients, if available as most MR scanners now have the capacity to automatically produce liver spectra without the need for off-line complex analysis. As for follow-up for patients with steatosis and assessment of response to therapy or lifestyle changes, only MRS and quantitative MRI techniques are sensitive for detection of small changes in hepatic fat. It is important to remember that in patients with NAFLD, the relationship between hepatic fat and fibrosis is a negative one and that reduction of hepatic fat may not always indicate response to therapy but worsening of hepatic fibrosis.

## References

1. Matteoni CA, Younossi ZM, Gramlich T, Boparai N, Liu YC, McCullough AJ. Nonalcoholic fatty liver disease: a spectrum of clinical and pathological severity. Gastroenterology. 1999;116(6):1413–9.
2. Sanyal AJ, Banas C, Sargeant C, et al. Similarities and differences in outcomes of cirrhosis due to nonalcoholic steatohepatitis and hepatitis C. Hepatology. 2006;43(4):682–9.
3. Adams LA, Waters OR, Knuiman MW, Elliott RR, Olynyk JK. NAFLD as a risk factor for the development of diabetes and the metabolic syndrome: an eleven-year follow-up study. The American Journal of Gastroenterology. 2009;104(4):861–7.
4. Dunn W, Xu R, Wingard DL, et al. Suspected nonalcoholic fatty liver disease and mortality risk in a population-based cohort study. The American Journal of Gastroenterology. 2008;103(9):2263–71.
5. Rubinstein E, Lavine JE, Schwimmer JB. Hepatic, cardiovascular, and endocrine outcomes of the histological subphenotypes of nonalcoholic fatty liver disease. Seminars in Liver Disease. 2008;28(4):380–5.
6. Targher G, Arcaro G. Non-alcoholic fatty liver disease and increased risk of cardiovascular disease. Atherosclerosis. 2007;191(2):235–40.
7. Reeder SB, Sirlin CB. Quantification of liver fat with magnetic resonance imaging. Magnetic Resonance Imaging Clinics of North America. 2010;18(3):337–57, ix.
8. Lok AS, Everhart JE, Chung RT, et al. Evolution of hepatic steatosis in patients with advanced hepatitis C: results from the hepatitis C antiviral long-term treatment against cirrhosis (HALT-C) trial. Hepatology. 2009;49(6):1828–37.
9. Guzman G, Brunt EM, Petrovic LM, Chejfec G, Layden TJ, Cotler SJ. Does nonalcoholic fatty liver disease predispose patients to hepatocellular carcinoma in the absence of cirrhosis? Archives of Pathology & Laboratory Medicine. 2008;132(11):1761–6.
10. Ioannou GN. Development and validation of a model predicting graft survival after liver transplantation. Liver Transplantation. 2006;12(11):1594–606.
11. Yoong KF, Gunson BK, Neil DA, et al. Impact of donor liver microvesicular steatosis on the outcome of liver retransplantation. Transplantation Proceedings. 1999;31(1–2):550–1.

12. Bravo AA, Sheth SG, Chopra S. Liver biopsy. The New England Journal of Medicine. 2001;344(7):495–500.

13. Vuppalanchi R, Unalp A, Van Natta ML, et al. Effects of liver biopsy sample length and number of readings on sampling variability in nonalcoholic Fatty liver disease. Clinical Gastroenterology and Hepatology. 2009;7(4):481–6.

14. Schwenzer NF, Springer F, Schraml C, Stefan N, Machann J, Schick F. Non-invasive assessment and quantification of liver steatosis by ultrasound, computed tomography and magnetic resonance. Journal of Hepatology. 2009;51(3):433–45.

15. Ma X, Holalkere NS, Kambadakone RA, Mino-Kenudson M, Hahn PF, Sahani DV. Imaging-based quantification of hepatic fat: methods and clinical applications. Radiographics. 2009;29(5):1253–77.

16. Saadeh S, Younossi ZM, Remer EM, et al. The utility of radiological imaging in nonalcoholic fatty liver disease. Gastroenterology. 2002;123(3):745–50.

17. Karcaaltincaba M, Akhan O. Imaging of hepatic steatosis and fatty sparing. European Journal of Radiology. 2007;61(1):33–43.

18. Lee SS, Park SH. Radiologic evaluation of nonalcoholic fatty liver disease. World Journal of Gastroenterology. 2014;20 (23):7392–402.

19. Lupsor-Platon M, Stefanescu H, Muresan D, et al. Noninvasive assessment of liver steatosis using ultrasound methods. Medical Ultrasonography. 2014;16(3):236–45.

20. Mazhar SM, Shiehmorteza M, Sirlin CB. Noninvasive assessment of hepatic steatosis. Clinical Gastroenterology and Hepatology. 2009;7(2):135–40.

21. Valls C, Iannaccone R, Alba E, et al. Fat in the liver: diagnosis and characterization. European Radiology. 2006;16(10): 2292–308.

22. Mathiesen UL, Franzen LE, Aselius H, et al. Increased liver echogenicity at ultrasound examination reflects degree of steatosis but not of fibrosis in asymptomatic patients with mild/moderate abnormalities of liver transaminases. Digestive and Liver Disease. 2002;34(7):516–22.

23. Hernaez R, Lazo M, Bonekamp S, et al. Diagnostic accuracy and reliability of ultrasonography for the detection of fatty liver: a meta-analysis. Hepatology. 2011;54(3):1082–90.

24. Dasarathy S, Dasarathy J, Khiyami A, Joseph R, Lopez R, McCullough AJ. Validity of real time ultrasound in the diagnosis of hepatic steatosis: a prospective study. Journal of Hepatology. 2009;51(6):1061–7.

25. Lee SS, Park SH, Kim HJ, et al. Non-invasive assessment of hepatic steatosis: prospective comparison of the accuracy of imaging examinations. Journal of Hepatology. 2010;52(4): 579–85.

26. Needleman L, Kurtz AB, Rifkin MD, Cooper HS, Pasto ME, Goldberg BB. Sonography of diffuse benign liver disease: accuracy of pattern recognition and grading. American Journal of Roentgenology. 1986;146(5):1011–5.

27. Saverymuttu SH, Joseph AE, Maxwell JD. Ultrasound scanning in the detection of hepatic fibrosis and steatosis. British Medical Journal. 1986;292(6512):13–5.

28. Hepburn MJ, Vos JA, Fillman EP, Lawitz EJ. The accuracy of the report of hepatic steatosis on ultrasonography in patients infected with hepatitis C in a clinical setting: a retrospective observational study. BMC Gastroenterology. 2005;5:14.

29. Palmentieri B, de Sio I, La Mura V, et al. The role of bright liver echo pattern on ultrasound B-mode examination in the diagnosis of liver steatosis. Digestive and Liver Disease. 2006;38(7):485–9.

30. Mottin CC, Moretto M, Padoin AV, et al. The role of ultrasound in the diagnosis of hepatic steatosis in morbidly obese patients. Obesity Surgery. 2004;14(5):635–7.

31. Festi D, Schiumerini R, Marzi L, et al. Review article: the diagnosis of non-alcoholic fatty liver disease—availability and accuracy of non-invasive methods. Alimentary Pharmacology & Therapeutics. 2013;37(4):392–400.

32. Qayyum A, Chen DM, Breiman RS, et al. Evaluation of diffuse liver steatosis by ultrasound, computed tomography, and magnetic resonance imaging: which modality is best? Clinical Imaging. 2009;33(2):110–5.

33. Strauss S, Gavish E, Gottlieb P, Katsnelson L. Interobserver and intraobserver variability in the sonographic assessment of fatty liver. American Journal of Roentgenology. 2007;189(6): W320–W323.

34. Fishbein M, Castro F, Cheruku S, et al. Hepatic MRI for fat quantitation: its relationship to fat morphology, diagnosis, and ultrasound. Journal of Clinical Gastroenterology. 2005;39(7):619–25.

35. Graif M, Yanuka M, Baraz M, et al. Quantitative estimation of attenuation in ultrasound video images: correlation with histology in diffuse liver disease. Investigative Radiology. 2000;35(5):319–24.

36. Kim SH, Lee JM, Kim JH, et al. Appropriateness of a donor liver with respect to macrosteatosis: application of artificial neural networks to US images—initial experience. Radiology. 2005;234(3):793–803.

37. Gaitini D, Baruch Y, Ghersin E, et al. Feasibility study of ultrasonic fatty liver biopsy: texture vs. attenuation and backscatter. Ultrasound in Medicine & Biology. 2004;30(10):1321–7.

38. van Werven JR, Marsman HA, Nederveen AJ, et al. Assessment of hepatic steatosis in patients undergoing liver resection: comparison of US, CT, T1-weighted dual-echo MR imaging, and point-resolved 1H MR spectroscopy. Radiology. 2010;256(1):159–68.

39. Park SH, Kim PN, Kim KW, et al. Macrovesicular hepatic steatosis in living liver donors: use of CT for quantitative and qualitative assessment. Radiology. 2006;239(1):105–12.

40. Park YS, Park SH, Lee SS, et al. Biopsy-proven nonsteatotic liver in adults: estimation of reference range for difference in

attenuation between the liver and the spleen at nonenhanced CT. Radiology. 2011;258(3):760–6.

41. Johnston RJ, Stamm ER, Lewin JM, Hendrick RE, Archer PG. Diagnosis of fatty infiltration of the liver on contrast enhanced CT: limitations of liver-minus-spleen attenuation difference measurements. Abdominal Imaging. 1998;23(4): 409–15.

42. Limanond P, Raman SS, Lassman C, et al. Macrovesicular hepatic steatosis in living related liver donors: correlation between CT and histologic findings. Radiology. 2004;230(1): 276–80.

43. Piekarski J, Goldberg HI, Royal SA, Axel L, Moss AA. Difference between liver and spleen CT numbers in the normal adult: its usefulness in predicting the presence of diffuse liver disease. Radiology. 1980;137(3):727–9.

44. Pickhardt PJ, Park SH, Hahn L, Lee SG, Bae KT, Yu ES. Specificity of unenhanced CT for non-invasive diagnosis of hepatic steatosis: implications for the investigation of the natural history of incidental steatosis. European Radiology. 2012;22(5):1075–82.

45. Birnbaum BA, Hindman N, Lee J, Babb JS. Multi-detector row CT attenuation measurements: assessment of intra- and interscanner variability with an anthropomorphic body CT phantom. Radiology. 2007;242(1):109–19.

46. Qayyum A, Goh JS, Kakar S, Yeh BM, Merriman RB, Coakley FV. Accuracy of liver fat quantification at MR imaging: comparison of out-of-phase gradient-echo and fat-saturated fast spin-echo techniques—initial experience. Radiology. 2005;237(2):507–11.

47. Hussain HK, Chenevert TL, Londy FJ, et al. Hepatic fat fraction: MR imaging for quantitative measurement and display—early experience. Radiology. 2005;237(3):1048–55.

48. Westphalen AC, Qayyum A, Yeh BM, et al. Liver fat: effect of hepatic iron deposition on evaluation with opposed-phase MR imaging. Radiology. 2007;242(2):450–5.

49. Kim SH, Lee JM, Han JK, et al. Hepatic macrosteatosis: predicting appropriateness of liver donation by using MR imaging—correlation with histopathologic findings. Radiology. 2006;240(1):116–29.

50. Wells SA. Quantification of hepatic fat and iron with magnetic resonance imaging. Magnetic Resonance Imaging Clinics of North America. 2014;22(3):397–416.

51. Yu H, Shimakawa A, McKenzie CA, Brodsky E, Brittain JH, Reeder SB. Multiecho water-fat separation and simultaneous $R2^*$ estimation with multifrequency fat spectrum modeling. Magnetic Resonance in Medicine. 2008;60(5):1122–34.

52. Bydder M, Yokoo T, Hamilton G, et al. Relaxation effects in the quantification of fat using gradient echo imaging. Magnetic Resonance Imaging. 2008;26(3):347–59.

53. Yu H, McKenzie CA, Shimakawa A, et al. Multiecho reconstruction for simultaneous water-fat decomposition and T2*

estimation. Journal of Magnetic Resonance Imaging. 2007;26(4):1153–61.

54. O'Regan DP, Callaghan MF, Wylezinska-Arridge M, et al. Liver fat content and T2*: simultaneous measurement by using breath-hold multiecho MR imaging at 3.0 T—feasibility. Radiology. 2008;247(2):550–7.

55. Guiu B, Petit JM, Loffroy R, et al. Quantification of liver fat content: comparison of triple-echo chemical shift gradient-echo imaging and in vivo proton MR spectroscopy. Radiology. 2009;250(1):95–102.

56. Hamilton G, Yokoo T, Bydder M, et al. In vivo characterization of the liver fat (1)H MR spectrum. NMR in Biomedicine. 2011;24(7):784–90.

57. Liu CY, McKenzie CA, Yu H, Brittain JH, Reeder SB. Fat quantification with IDEAL gradient echo imaging: correction of bias from T(1) and noise. Magnetic Resonance in Medicine. 2007;58(2):354–64.

58. Hernando D, Hines CD, Yu H, Reeder SB. Addressing phase errors in fat-water imaging using a mixed magnitude/complex fitting method. Magnetic Resonance in Medicine. 2012;67(3):638–44.

59. Yu H, Shimakawa A, Hines CD, et al. Combination of complex-based and magnitude-based multiecho water-fat separation for accurate quantification of fat-fraction. Magnetic Resonance in Medicine. 2011;66(1):199–206.

60. Yu H, Shimakawa A, McKenzie CA, et al. Phase and amplitude correction for multi-echo water-fat separation with bipolar acquisitions. Journal of Magnetic Resonance Imaging. 2010;31(5):1264–71.

61. Yokoo T, Bydder M, Hamilton G, et al. Nonalcoholic fatty liver disease: diagnostic and fat-grading accuracy of low-flip-angle multiecho gradient-recalled-echo MR imaging at 1.5 T. Radiology. 2009;251(1):67–76.

62. Yokoo T, Shiehmorteza M, Hamilton G, et al. Estimation of hepatic proton-density fat fraction by using MR imaging at 3.0 T. Radiology. 2011;258(3):749–59.

63. Tang A, Tan J, Sun M, et al. Nonalcoholic fatty liver disease: MR imaging of liver proton density fat fraction to assess hepatic steatosis. Radiology. 2013;267(2):422–31.

64. Permutt Z, Le TA, Peterson MR, et al. Correlation between liver histology and novel magnetic resonance imaging in adult patients with non-alcoholic fatty liver disease—MRI accurately quantifies hepatic steatosis in NAFLD. Alimentary Pharmacology & Therapeutics. 2012;36(1):22–9.

65. Meisamy S, Hines CD, Hamilton G, et al. Quantification of hepatic steatosis with T1-independent, T2-corrected MR imaging with spectral modeling of fat: blinded comparison with MR spectroscopy. Radiology. 2011;258(3):767–75.

66. Idilman IS, Aniktar H, Idilman R, et al. Hepatic steatosis: quantification by proton density fat fraction with MR imaging versus liver biopsy. Radiology. 2013;267(3):767–75.

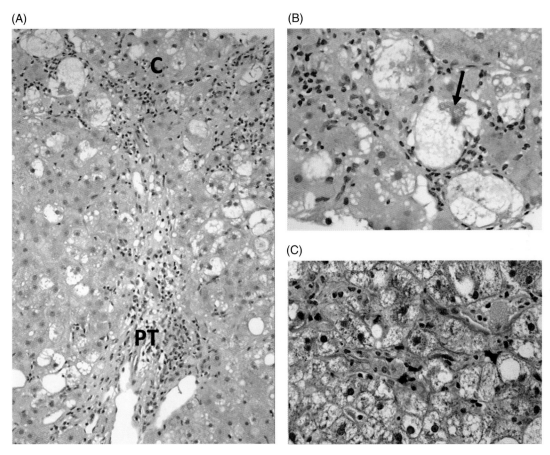

**FIG 5.1** Classical non-alcoholic steatohepatitis (NASH). (A) Steatosis, hepatocyte ballooning, and inflammation (the trio of changes representing the minimal histological criteria of steatohepatitis) are evident in the centrilobular region (C). (B) Hepatocyte ballooning and intracellular Mallory–Denk bodies (arrow) are shown at high magnification. (C) The characteristic pericellular/perisinusoidal "chicken-wire" pattern of fibrosis surrounding centrilobular hepatocytes is seen on this trichrome stain (A and B, hematoxylin and eosin stain; C: Masson trichrome stain).

*Clinical Dilemmas in Non-Alcoholic Fatty Liver Disease,* First Edition. Edited by Roger Williams and Simon D. Taylor-Robinson.
© 2016 John Wiley & Sons, Ltd. Published 2016 by John Wiley & Sons, Ltd.

(A)

(B)

(C)

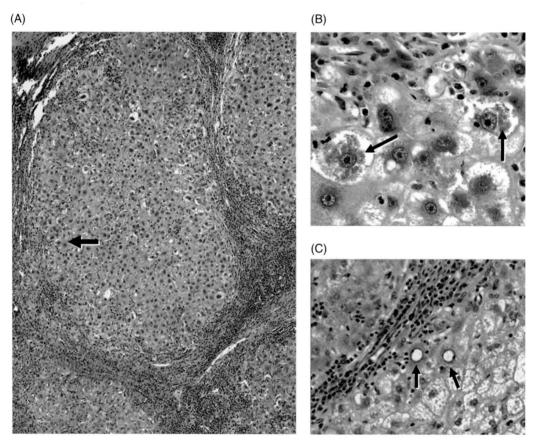

**FIG 5.2** "Cryptogenic cirrhosis" due to NAFLD. (A) Cirrhosis without fat is seen at low magnification. Portal tracts and fibrous septa contain mild to moderate chronic inflammatory cell infiltrates, rendering a superficial resemblance to chronic hepatitis. However, careful examination of the hepatocytes located at the periphery of the nodules (arrow) allows recognition of remaining NASH features (seen at high power in panel B). (B) High magnification of the parenchyma near the arrow in panel A. Hepatocytes are variably ballooned and there is robust Mallory–Denk body formation (arrows). (C): Occasional periportal/periseptal hepatocytes show glycogenated nuclei (arrows) (A, B, and C: hematoxylin and eosin stain).

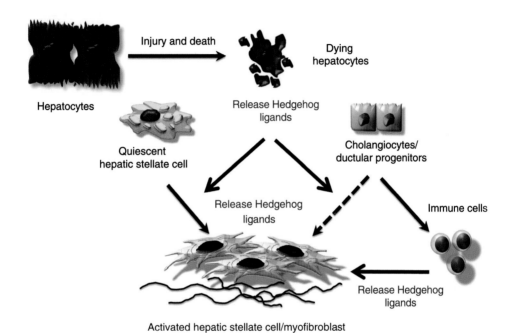

**Injury and death**

**Dying hepatocytes**

**Hepatocytes**

**Quiescent hepatic stellate cell**

**Release Hedgehog ligands**

**Cholangiocytes/ ductular progenitors**

**Release Hedgehog ligands**

**Immune cells**

**Release Hedgehog ligands**

**Activated hepatic stellate cell/myofibroblast**

**FIG 8.1** Link between cell death and fibrogenic liver repair. Liver cell injury or death from lipotoxicity, oxidative stress and immune imbalance leads to the release of signalling factors (such as Hedgehog ligands), which promote the proliferation of ductular progenitors and liver pericytes (hepatic stellate cells) as part of the repair response. Stimulated hepatic stellate cells transition into collagen-producing myofibroblasts, and ductular progenitor cells secrete high levels of cytokines and growth factors that recruit immune cells into the liver. In turn, recruited immune cells secrete even more cytokines and growth factors that perpetuate the inflammatory and fibrogenic response. Ductular progenitors may also undergo direct differentiation into scar-producing myofibroblasts.

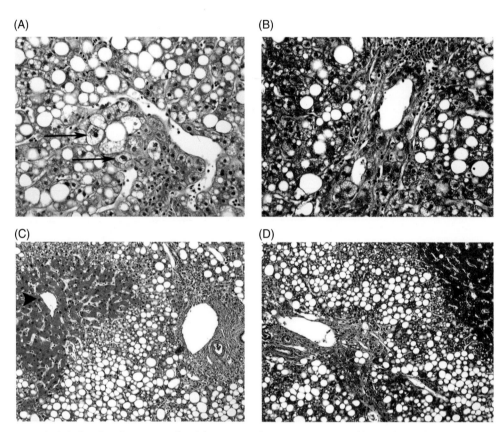

**FIG 9.1** Non-alcoholic fatty liver disease. Examples of the zone 3 and zone 1 injury patterns. (A) Typical steatohepatitis with perivenular inflammation and ballooning (arrows). (B) Masson trichrome stain from the same case showing delicate zone 3 perisinusoidal fibrosis. (C) Zone 1 borderline pattern with periportal steatosis and portal inflammation. No injury is seen around the terminal hepatic venule (arrowhead). (D) Masson trichrome stain from the same case showing periportal fibrosis but no perivenular fibrosis (arrowhead).

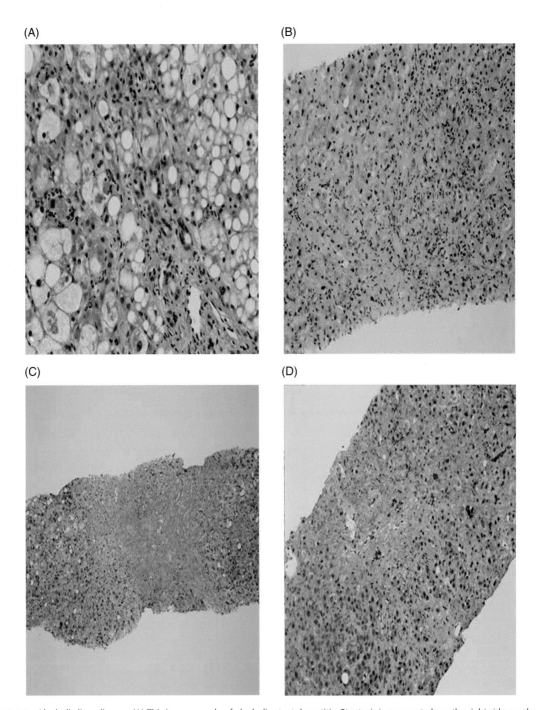

**FIG 9.2** Alcoholic liver disease. (A) This is an example of alcoholic steatohepatitis. Steatosis is apparent along the right side; marked ballooning and Mallory–Denk bodies are noted in hepatocytes along the left. Satellitosis is also seen as well as ductular reaction. (B–D) These figures are from a patient who presented with signs and symptoms of venous outflow obstruction. (B) In this example of several alcoholic hepatitis, there is very little steatosis, and one can appreciate near obliteration of all vascular (terminal hepatic venule and portal tract) structures. The primary component of the cellular infiltrate is neutrophils. With close inspection, Mallory–Denk bodies can be seen, as well as bile-stained hepatocytes. This is an example of sclerosing hyaline necrosis and would not be seen in NAFLD/NASH. (C) A low-power trichrome stain shows obliterative fibrosis of a centrilobular region; this extent and type of fibrotic response are not described in NAFLD/NASH. (D) The high-power view of the Masson trichrome highlights the remnant of a terminal hepatic venule centrally and dense sinusoidal fibrosis in the lobules. Capillarization to this extent in alcoholic liver disease results in portal hypertension without the classic histologic features of cirrhosis.

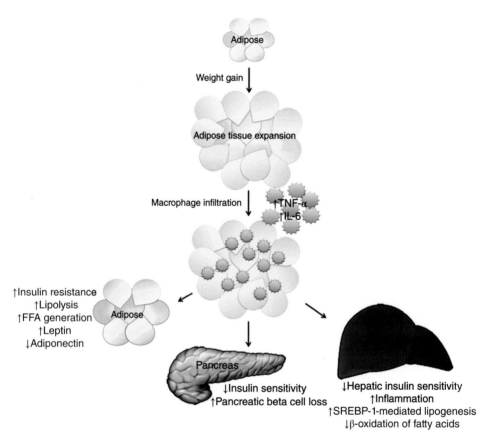

**FIG 10.1** Weight gain leads to adipose tissue expansion and inflammation, which results in a proinflammatory state. These adipokines worsen adipose tissue and hepatic and systemic insulin resistance. The deterioration in insulin sensitivity leads to pancreatic β-cell loss, de novo lipogenesis, and hepatic steatosis.

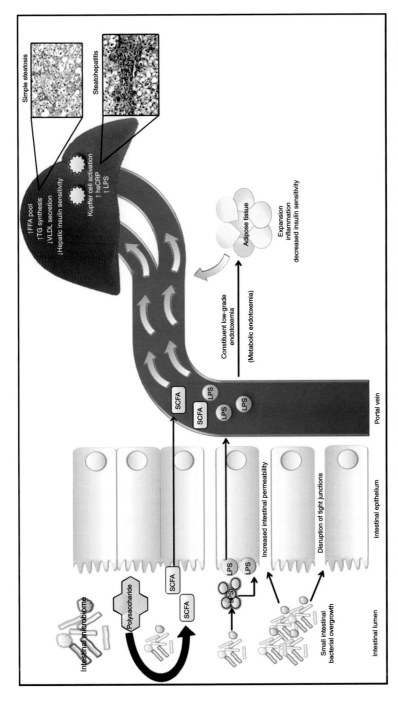

**FIG 10.2** NAFLD is associated with an increase in small intestinal bacterial overgrowth (SIBO). The intestinal microbiome breaks down polysaccharides into short-chain fatty acids (SCFAs), and increased bacterial productions (i.e., LPS) are then readily absorbed into the portal circulation. These by-products of digestion and intestinal microbiome subsequently influence insulin resistance and impair hepatic triglyceride synthesis leading to hepatic steatosis.

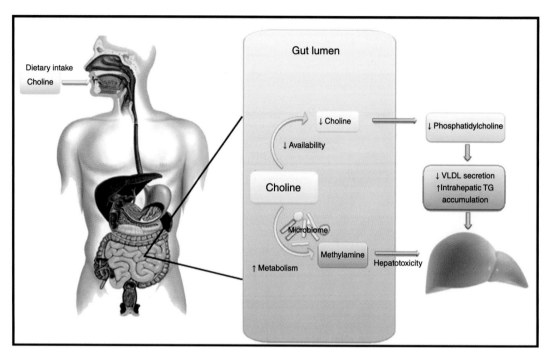

**FIG 10.3** The gut microbiota catalyzes the conversion of dietary choline into methylamines, which enter the portal circulation and promote hepatocellular injury. The conversion of choline to methylamines also reduces the bioavailability of choline, leading to phosphatidylcholine deficiency, which impairs VLDL secretion and promotes steatosis.

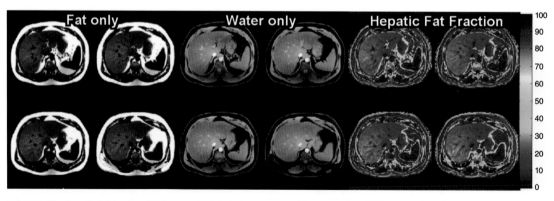

**FIG 16.7** The hepatic fat fraction (HFF) map calculated using water and fat separation GRE images. The color scale on the side indicates the percent HFF.

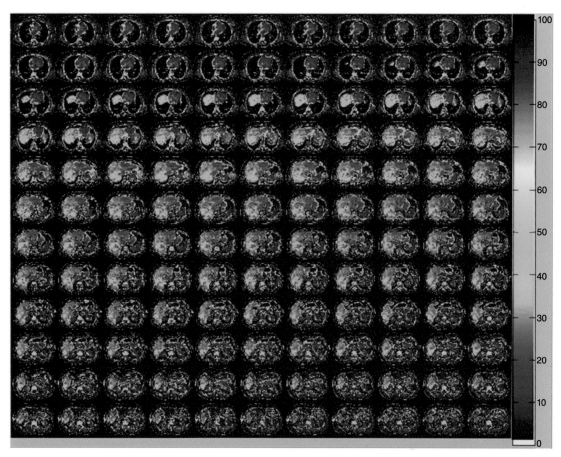

**FIG 16.8** Proton density hepatic fat fraction (PD-HFF) map of the entire liver. The color scale on the side indicates the percent HFF.

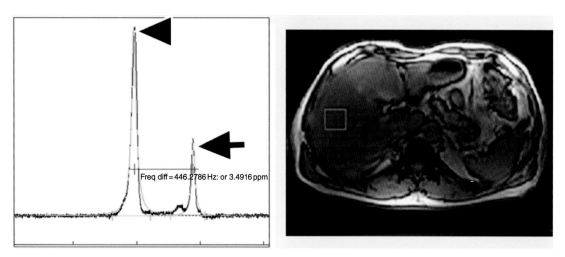

Freq diff = 446.2786 Hz: or 3.4916 ppm

**FIG 16.10** Single-voxel proton MR spectroscopy of a fatty liver at 1.5 T. Note the small red voxel placed in the right lobe of the liver and the water (arrowhead) and dominant fat (methylene) (arrow) peaks in the sampled parenchyma.

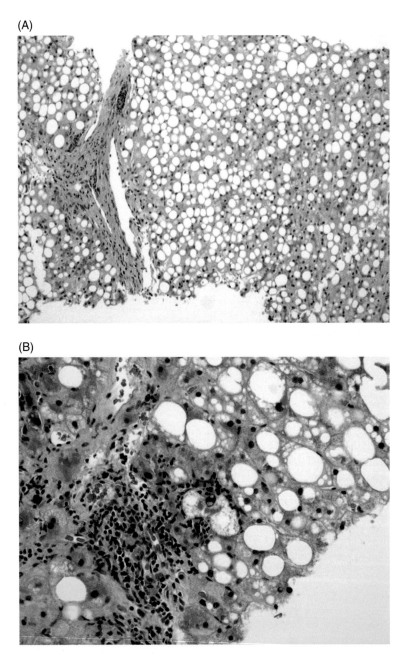

**FIG 17.1** (A) Liver biopsy section with H&E staining at ×200 magnification, showing simple severe steatosis. (B) Liver biopsy section with H&E staining at ×400 magnification, showing non-alcoholic steatohepatitis with ballooning, Mallory's hyaline, glycogenated nuclei, portal and lobular inflammation (*Source*: Courtesy of Dr Eve Fryer, Oxford University Hospitals NHS Trust).

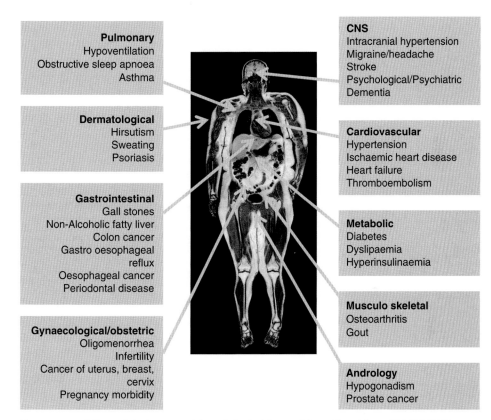

**Pulmonary**
Hypoventilation
Obstructive sleep apnoea
Asthma

**Dermatological**
Hirsutism
Sweating
Psoriasis

**Gastrointestinal**
Gall stones
Non-Alcoholic fatty liver
Colon cancer
Gastro oesophageal
reflux
Oesophageal cancer
Periodontal disease

**Gynaecological/obstetric**
Oligomenorrhea
Infertility
Cancer of uterus, breast,
cervix
Pregnancy morbidity

**CNS**
Intracranial hypertension
Migraine/headache
Stroke
Psychological/Psychiatric
Dementia

**Cardiovascular**
Hypertension
Ischaemic heart disease
Heart failure
Thromboembolism

**Metabolic**
Diabetes
Dyslipaemia
Hyperinsulinaemia

**Musculo skeletal**
Osteoarthritis
Gout

**Andrology**
Hypogonadism
Prostate cancer

**FIG 19.1** The spectrum of disease linked to overweight and obesity ( *Source*: Science Photo Library C007/2245 (Obese woman, MRI scan). Reproduced with permission from Science Photo Library).

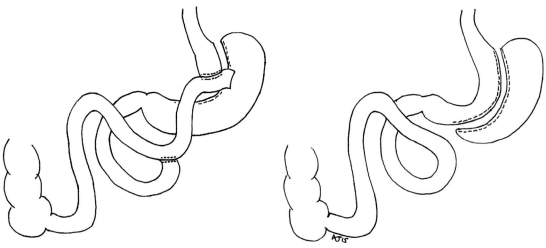

**FIG 22.1** Gastric bypass.

**FIG 22.2** Sleeve gastrectomy.

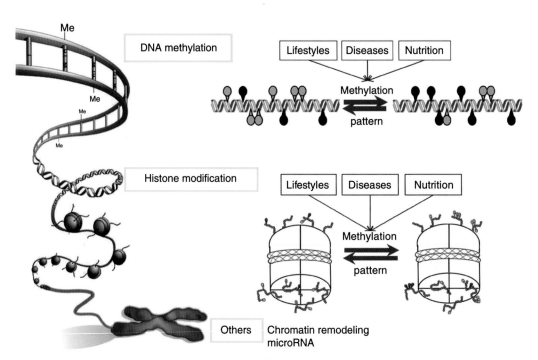

**FIG 26.1** The main epigenetic reactions are the methylation of CpG sites and the modifications on amino acidic tails of histones such as by methylation, acetylation or phosphorylation. These reactions could be influenced by factors such as lifestyles, diseases and diet, and the final conformation of DNA could facilitate joining of the transcription factors (*Source*: (left) Qiu [40], reproduced with permission of Nature Publishing Group and (right) Cordero et al. [41]).

67. Negrete LM, Middleton MS, Clark L, et al. Inter-examination precision of magnitude-based MRI for estimation of segmental hepatic proton density fat fraction in obese subjects. Journal of Magnetic Resonance Imaging. 2014;39(5):1265–71.

68. Kang GH, Cruite I, Shiehmorteza M, et al. Reproducibility of MRI-determined proton density fat fraction across two different MR scanner platforms. Journal of Magnetic Resonance Imaging. 2011;34(4):928–34.

69. Noureddin M, Lam J, Peterson MR, et al. Utility of magnetic resonance imaging versus histology for quantifying changes in liver fat in nonalcoholic fatty liver disease trials. Hepatology. 2013;58(6):1930–40.

70. Szczepaniak LS, Nurenberg P, Leonard D, et al. Magnetic resonance spectroscopy to measure hepatic triglyceride content: prevalence of hepatic steatosis in the general population. American Journal of Physiology. Endocrinology and Metabolism. 2005;288(2):E462–E468.

71. Hamilton G, Middleton MS, Bydder M, et al. Effect of PRESS and STEAM sequences on magnetic resonance spectroscopic liver fat quantification. Journal of Magnetic Resonance Imaging. 2009;30(1):145–52.

72. Reeder SB, Cruite I, Hamilton G, Sirlin CB. Quantitative assessment of liver fat with magnetic resonance imaging and spectroscopy. Journal of Magnetic Resonance Imaging. 2011; 34(4):spcone.

73. Kang BK, Yu ES, Lee SS, et al. Hepatic fat quantification: a prospective comparison of magnetic resonance spectroscopy and analysis methods for chemical-shift gradient echo magnetic resonance imaging with histologic assessment as the reference standard. Investigative Radiology. 2012;47(6): 368–75.

74. Pineda N, Sharma P, Xu Q, Hu X, Vos M, Martin DR. Measurement of hepatic lipid: high-speed T2-corrected multiecho acquisition at 1H MR spectroscopy—a rapid and accurate technique. Radiology. 2009;252(2):568–76.

75. Lee SS, Lee Y, Kim N, et al. Hepatic fat quantification using chemical shift MR imaging and MR spectroscopy in the presence of hepatic iron deposition: validation in phantoms and in patients with chronic liver disease. Journal of Magnetic Resonance Imaging. 2011;33(6): 1390–8.

76. Urdzik J, Bjerner T, Wanders A, et al. The value of preoperative magnetic resonance spectroscopy in the assessment of steatohepatitis in patients with colorectal liver metastasis. Journal of Hepatology. 2012;56(3):640–6.

77. Roldan-Valadez E, Favila R, Martinez-Lopez M, Uribe M, Rios C, Mendez-Sanchez N. In vivo 3 T spectroscopic quantification of liver fat content in nonalcoholic fatty liver disease: correlation with biochemical method and morphometry. Journal of Hepatology. 2010;53(4): 732–7.

78. Raptis DA, Fischer MA, Graf R, et al. MRI: the new reference standard in quantifying hepatic steatosis? Gut. 2012; 61(1):117–27.

# 17 Are the advantages of obtaining a liver biopsy outweighed by the disadvantages?

## Jeremy F. L. Cobbold[1] and Simon D. Taylor-Robinson[2]

[1] Oxford University Hospitals NHS Trust, Oxford, UK
[2] Digestive Diseases Division, Imperial College London, London, UK

## LEARNING POINTS

- Liver biopsy is subject to sampling error as it represents less than 1/50 000 of the liver.

- However, histological assessment of hepatic fat content is still the gold standard (although ultrasound or MR imaging techniques are good for uncomplicated NAFLD).

- Non-invasive methodologies for assessing liver fibrosis (ultrasound-based elastography techniques and MR elastography) are robust, but liver biopsy should be performed where there is diagnostic doubt.

- Non-invasive assessment of hepatic inflammation remains uncertain, and where diagnosis is in doubt in NASH, then liver biopsy remains the best option.

## Introduction

Fatty infiltration of the liver, seen histologically in the absence of excessive alcohol intake and in association with obesity and/or type 2 diabetes, has long been described and latterly termed non-alcoholic fatty liver disease (NAFLD) [1, 2]. NAFLD encompasses a range of liver pathology ranging from steatosis, without significant inflammation ('simple steatosis' (SS) or non-alcoholic fatty liver (NAFL); Figure 17.1A), through non-alcoholic steatohepatitis (NASH; Figure 17.1B), with or without associated hepatic fibrosis, to cirrhosis and its complications [3]. NAFLD is closely associated the metabolic syndrome of abdominal obesity, type 2 diabetes or impaired fasting glucose, dyslipidaemia and hypertension [4], and its global prevalence of 15–50% reflects the worsening

pandemic of obesity [5]. Such is the prevalence of NAFLD that in some populations, hepatic steatosis may be considered normal, yet in a substantial minority of patients, NAFLD has the potential to progress to advanced liver disease and NASH is associated with increased liver-related and all-cause mortality [6]. Diagnosis and assessment of disease severity are central to the allocation of resources, delivery of established and novel therapies and our greater understanding of the condition. In this chapter, the utility of histological examination of liver biopsy is discussed in the context of possible non-invasive alternatives.

## Diagnosis and assessment of disease severity

### Diagnosis of NAFLD

NAFLD is histologically defined as the presence of steatosis, of a predominantly macrovesicular pattern, in >5% of hepatocytes, causing displacement of the nucleus, in the absence of excessive alcohol intake. Steatosis is required to diagnose all categories within the NAFLD spectrum. Secondary causes of hepatic steatosis including drugs (such as highly active antiretroviral therapy, amiodarone and tamoxifen), viruses (such as hepatitis C) and jejunal bypass surgery conventionally preclude the diagnosis [3]. Cryptogenic cirrhosis lacks characteristics of NAFLD, in that significant steatosis is not evident (or has been considered 'burnt out'). In this situation, a substantial proportion of patients with cryptogenic cirrhosis are considered to have NAFLD as the primary aetiology, based on concomitant metabolic risk

*Clinical Dilemmas in Non-Alcoholic Fatty Liver Disease*, First Edition. Edited by Roger Williams and Simon D. Taylor-Robinson.
© 2016 John Wiley & Sons, Ltd. Published 2016 by John Wiley & Sons, Ltd.

(A)

(B)

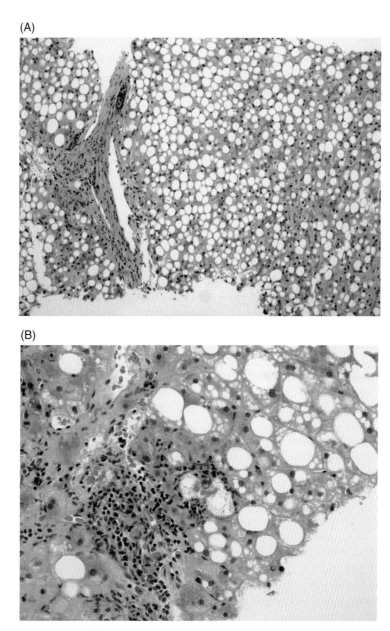

**FIG 17.1** (A) Liver biopsy section with H&E staining at ×200 magnification, showing simple severe steatosis. (B) Liver biopsy section with H&E staining at ×400 magnification, showing non-alcoholic steatohepatitis with ballooning, Mallory's hyaline, glycogenated nuclei, portal and lobular inflammation (*Source*: Courtesy of Dr Eve Fryer, Oxford University Hospitals NHS Trust). (*See insert for color representation of the figure.*)

factors and subtle histological features [7]. Morphological features typically observed in NASH in addition to steatosis include ballooning degeneration of hepatocytes, lobular and portal inflammation and other features, such as the presence of Mallory's hyaline, glycogenated nuclei and a degree of siderosis, with or without fibrosis [8] (Figure 17.1B).

With such a high global prevalence of NAFLD, a strictly histological definition is not practical. The diagnosis may be suspected in patients with mild elevations of aminotransferase values (typically <3× upper limit of normal) or increased echogenicity of the hepatic parenchyma on ultrasound, often found incidentally, without excessive alcohol intake or contributory drugs, particularly in those with features of the metabolic syndrome [9, 10]. Indeed, NASH or SS was found in 66% of a series of over 350 patients with elevated aminotransferase values, who underwent liver biopsy following exclusion of alcohol and a negative chronic liver disease screen [11]. However, aminotransferase values may also be within normal limits for any degree of disease severity [12, 13].

Abdominal ultrasound is a widely available clinical tool with good sensitivity (91%) and specificity (93%) for the detection of moderate steatosis, but the technique is operator dependent, is not quantitative and is less sensitive in obese subjects and those with mild steatosis [14]. Serological testing is used to exclude other causes of chronic liver disease including hepatitis B and C, autoimmune hepatitis and primary biliary cirrhosis, while iron indices, caeruloplasmin and alpha-1 antitrypsin levels may be determined to exclude metabolic causes or co-morbidities [15]. Elevated serum ferritin concentrations are commonly seen in NAFLD/NASH and are associated with greater severity of disease [16]. Where ultrasound is unavailable, a 'fatty liver index' has been derived to predict fatty liver, as seen on ultrasound with components including gamma-glutamyl transferase, waist circumference, body mass index and serum triglyceride concentration, which predicted fatty liver with an accuracy of 0.84 [17].

Thus, in the majority of cases, a diagnosis of NAFLD can be made without liver biopsy. However, there may be diagnostic uncertainty in patients who do not present conventionally, for example: in patients taking multiple medications; in patients with low titres of the anti-nuclear antibody or mildly elevated immunoglobulin G or A values; or where serum ferritin, commonly mildly elevated in NAFL/NASH, is moderately elevated. Histological examination of liver biopsy may aid confirmation of a suspected diagnosis of NAFLD or exclusion of alternative diagnoses not clearly or readily excluded by a non-invasive chronic liver disease screen, such as drug-induced liver injury, granulomatous disease, primary sclerosing cholangitis or even normal liver [11].

### Diagnosis of hepatic co-morbidity

With the rising prevalence of obesity and type 2 diabetes, there is an increased likelihood of dual pathology with other liver diseases including hepatitis C and hepatitis B,

haemochromatosis and autoimmune liver diseases. Although dual pathology may yet be suspected on the basis of non-invasive assessment as described previously, dual pathology may be associated with more rapid progression of disease [18], providing further indication for biopsy to establish a contribution from non-alcoholic or metabolic fatty liver disease.

### Quantification of steatosis

The relationship between the quantity of steatosis and disease progression is unclear. Severe steatosis may occur in mild disease but can decrease with advanced fibrosis. A study of paired biopsies suggested that the degree of steatosis was the only independent histological factor in disease progression [19]. However, a murine model demonstrated that inhibition of triglyceride synthesis decreased steatosis but worsened inflammation [20], raising the possibility that steatosis represents an adaptive response to inflammatory and oxidative stress [21]. Accordingly, it is not clear how the quantification of steatosis may help in diagnosis or assessment of severity, but serial analysis may aid assessment of response to therapy.

Quantification of steatosis by histology usually involves counting the proportion of hepatocytes containing triglyceride droplets, categorised as <5; 5–33%; 33–66; >66% and incorporated into the NAFLD activity score (NAS) as 0–3, described in the following [22]. This is a robust, pragmatic measure with good inter-observer agreement but correlates poorly with tissue triglyceride assessed biochemically. However, Oil Red-O staining (requiring snap freezing of liver tissue) and digital image analysis correlated closely with the biochemical assessment [23].

Non-invasive alternatives can quantify liver fat with high accuracy. In particular, appropriately calibrated proton magnetic resonance spectroscopy ($^1$H MRS) and multi-echo magnetic resonance imaging (MRI) enable the quantitation of hepatic triglyceride [24]. Although not yet widely clinically available, most MRI scanners have capability to perform MRS with appropriate sequences and software. Being non-invasive, it is appropriate for research studies, including studies establishing the prevalence of hepatic steatosis [25, 26] and repeated measurement. Although conventional B-mode ultrasound scanning is unable to quantify steatosis [24], a derivation of the information obtained during transient elastography (TE), the controlled attenuation parameter (CAP) also provides a measure of steatosis [27], with further validation ongoing.

## Diagnosis of steatohepatitis

NASH is considered to be the progressive form of NAFLD (Figure 17.1) and is defined histologically [6, 28]. A standardised method for the semi-quantitative description of these lesions was described by Brunt in 1999 [29] and revised by the NASH CRN, resulting in the NAS [22]. This system, in which the features of steatosis, lobular inflammation and hepatocyte ballooning are score from 0–3, 0–3 and 0–2, respectively, was originally designed to detect change in a quantitative manner for the purposes of clinical trials. The unweighted sum of scores was grouped into categories: non-NASH (0–2), borderline NASH [3, 4] and NASH (≥5), which correlated with the histologists' diagnoses of NASH or non-NASH. However, the authors emphasise that such a scoring system does not replace a histological diagnosis that considers the overall picture of pathological lesions [30]. The steatosis, activity and fibrosis (SAF) score, which employs an algorithm in which ballooning of hepatocytes is necessary but not sufficient for the diagnosis of NASH, was validated in patients with morbid obesity with biopsy material collected at the time of bariatric surgery. In this cohort, and a smaller retrospective review of non-obese subjects, there was clearer separation of NASH and not-NASH entities [31, 32].

Standard clinical indices and routine biochemistry are unable to diagnose NASH [13], despite correlation between ALT values and NAS score and SAF score [31]. However, accurate non-invasive identification of patients with NASH has been the subject of much research. For example, measurement of plasma CK-18 fragments, a marker of apoptosis and cell death, yielded significant differences between patients with and without NASH [33], yet in a larger validation cohort, the diagnostic accuracy as described by the area under the receiver operator characteristic curve (AUROC) for detection of biopsy-proven NASH was just 0.65, limiting its clinical utility for this purpose [34]. Measurement of the terminal peptide of procollagen III (PIIINP) was found to distinguish SS from NASH in the absence of advanced fibrosis with an AUROC of 0.83 in a derivation set and 0.78 in a validation set [35], although further validation is awaited. Non-invasive assessment is discussed further in Chapter 14 and reviewed elsewhere [36].

## Staging of fibrosis

In NAFLD, like in other chronic liver diseases, the presence of advanced fibrosis stage is the best predictor of the development of liver-related and all-cause mortality and so of prognostic value [37, 38]. Histological staging of fibrosis is, strictly speaking, an ordinal description of the pattern of distribution of fibrosis within the tissue architecture. There is correlation between staging (according to Ishak) and fibrosis, quantified in two dimensions by collagen proportionate area and furthermore with hepatic venous pressure gradient (HVPG) measurement [39]. The NAS system, which stages fibrosis from 0 to 4, is analogous to other staging systems for chronic liver diseases and has excellent intra- and inter-rater variability [22].

Over the last decade, however, progress has been made in the development and validation of non-invasive markers of chronic liver disease and, in particular, biomarkers of fibrosis [36, 40]. Initially shown simply to correlate with histological staging, these have been sufficiently validated so as to reduce the necessity for liver biopsy to exclude advanced fibrosis. Markers include blood and clinical based markers, which in turn may be direct or indirect, and imaging-based markers including elastography-based techniques (including TE and acoustic force radiation imaging (ARFI)) and magnetic resonance (MR) scanning (including MR elastography and multiparametric approaches [40, 41]). Most such techniques have been validated using fibrosis staging from liver biopsy as a reference standard. Diagnostic accuracy, derived from the area under the receiver operator curve, exceeds 90% for many techniques in the diagnosis of cirrhosis [40, 42] and also exceeds 90% NPV for excluding advanced fibrosis (i.e. bridging fibrosis and cirrhosis). As liver biopsy itself has inherent inaccuracies in up to 20% of cases, this approaches the theoretical diagnostic limit for modelling histological features, so in clinical practice, close attention to discordant information (e.g. among clinical findings, blood markers, imaging and any histology) is required [43].

Reliable delineation of intermediate fibrosis stages by non-invasive techniques is limited because histological staging is a descriptive, morphological, ordinal, categorical variable, which is semi-quantitative at best [44]. Thus, techniques that measure a quantitative continuous variable should not be expected to model this reliably. However, it may also be argued that in clinical practice, the determination of intermediate stages of fibrosis is not clinically useful but that the diagnosis of cirrhosis and the exclusion of advanced fibrosis are of greatest utility, both of which are achievable with a high degree of diagnostic accuracy with a number of non-invasive techniques. When considering the advantages and disadvantages of liver biopsy in staging

NAFLD, it should be borne in mind that liver biopsy too remains a surrogate marker of disease, which does not provide precise prognostic information. Long-term follow-up studies using non-invasive markers including TE, enhanced liver fibrosis test (ELF) and FibroTest, albeit not yet in NAFLD-specific populations, are now demonstrating the ability to stratify patients by hard outcome measures such as hepatic decompensation and death [45–47].

## Technical and logistical matters

### Techniques

Liver biopsy of hepatic parenchyma may be performed as a needle biopsy: percutaneous (transthoracic), via the transjugular route or as a needle biopsy or wedge biopsy intraoperatively (frequently during bariatric surgery). Percutaneous techniques are usually performed with ultrasound assistance or under direct ultrasound guidance, as a day case performed using infiltration of local anaesthetic, with or without conscious sedation. The procedure is brief and causes little discomfort in the majority of cases [48, 49]. Commonly, patients are observed for pain or signs of complications for up to 6 h afterwards. Patients are usually able to return to work the following day but are advised to avoid heavy lifting so as not to increase intra-abdominal pressure, which might lead to bleeding.

### Patient safety

Patient safety is an overriding priority in healthcare provision and the invasiveness of liver biopsy is a disadvantage in its use. Complications of percutaneous liver biopsy include pain, bleeding and perforation of a viscus. Mild pain is frequently encountered (between 30 and 84% of patients) and may be treated by short-term administration of simple oral analgesia [48, 50]. In an up-to-date series of 2229 ultrasound-guided percutaneous liver biopsies, there were 12 major complications (0.5%), 17 minor complications (0.7%) and no deaths. Of note, in approximately half of the cases, the biopsy was of a focal lesion and, of eight major complications in which bleeding required transfusion, the indication for biopsy was investigation of a potentially malignant lesion in six [51]. A review of previous case series for the AASLD concluded that the risk of severe bleeding requiring hospitalisation was between 1:2 500 and 1:10 000 [48]. These considerations are set against the minimal discomfort of blood testing for non-invasive markers or the complete safety and real-time results obtained by TE.

### Cost considerations

Liver biopsy incurs costs related to equipment, operator and support staff, day case or ward admission, pre-biopsy investigations, the possibility of complications, sample preparation and sample analysis. A further consideration is whether the result changes the cost of subsequent patient management, such as prescription of further medication, or further consultation. Non-invasive alternatives incur costs, which include capital costs of equipment purchase, running costs/maintenance and operator costs. Formal cost–benefit analyses in the context of NAFLD are awaited.

### Sample size and quality

The advantages of histological analysis assume the availability of an adequate sample. Whether a sample is adequate depends in part on the question being asked. For example, if diagnostic features of a suspected condition are seen in a small biopsy, the sample may be considered adequate. However, for staging of fibrosis, digital image analysis data from resected liver from patients with hepatitis C demonstrated that the coefficient of variation for fibrosis area measurement decreased with increasing sample length (from 55% at 15 mm to 45% at 25 mm), while the percentage of samples that were scored correctly by the METAVIR system increased from 65% at 15 mm to 75% at 25 mm [52]. The AASLD guidelines on liver biopsy recommend that a sample containing 11 portal tracts is adequate, based on data from Colloredo and colleagues in patients with viral hepatitis, in which smaller samples were found to 'understage' the disease [48, 53]. The technique used (aspiration needle vs. cutting needle) may influence sample quality and the site of the sample may also affect the information obtained, as subcapsular samples may be more fibrous and thus may not be representative of underlying liver. Non-invasive imaging-based techniques are less affected by sampling variability than liver biopsy and so may be considered more representative of the liver tissue, while blood markers are unaffected by sampling variability but may be affected by extra-hepatic processes.

### Contraindications

The applicability of percutaneous liver biopsy is limited in some patients, in whom the procedure is contraindicated, including those with clotting abnormalities, ascites and morbid obesity [48, 49]. A transjugular approach enables a sample to be obtained in many of these cases, but the availability of this technique is not so widespread. It should

**TABLE 17.1** Table with examples of when the pros of liver biopsy outweigh the cons, and *vice versa*

| Liver biopsy desirable (pros outweigh cons) | Clinical equipoise (grey area) | Liver biopsy may be unnecessary (cons may outweigh pros, alternatives exist) |
|---|---|---|
| Diagnostic uncertainty | Diagnosis of NASH (*will it change management?*) | Confirmation of a clinical diagnosis of NAFLD |
| Assessment of dual pathology | Diagnosis of advanced fibrosis in absence of overt cirrhosis (*high-risk group*) | Exclusion of advanced fibrosis in clinically diagnosed NAFLD (*possible with non-invasive markers*) |
| Indeterminate or conflicting non-invasive markers | Fibrosis staging | Diagnosis of cirrhosis in the presence of typical clinical and radiological findings |
| Endpoints in clinical trials (NAS and fibrosis) | Routine follow-up biopsy (3–5-year intervals) | Quantitation of steatosis |
| Patient motivation, patient choice | Quantitation of siderosis (*can be determined by MR techniques*) | Patient choice |

These examples are the opinion of the authors and do not constitute guidelines.

be noted that morbid obesity also reduces the likelihood of successful assessment with TE [54], while TE is usually not possible in the setting of significant ascites. Blood markers and ARFI are technically limited in very few patients, while contraindications to MR scanning are well known.

### Clinical trials and natural history

In the absence of full validation of non-invasive markers for longitudinal analysis, histological definitions of resolution of steatohepatitis, without worsening of fibrosis, remain a recommended primary endpoint in phase 2 and 3 clinical trials of investigational medicinal products in NAFLD, while MR spectroscopy and liver biochemistry may serve as a primary endpoint in early phase studies of shorter duration [55]. Studies of natural history have used paired biopsy [19, 56]. However, there is a considerable risk of selection bias for any such study where the criteria for biopsy define the cohort studied and non-invasive endpoints will be used increasingly as they are validated further.

### Does liver biopsy change management?

Confirmation of the diagnosis of NAFLD or of hepatic co-morbidity clearly has the potential to change management. The diagnosis of cirrhosis is of prognostic importance and will influence initiation of screening programmes for varices and for hepatocellular carcinoma. However, cirrhosis may be diagnosed with confidence in many patients using routine clinical information and non-invasive markers of fibrosis. Here, biopsy might be limited to those patients in whom biomarkers are borderline, indeterminate or contradictory. At the other end of the scale, exclusion of advanced disease may allow lower-intensity

follow-up. Identification of NASH may influence treatment in the selection of patients who might benefit from therapy with pioglitazone or vitamin E within the bounds of evidence from clinical trials and guidelines [10, 57]. It also identifies a subgroup considered to be at increased risk of disease progression, which may provide motivation for lifestyle changes to aid weight loss. The age of the patient affected may also determine the importance of making a diagnosis of intermediate disease severity, with younger patients more likely to be affected by complications of NAFLD/NASH during their lifetime. There is no consensus as to which patients with suspected NAFLD should undergo liver biopsy [9, 10], but instances where liver biopsy may be more or less desirable are presented in Table 17.1 and are informed by whether the information obtained will change management, risk to the patient and whether alternatives exist to answer the clinical question.

### Conclusions

In conclusion, whether the pros of obtaining a liver biopsy are outweighed by the cons depends on the individual clinical case, the information sought, whether that information will change management, whether alternatives are available and patient choice. These matters are weighed up in the context of the diagnostic performance of histology and the ability to determine disease severity, the performance of non-invasive alternatives and local resources. Ultimately, histological analysis of liver biopsy remains a clinical tool to complement comprehensive, patient-centred, holistic clinical decision making and a research tool to improve our understanding of NAFLD, its natural history and therapy.

## References

1. Zelman S. The liver in obesity. AMA Arch Intern Med 1952;90:141–156.
2. Ludwig J, Viggiano TR, McGill DB, Oh BJ. Nonalcoholic steatohepatitis: Mayo Clinic experiences with a hitherto unnamed disease. Mayo Clin Proc 1980;55:434–438.
3. Angulo P. Nonalcoholic fatty liver disease. N Engl J Med 2002;346:1221–1231.
4. Alberti KG, Zimmet P, Shaw J; Group IDFETFC. The metabolic syndrome – a new worldwide definition. Lancet 2005;366:1059–1062.
5. Vernon G, Baranova A, Younossi ZM. Systematic review: the epidemiology and natural history of non-alcoholic fatty liver disease and non-alcoholic steatohepatitis in adults. Aliment Pharmacol Ther 2011;34:274–285.
6. Ekstedt M, Franzen LE, Mathiesen UL, Thorelius L, Holmqvist M, Bodemar G, Kechagias S. Long-term follow-up of patients with NAFLD and elevated liver enzymes. Hepatology 2006;44:865–873.
7. Caldwell SH, Lee VD, Kleiner DE, Al-Osaimi AM, Argo CK, Northup PG, Berg CL. NASH and cryptogenic cirrhosis: a histological analysis. Ann Hepatol 2009;8:346–352.
8. Yeh MM, Brunt EM. Pathological features of fatty liver disease. Gastroenterology 2014;147:754–764.
9. Ratziu V, Bellentani S, Cortez-Pinto H, Day C, Marchesini G. A position statement on NAFLD/NASH based on the EASL 2009 special conference. J Hepatol 2010;53:372–384.
10. Chalasani N, Younossi Z, Lavine JE, Diehl AM, Brunt EM, Cusi K, Charlton M, et al. The diagnosis and management of non-alcoholic fatty liver disease: practice guideline by the American Gastroenterological Association, American Association for the Study of Liver Diseases, and American College of Gastroenterology. Gastroenterology 2012;142:1592–1609.
11. Skelly MM, James PD, Ryder SD. Findings on liver biopsy to investigate abnormal liver function tests in the absence of diagnostic serology. J Hepatol 2001;35:195–199.
12. Mofrad P, Contos MJ, Haque M, Sargeant C, Fisher RA, Luketic VA, Sterling RK, et al. Clinical and histologic spectrum of nonalcoholic fatty liver disease associated with normal ALT values. Hepatology 2003;37:1286–1292.
13. Wong VW, Wong GL, Tsang SW, Hui AY, Chan AW, Choi PC, Chim AM, et al. Metabolic and histological features of non-alcoholic fatty liver disease patients with different serum alanine aminotransferase levels. Aliment Pharmacol Ther 2009;29:387–396.
14. Palmentieri B, de Sio I, La Mura V, Masarone M, Vecchione R, Bruno S, Torella R, et al. The role of bright liver echo pattern on ultrasound B-mode examination in the diagnosis of liver steatosis. Dig Liver Dis 2006;38:485–489.
15. Cobbold JF, Anstee QM, Thomas HC. Investigating mildly abnormal serum aminotransferase values. BMJ 2010;341:c4039.
16. Kowdley KV, Belt P, Wilson LA, Yeh MM, Neuschwander-Tetri BA, Chalasani N, Sanyal AJ, et al. Serum ferritin is an independent predictor of histologic severity and advanced fibrosis in patients with nonalcoholic fatty liver disease. Hepatology 2012;55:77–85.
17. Bedogni G, Bellentani S, Miglioli L, Masutti F, Passalacqua M, Castiglione A, Tiribelli C. The Fatty Liver Index: a simple and accurate predictor of hepatic steatosis in the general population. BMC Gastroenterol 2006;6:33.
18. Powell EE, Jonsson JR, Clouston AD. Metabolic factors and non-alcoholic fatty liver disease as co-factors in other liver diseases. Dig Dis 2010;28:186–191.
19. Pais R, Charlotte F, Fedchuk L, Bedossa P, Lebray P, Poynard T, Ratziu V, et al. A systematic review of follow-up biopsies reveals disease progression in patients with non-alcoholic fatty liver. J Hepatol 2013;59:550–556.
20. Yamaguchi K, Yang L, McCall S, Huang J, Yu XX, Pandey SK, Bhanot S, et al. Inhibiting triglyceride synthesis improves hepatic steatosis but exacerbates liver damage and fibrosis in obese mice with nonalcoholic steatohepatitis. Hepatology 2007;45:1366–1374.
21. Tilg H, Moschen AR. Evolution of inflammation in nonalcoholic fatty liver disease: the multiple parallel hits hypothesis. Hepatology 2010;52:1836–1846.
22. Kleiner DE, Brunt EM, Van Natta M, Behling C, Contos MJ, Cummings OW, Ferrell LD, et al. Design and validation of a histological scoring system for nonalcoholic fatty liver disease. Hepatology 2005;41:1313–1321.
23. Levene AP, Kudo H, Armstrong MJ, Thursz MR, Gedroyc WM, Anstee QM, Goldin RD. Quantifying hepatic steatosis – more than meets the eye. Histopathology 2012;60:971–981.
24. Schwenzer NF, Springer F, Schraml C, Stefan N, Machann J, Schick F. Non-invasive assessment and quantification of liver steatosis by ultrasound, computed tomography and magnetic resonance. J Hepatol 2009;51:433–445.
25. Szczepaniak LS, Nurenberg P, Leonard D, Browning JD, Reingold JS, Grundy S, Hobbs HH, et al. Magnetic resonance spectroscopy to measure hepatic triglyceride content: prevalence of hepatic steatosis in the general population. Am J Physiol Endocrinol Metab 2005;288:E462–E468.
26. Wong VW, Chu WC, Wong GL, Chan RS, Chim AM, Ong A, Yeung DK, et al. Prevalence of non-alcoholic fatty liver disease and advanced fibrosis in Hong Kong Chinese: a population study using proton-magnetic resonance spectroscopy and transient elastography. Gut 2012;61:409–415.
27. Sasso M, Beaugrand M, de Ledinghen V, Douvin C, Marcellin P, Poupon R, Sandrin L, et al. Controlled attenuation parameter (CAP): a novel VCTE guided ultrasonic attenuation measurement for the evaluation of hepatic steatosis: preliminary study and validation in a cohort of patients with chronic liver disease from various causes. Ultrasound Med Biol 2010;36:1825–1835.

28. Matteoni CA, Younossi ZM, Gramlich T, Boparai N, Liu YC, McCullough AJ. Nonalcoholic fatty liver disease: a spectrum of clinical and pathological severity. Gastroenterology 1999;116:1413–1419.

29. Brunt EM, Janney CG, Di Bisceglie AM, Neuschwander-Tetri BA, Bacon BR. Nonalcoholic steatohepatitis: a proposal for grading and staging the histological lesions. Am J Gastroenterol 1999;94:2467–2474.

30. Kleiner DE, Brunt EM. Nonalcoholic fatty liver disease: pathologic patterns and biopsy evaluation in clinical research. Semin Liver Dis 2012;32:3–13.

31. Bedossa P, Poitou C, Veyrie N, Bouillot JL, Basdevant A, Paradis V, Tordjman J, et al. Histopathological algorithm and scoring system for evaluation of liver lesions in morbidly obese patients. Hepatology 2012;56:1751–1759.

32. Bedossa P, Consortium FP. Utility and appropriateness of the fatty liver inhibition of progression (FLIP) algorithm and steatosis, activity, and fibrosis (SAF) score in the evaluation of biopsies of nonalcoholic fatty liver disease. Hepatology 2014;60:565–575.

33. Feldstein AE, Wieckowska A, Lopez AR, Liu YC, Zein NN, McCullough AJ. Cytokeratin-18 fragment levels as noninvasive biomarkers for nonalcoholic steatohepatitis: a multicenter validation study. Hepatology 2009;50:1072–1078.

34. Cusi K, Chang Z, Harrison S, Lomonaco R, Bril F, Orsak B, Ortiz-Lopez C, et al. Limited value of plasma cytokeratin-18 as a biomarker for NASH and fibrosis in patients with non-alcoholic fatty liver disease. J Hepatol 2014;60:167–174.

35. Tanwar S, Trembling PM, Guha IN, Parkes J, Kaye P, Burt AD, Ryder SD, et al. Validation of terminal peptide of procollagen III for the detection and assessment of nonalcoholic steatohepatitis in patients with nonalcoholic fatty liver disease. Hepatology 2013;57:103–111.

36. Dowman JK, Tomlinson JW, Newsome PN. Systematic review: the diagnosis and staging of non-alcoholic fatty liver disease and non-alcoholic steatohepatitis. Aliment Pharmacol Ther 2011;33:525–540.

37. Bhala N, Angulo P, van der Poorten D, Lee E, Hui JM, Saracco G, Adams LA, et al. The natural history of non-alcoholic fatty liver disease with advanced fibrosis or cirrhosis: an international collaborative study. Hepatology 2011;54:1208–1216.

38. Ekstedt M, Hagstrom H, Nasr P, Fredrikson M, Stal P, Kechagias S, Hultcrantz R. Fibrosis stage is the strongest predictor for disease-specific mortality in NAFLD after up to 33 years of follow-up. Hepatology 2015;61:1547–1557.

39. Calvaruso V, Burroughs AK, Standish R, Manousou P, Grillo F, Leandro G, Maimone S, et al. Computer-assisted image analysis of liver collagen: relationship to Ishak scoring and hepatic venous pressure gradient. Hepatology 2009;49:1236–1244.

40. Cobbold JF, Patel D, Taylor-Robinson SD. Assessment of inflammation and fibrosis in non-alcoholic fatty liver disease by imaging-based techniques. J Gastroenterol Hepatol 2012;27:1281–1292.

41. Banerjee R, Pavlides M, Tunnicliffe EM, Piechnik SK, Sarania N, Philips R, Collier JD, et al. Multiparametric magnetic resonance for the non-invasive diagnosis of liver disease. J Hepatol 2014;60:69–77.

42. McPherson S, Stewart SF, Henderson E, Burt AD, Day CP. Simple non-invasive fibrosis scoring systems can reliably exclude advanced fibrosis in patients with non-alcoholic fatty liver disease. Gut 2010;59:1265–1269.

43. Manning DS, Afdhal NH. Diagnosis and quantitation of fibrosis. Gastroenterology 2008;134:1670–1681.

44. Standish RA, Cholongitas E, Dhillon A, Burroughs AK, Dhillon AP. An appraisal of the histopathological assessment of liver fibrosis. Gut 2006;55:569–578.

45. Parkes J, Roderick P, Harris S, Day C, Mutimer D, Collier J, Lombard M, et al. Enhanced liver fibrosis test can predict clinical outcomes in patients with chronic liver disease. Gut 2010;59:1245–1251.

46. Klibansky DA, Mehta SH, Curry M, Nasser I, Challies T, Afdhal NH. Transient elastography for predicting clinical outcomes in patients with chronic liver disease. J Viral Hepat 2012;19:e184–e193.

47. Perazzo H, Munteanu M, Ngo Y, Lebray P, Seurat N, Rutka F, Couteau M, et al. Prognostic value of liver fibrosis and steatosis biomarkers in type-2 diabetes and dyslipidaemia. Aliment Pharmacol Ther 2014;40:1081–1093.

48. Rockey DC, Caldwell SH, Goodman ZD, Nelson RC, Smith AD; American Association for the Study of Liver D. Liver biopsy. Hepatology 2009;49:1017–1044.

49. Grant A, Neuberger J. Guidelines on the use of liver biopsy in clinical practice. British Society of Gastroenterology. Gut 1999;45(Suppl 4):IV1–IV11.

50. Gilmore IT, Burroughs A, Murray-Lyon IM, Williams R, Jenkins D, Hopkins A. Indications, methods, and outcomes of percutaneous liver biopsy in England and Wales: an audit by the British Society of Gastroenterology and the Royal College of Physicians of London. Gut 1995;36:437–441.

51. Mueller M, Kratzer W, Oeztuerk S, Wilhelm M, Mason RA, Mao R, Haenle MM. Percutaneous ultrasonographically guided liver punctures: an analysis of 1961 patients over a period of ten years. BMC Gastroenterol 2012;12:173.

52. Bedossa P, Dargere D, Paradis V. Sampling variability of liver fibrosis in chronic hepatitis C. Hepatology 2003;38:1449–1457.

53. Colloredo G, Guido M, Sonzogni A, Leandro G. Impact of liver biopsy size on histological evaluation of chronic viral hepatitis: the smaller the sample, the milder the disease. J Hepatol 2003;39:239–244.

54. Myers RP, Pomier-Layrargues G, Kirsch R, Pollett A, Beaton M, Levstik M, Duarte-Rojo A, et al. Discordance in fibrosis staging between liver biopsy and transient elastography using the FibroScan XL probe. J Hepatol 2012;56:564–570.

55. Sanyal AJ, Brunt EM, Kleiner DE, Kowdley KV, Chalasani N, Lavine JE, Ratziu V, et al. Endpoints and clinical trial design for nonalcoholic steatohepatitis. Hepatology 2011; 54:344–353.

56. Adams LA, Sanderson S, Lindor KD, Angulo P. The histo-logical course of nonalcoholic fatty liver disease: a longitudi-nal study of 103 patients with sequential liver biopsies. J Hepatol 2005;42:132–138.

57. Sanyal AJ, Chalasani N, Kowdley KV, McCullough A, Diehl AM, Bass NM, Neuschwander-Tetri BA, et al. Pioglitazone, vitamin E, or placebo for nonalcoholic steatohepatitis. N Engl J Med 2010;362:1675–1685.

# 18 Screening for NAFLD in high-risk populations

**Nader Lessan**

Imperial College London Diabetes Centre, Abu Dhabi, United Arab Emirates, Imperial College London, United Kingdom

## LEARNING POINTS

- The high prevalence and potential serious consequences of non-alcoholic fatty liver disease (NAFLD) may justify screening, particularly in high-risk groups, which include obesity and type 2 diabetes.

- Currently, there is no ideal screening method for NAFLD and as such screening is not recommended by AASLD.

- Prevalence of NAFLD in insulin-resistant populations is very high. NAFLD is more likely to be progressive and is associated with higher mortality in these populations.

- Simple blood tests including ALT and AST may be useful simple initial tests when above a certain threshold. These are lower than the currently used upper limit of normal values used by most laboratories. Normal liver enzymes do not exclude a diagnosis of NAFLD.

- Other proposed screening tests include scoring systems such as the fatty liver index (FLI) and the hepatic steatosis index (HSI). Studies on most scoring systems are limited to specific populations.

- Radiological tests include liver ultrasound, but the cost precludes their use as screening tools.

## Introduction

The aim of screening is to identify disease in its asymptomatic phase. As such, screening is distinct from the diagnostic process, which is applied to symptomatic disease [1]. This distinction is important in the context of NAFLD, which is largely asymptomatic. It is useful to consider the principles of early disease detection (Table 18.1), initially proposed by Wilson and Jungner in 1971 in relation to NAFLD screening [2]. For screening to be useful, four major factors need to be considered: the disease itself, the test, the treatment and the cost. Some of these have been discussed in the previous chapters. Only aspects relevant to screening will be addressed in this chapter.

## Nature of NAFLD: Relevance to screening

'Simple steatosis' represents the early part of the natural history and affects between 20 and 30% of the adult population in Western countries [3–5]. In a minority of cases, this progresses to non-alcoholic steatohepatitis (NASH), an inflammatory condition with a more aggressive nature. This can lead to fibrosis, cirrhosis and hepatocellular carcinoma in a smaller percentage of patients [6–8]. While there is no doubt about the morbidity and the mortality associated with NASH, simple steatosis without inflammation tends to be a more indolent condition [9]. NAFLD is associated with cardiovascular (CV) risk. However, the increased CV risk in the absence of steatohepatitis is thought to be minimal. NASH is also associated with increased mortality [10]. This distinction in behaviour of simple steatosis and NASH is important in the context of screening.

## Current opinion and guidelines

Opinion is divided as to the value of screening for NAFLD, both in the general population and in the populations considered to be at high risk. Direct evidence on screening

*Clinical Dilemmas in Non-Alcoholic Fatty Liver Disease*, First Edition. Edited by Roger Williams and Simon D. Taylor-Robinson.
© 2016 John Wiley & Sons, Ltd. Published 2016 by John Wiley & Sons, Ltd.

**TABLE 18.1** Screening principles [2] as applied to NAFLD

Condition
  Important health problem
    Common, associated morbidity (liver, cardiac) and increased mortality (especially with NASH)
  Recognisable latent asymptomatic phase
    NAFLD has a long mostly asymptomatic phase
  Natural history adequately understood
Test
  Suitable test available and acceptable to population
    Questionable. Widely available tests such as ALT have poor sensitivity and specificity for NAFLD at currently accepted normal
      ranges.
    No other simple widely available biomarker is available
    Imaging techniques including ultrasonography may not be suitable for mass screening as the target 'at-risk' population is
      large
    Other tests are less widely available or not validated
Treatment
  Accepted treatment for patients available/Agreed policy on whom to treat
    Treatment for patients with diabetes and obesity may not be very different from a patient not confirmed to have NAFLD
Other
  Cost balanced against medical expenditure as a whole
    No cost-benefit analyses available
  Facilities for diagnosis and treatment available
    Variable in different parts of the world
  Case finding continuous process
May be limited by above factors and magnitude of the problem

relevant to NAFLD is scant. Nomura et al. investigated the effectiveness and efficacy of a liver screening programme to detect fatty liver in periodic check-ups and concluded that monitoring BMI alone might provide a more suitable inexpensive alternative [11]. Notably, the programme was conducted on 411 Japanese workers and included liver function tests and was estimated to cost around $4 per person.

The joint practice guidelines on diagnosis and management of NAFLD by AASLD, ACG and AGA advised against screening for NAFLD in adults attending primary care clinics, or high-risk groups attending diabetes or obesity clinics, citing 'uncertainties surrounding diagnostic tests and treatment options' and 'lack of knowledge related to long-term benefits and cost-effectiveness of screening' [12]. The EASL position statement [13] does advocate screening for NAFLD/NASH in patients with metabolic risk factors characterised by insulin resistance. However, it does not recommend screening in the general adult population. The evidence for NAFLD screening in children seems to be different, however. Indeed, paediatric guidelines recommend overweight or obese children over 10 years of age should be screened for NAFLD using ALT and AST [14].

## The high-risk population

The close association of insulin resistance and NAFLD has been discussed in the previous chapters. In normal-weight individuals without any metabolic risk factors, NAFLD prevalence is 16% [15, 16]. In contrast, 60% of patients with obesity and type 2 diabetes exhibit hepatic steatosis; in severe obesity, even higher prevalence rates for NAFLD, NASH and fibrosis have been reported (Figure 18.1) [16–19]. Furthermore, progression from simple steatosis to NASH, cirrhosis and hepatocellular carcinoma is more likely and more rapid in these patients [7, 20, 21]. Patients with diabetes and NAFLD are also at a greater risk of ischaemic heart disease and have a higher mortality risk [21]. Screening and identification of patients with NAFLD and NASH in metabolic syndrome is therefore very important.

Several other conditions are also associated with an increased risk of developing NAFLD. These include hypothyroidism, hypopituitarism and HIV/AIDS (Table 18.2). Among these, conditions associated with insulin resistance, obesity, type 2 diabetes and metabolic syndrome are the most prevalent and hence will be the main focus of this chapter. Obesity, diabetes and other insulin resistance syndromes constitute a large population

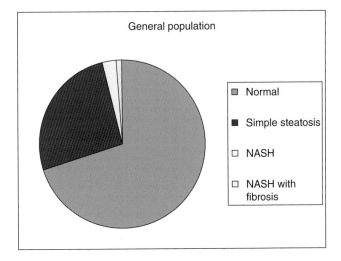

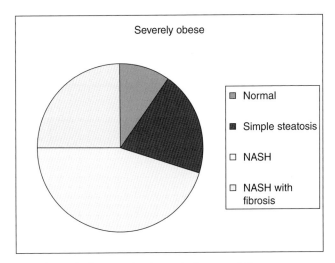

**FIG 18.1** Prevalence of NAFLD and NASH in the general and severely obese populations.

in Western and many other countries with major implications for NAFLD screening.

## Potential screening tests

Several blood tests and imaging modalities are used for diagnosing liver disease in general [36, 37]. Other potential tests and scoring systems, some with great promise, are also emerging. However, only a handful has been studied in the context of screening for NAFLD (Table 18.3).

A screening test needs to be highly sensitive; ideally the test should also be highly specific where possible. It needs to be simple, cheap and acceptable by the population being screened. In the setting of a common disease such as NAFLD, high specificity becomes even more important. In addition, a screening test should identify a condition where early intervention provides meaningful clinical benefit. These requirements automatically exclude many of the currently available diagnostic tests. As such, more complex imaging techniques such as magnetic resonance spectroscopy will not be suitable for screening purposes and will not be further discussed. A summary of tests relevant to NAFLD screening is given in Table 18.3. As well as some of the tests that are used more routinely, the list includes some

**TABLE 18.2** Risk factors for NAFLD

Gender
Age
Metabolic syndrome
  Obesity
    NAFLD affects up to 75% of the obese NAFLD [16]
    95% of morbidly obese awaiting bariatric surgery [22, 23]
    NAFLD more prevalent in childhood and adolescent obesity
    NASH affects 25–30% of the obese population [24, 25]
  Type 2 diabetes
    NAFLD prevalence 40–75% [18, 26, 27].
    NAFLD more likely to progress to NASH, fibrosis and hepatocellular carcinoma [21]
    Mortality increased more than twofold (cardiovascular and liver) [21]
    Poor glycaemic control correlates positively with steatosis [28]
  Hyperlipidaemia
  Insulin resistance
Race
  Hispanics- 33% NAFLD prevalence [29, 30]
  African Americans-lower NAFLD [29, 31, 32]
HIV
  NAFLD prevalence of 31%
  NAFLD behaves more aggressively with a more rapid progression to NASH, fibrosis and cirrhosis [33]
Hypothyroidism
Hypopituitarism
Some surgical procedures [34].
  Jejunoileal bypass
  Extensive small bowel resection
  Biliopancreatic diversion
  Gastroplasty for morbid obesity
  Pancreaticodudenectomy [35]

simple scoring systems, namely, the fatty liver index (FLI), hepatic steatosis index (HSI) and NAFLD index. Several other biomarkers and scoring systems (such as cytokeratin-18 fragments and NAFLD fibrosis score) have been proven more useful in fibrosis staging and diagnosing NASH and are of less relevance to screening [42–44].

### Can liver enzymes be useful in NAFLD screening?

As NAFLD is mostly an asymptomatic disease, the diagnosis is most commonly suspected when abnormalities of liver enzymes, chiefly serum alanine transaminase (ALT) and aspartate transaminase (AST), have been observed. Unlike AST, which can be increased in some non-liver-related conditions, ALT almost solely reflects hepatocyte injury. Typically, the elevation in NAFLD is mild with an AST to ALT ratio of <1. Several studies have focused on the former as a potential screening test. An elevated AST or ALT may be an indicator of NAFD if other causes are

excluded and features of metabolic syndrome are present [45, 46]. Liver enzymes in general and ALT specifically fluctuate with time and as such, a single measurement may be insufficient to make a decision on whether further investigation is required. Follow-up of abnormal results with a repeat ALT after 6 months has been shown to increase specificity [47].

ALT at current upper limit of normal (ULN) has a very low sensitivity for NAFLD [48]. As such, around 80% of patients with sonographically confirmed hepatic steatosis have 'normal' ALT [3]. Furthermore, ALT can be normal in 60% of patients who have actually progressed from NAFLD and developed NASH. The low sensitivity may improve by reducing the ULN cut-off. The currently used ULN for ALT of around 40 IU/L has been challenged [49–52], and lower thresholds have been proposed in several studies. Prati et al. showed that changing the ALT cut-off to 30 IU/L for men and 19 IU/L for women could improve its sensitivity to 76.3%, although specificity will be modestly reduced

**TABLE 18.3** Potential screening tests for NAFLD

| Test | Threshold | Sensitivity (%) | Specificity (%) | Study/Reference | Comment |
|---|---|---|---|---|---|
| ALT (IU/L) | >19 for women<br>>30 for men | 76.3 | 88.5 | Prati 2002 [38] | Study investigated use for Hepatitis c viraemia, not NAFLD. Western population. |
| ALT (IU/L) | >17 for women<br>>25 for men | 65.8<br>75.2 | 70.5<br>71.7 | Miyake 2011 [39] | Japanese population |
| Fatty liver index (FLI) | <30 for ruling out<br>≥60 for detecting NAFLD | 87 | 64 | Bedogni 2006 [40] | *FLI = $e^L/(1 + e^L) \times 100$<br>Studied and validated in different populations including Western, Chinese and Korean subjects. |
| Hepatic steatosis index (HSI) | <30 for ruling our<br>>36 for detecting NAFLD | 93.1 | 92.4 | Lee 2010 [41] | HSI = $8 \times$ ALT/AST ratio + BMI (+2 if DM; +2 if female)<br>Based on multivariate analysis in a Korean population. |
| NAFLD index | >−1.976 for women<br>>−0.4867 for men | 84.4<br>77.8 | 76.4<br>81.3 | Miyake 2011 [39] | Not validated in other populations. Japanese population |

BMI, body mass index; TG, triglyceride in mmol/L; WCirc, waist circumference in cm.

*L = $0.953 \times \log_e$(TG/0.0113) + $0.139 \times$ BMI + $0.718 \times \log_e$(GGT) + $0.053 \times$ WCirc−15.745.

NAFLD Index:

For male: −10.48 + 0.232 × BMI + 0.064 × ALT + 0.004TG − 0.022 × HDL + 0.164 × UA + 0.439 × HbA1c.

For female: −13.815 + 0.256 × BMI + 0.06 × ALT + 0.006 × TG − 0.016 × HDL + 0.3 × UA + 0.784 × HbA1c.

to 88.5% [38.49]. The ULN for ALT may be different in other populations; different ALT cut-offs of 21 U/L for men and 17 U/L for women were used in a study from Taiwan and showed sensitivity and specificity values of 74.5 and 63.6% for men and 67.0 and 63.0% for women, respectively (Table 18.3) [51].

Even with these lower ULN cut-off values, the sensitivity and specificity figures quoted make ALT a less than ideal test for NAFLD screening. However, it is relatively cheap, minimally invasive and widely available in many parts of the world and has been suggested in some screening algorithms for NAFLD [53].

Combining ALT with other readily available parameters may help improve diagnostic accuracy. Tomizawa et al. demonstrated that a combination of ALT >19 IU/L or triglyceride >101 mg/dL provided an increased specificity of 80.9% for the diagnosis of NAFLD in a Japanese population [54].

### Ultrasonography

Currently, ultrasonography is the investigation of choice in screening for NAFLD. However, as has been stated in the previous chapters, there are potential problems and shortcomings with ultrasonography. Ultrasound has a sensitivity of 60–94% and a specificity of 66–95% for detecting hepatic steatosis [55]. It is operator dependent and insensitive to milder fatty change [56]. Nevertheless, ultrasound is the most commonly used technique to confirm hepatic steatosis. However, performance in obesity is not good; in morbidly obese patients undergoing bariatric surgery, only around 50% of cases with hepatic steatosis had been confirmed by ultrasonography.

## A practical approach to NAFLD screening

Based on current evidence, no firm recommendation on NAFLD screening, even a high-risk population can be given. However, useful pathways can be suggested with careful consideration to current practice, commonly available tests and available evidence (Figure 18.2).

### Risk factor identification

- Does the patient have metabolic syndrome or any of the conditions associated with it?
  The main risk groups are patients with insulin resistance, diabetes, metabolic syndrome and obesity. The vast majority of patients with NAFLD will fall into

one or more of these categories (Table 18.1). Clinical and biochemical assessment of insulin resistance should be performed. Hypertension and hypertriglyceridaemia should also be noted. A very high percentage of patients in this group are likely to have NAFLD, and further workup should not be solely based on liver function test normality at current thresholds.

- Does the patient belong to any of the other high-risk groups? These will be smaller in number, and based on other clinical parameters, many of them will be having further investigations including hepatic ultrasound.

### Understanding liver enzymes in high-risk patients

- **ALT is a readily available** test and will help further risk stratify the high-risk patients. Many patients in high-risk groups will have had their liver function tests checked.
- **Using conventional ULN for ALT**, about 20% of patients with NAFLD have elevated ALT. The prevalence of hypertransaminasaemia in high-risk groups is even higher. Most patients with high ALT in this context will have NAFLD. Indeed, prevalence of NASH in this group was reported to be around 47% in one study. So, in high-risk groups, a persistently elevated ALT in the absence of other explanations does warrant further investigation. This should include workup to exclude other causes of raised liver enzymes as well as a hepatic ultrasound.
- **Using a lower cut-off value for ALT** will increase its sensitivity, although specificity will be reduced [54]. Different ALT cut-off values have been used in different studies [38, 39, 48–51]. Patients so identified will also have an increased risk of NAFLD and a closer follow-up and perhaps early investigation may be advisable if there is other cause for concern.
- **A repeat ALT after 6 months** to identify persistently 'elevated ALT' – above the lower threshold – will be a useful strategy. Those with 'normal values' can have less stringent follow-up.
- **High-risk patients with 'normal' liver function tests** should not be ignored as a significant percentage in this group will have NAFLD or even NASH.
- **Other causes of elevated ALT** need to be considered and excluded.

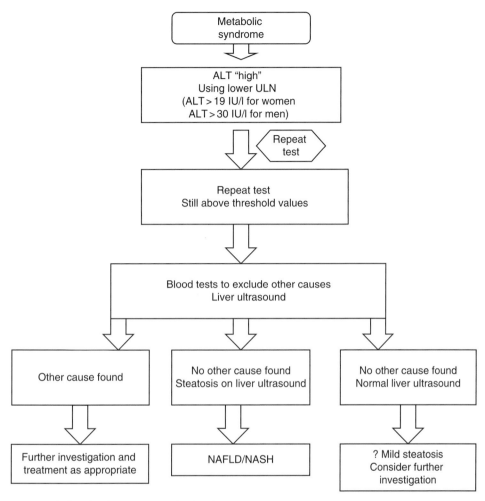

**FIG 18.2** Suggested Algorithm for NAFLD screening in risk groups.

### Use of scoring systems to identify NAFLD

These are useful, albeit less familiar than more conventional tests to most non-hepatologists (Table 18.2). Whether they are applicable to different ethnic groups may be debated. There have been no large-scale studies on the use of many of these scoring systems as screening tools for NAFLD. They can be incorporated into computerised patient management systems to help clinicians decide whether further investigation is needed. Some of the more extensively studied scoring systems (Table 18.3) include the FLI and the HSI.

### Ultrasonography

Ultrasonography should be done on patients suspected of having NAFLD. Ultrasound has good sensitivity and

specificity but important limitations in mild steatosis and obesity. Other imaging modalities including magnetic resonance imaging (MRI) and MR spectroscopy should be considered, if available.

### From NAFLD to NASH

Techniques that can be used here include transient elastography. By this stage, the patient should be having specialist care in a hepatology centre. Liver biopsy may need to be performed on some patients, especially those identified to have NASH or significant fibrosis on less invasive tests. Further discussion on management of patient with NASH is beyond the scope of this chapter, but it should be stressed that one important aim of any screening procedure for

NAFLD will in fact be identifying patients with NASH, fibrosis or cirrhosis.

## Summary

NAFLD is very common among patients with diabetes, obesity and other forms of insulin resistance. At present time, no simple and validated screening test with an acceptable sensitivity and specificity is available. Nonetheless, a combination of clinical assessment with available tests and scoring systems can be used to make an informed decision on further assessment and follow-up of patients with suspected NAFLD. As mortality and morbidity figures change significantly through transition from simple steatosis to NASH, it may make more sense for screening to target NASH rather than simple steatosis alone.

## References

1. Nielsen C, Lang RS. Principles of screening. Med Clin North Am. 1999;83(6):1323–37, v.

2. Wilson JM. Principles of screening for disease. Proc R Soc Med. 1971;64(12):1255–6.

3. Browning JD, Szczepaniak LS, Dobbins R, et al. Prevalence of hepatic steatosis in an urban population in the United States: impact of ethnicity. Hepatology. 2004;40(6):1387–95.

4. Bedogni G, Miglioli L, Masutti F, et al. Prevalence of and risk factors for nonalcoholic fatty liver disease: the Dionysos nutrition and liver study. Hepatology. 2005;42(1):44–52.

5. Bedogni G, Nobili V, Tiribelli C. Epidemiology of fatty liver: an update. World J Gastroenterol. 2014;20(27):9050–4.

6. Milic S, Lulic D, Stimac D. Non-alcoholic fatty liver disease and obesity: biochemical, metabolic and clinical presentations. World J Gastroenterol. 2014;20(28):9330–7.

7. Ekstedt M, Franzen LE, Mathiesen UL, et al. Long-term follow-up of patients with NAFLD and elevated liver enzymes. Hepatology. 2006;44(4):865–73.

8. White DL, Kanwal F, El-Serag HB. Association between nonalcoholic fatty liver disease and risk for hepatocellular cancer, based on systematic review. Clin Gastroenterol Hepatol. 2012;10(12):1342–59.e2.

9. LaBrecque DR, Abbas Z, Anania F, et al. World Gastroenterology Organisation global guidelines: nonalcoholic fatty liver disease and nonalcoholic steatohepatitis. J Clin Gastroenterol. 2014;48(6):467–73.

10. Sullivan PB, Alder N, Bachlet AM, et al. Gastrostomy feeding in cerebral palsy: too much of a good thing? Dev Med Child Neurol. 2006;48(11):877–82.

11. Nomura K, Yano E, Shinozaki T, et al. Efficacy and effectiveness of liver screening program to detect fatty liver in the periodic health check-ups. J Occup Health. 2004;46(6): 423–8.

12. Chalasani N, Younossi Z, Lavine JE, et al. The diagnosis and management of non-alcoholic fatty liver disease: practice guideline by the American Gastroenterological Association, American Association for the Study of Liver Diseases, and American College of Gastroenterology. Gastroenterology. 2012;142(7):1592–609.

13. Ratziu V, Bellentani S, Cortez-Pinto H, et al. A position statement on NAFLD/NASH based on the EASL 2009 special conference. J Hepatol. 2010;53(2):372–84.

14. Krebs NF, Himes JH, Jacobson D, et al. Assessment of child and adolescent overweight and obesity. Pediatrics 2007; 120(Suppl 4):S193–228.

15. Williams CD, Stengel J, Asike MI, et al. Prevalence of nonalcoholic fatty liver disease and nonalcoholic steatohepatitis among a largely middle-aged population utilizing ultrasound and liver biopsy: a prospective study. Gastroenterology. 2011;140(1):124–31.

16. Bellentani S, Saccoccio G, Masutti F, et al. Prevalence of and risk factors for hepatic steatosis in Northern Italy. Ann Intern Med. 2000;132(2):112–7.

17. Bellentani S, Scaglioni F, Marino M, et al. Epidemiology of non-alcoholic fatty liver disease. Dig Dis. 2010;28(1): 155–61.

18. Williamson RM, Price JF, Glancy S, et al. Prevalence of and risk factors for hepatic steatosis and nonalcoholic fatty liver disease in people with type 2 diabetes: the Edinburgh Type 2 Diabetes Study. Diabetes Care. 2011;34(5):1139–44.

19. Targher G, Bertolini L, Padovani R, et al. Prevalence of non-alcoholic fatty liver disease and its association with cardiovascular disease in patients with type 1 diabetes. J Hepatol. 2010;53(4):713–8.

20. Adams LA. Nonalcoholic fatty liver disease and diabetes mellitus. Endocr Res. 2007;32(3):59–69.

21. Adams LA, Harmsen S, St Sauver JL, et al. Nonalcoholic fatty liver disease increases risk of death among patients with diabetes: a community-based cohort study. Am J Gastroenterol. 2010;105(7):1567–73.

22. Dixon JB, Bhathal PS, O'Brien PE. Nonalcoholic fatty liver disease: predictors of nonalcoholic steatohepatitis and liver fibrosis in the severely obese. Gastroenterology. 2001;121(1):91–100.

23. Losekann A, Weston AC, Carli LA, et al. Nonalcoholic fatty liver disease in severe obese patients, subjected to bariatric surgery. Arq Gastroenterol. 2013;50(4):285–9.

24. Angulo P, Keach JC, Batts KP, et al. Independent predictors of liver fibrosis in patients with nonalcoholic steatohepatitis. Hepatology. 1999;30(6):1356–62.

25. Powell EE, Cooksley WG, Hanson R, et al. The natural history of nonalcoholic steatohepatitis: a follow-up study of forty-two patients for up to 21 years. Hepatology. 1990; 11(1):74–80.

26. Agarwal AK, Jain V, Singla S, et al. Prevalence of non-alcoholic fatty liver disease and its correlation with coronary risk factors in patients with type 2 diabetes. J Assoc Physicians India 2011;59:351–4.

27. Targher G, Byrne CD. Clinical Review: nonalcoholic fatty liver disease: a novel cardiometabolic risk factor for type 2 diabetes and its complications. J Clin Endocrinol Metab. 2013;98(2):483–95.

28. Toledo FG, Sniderman AD, Kelley DE. Influence of hepatic steatosis (fatty liver) on severity and composition of dyslipidemia in type 2 diabetes. Diabetes Care. 2006;29(8): 1845–50.

29. North KE, Graff M, Franceschini N, et al. Sex and race differences in the prevalence of fatty liver disease as measured by computed tomography liver attenuation in European American and African American participants of the NHLBI family heart study. Eur J Gastroenterol Hepatol. 2012;24(1):9–16.

30. Pan JJ, Fallon MB. Gender and racial differences in non-alcoholic fatty liver disease. World J Hepatol. 2014;6(5): 274–83.

31. Giday SA, Ashiny Z, Naab T, et al. Frequency of nonalcoholic fatty liver disease and degree of hepatic steatosis in African-American patients. J Natl Med Assoc. 2006;98(10): 1613–5.

32. Foster T, Anania FA, Li D, et al. The prevalence and clinical correlates of nonalcoholic fatty liver disease (NAFLD) in African Americans: the multiethnic study of atherosclerosis (MESA). Dig Dis Sci. 2013;58(8):2392–8.

33. Vodkin I, Valasek MA, Bettencourt R, et al. Clinical, biochemical and histological differences between HIV-associated NAFLD and primary NAFLD: a case-control study. Aliment Pharmacol Ther. 2015;41:368–78.

34. Allard JP. Other disease associations with non-alcoholic fatty liver disease (NAFLD). Best Pract Res Clin Gastroenterol. 2002;16(5):783–95.

35. Kato H, Isaji S, Azumi Y, et al. Development of nonalcoholic fatty liver disease (NAFLD) and nonalcoholic steatohepatitis (NASH) after pancreaticoduodenectomy: proposal of a postoperative NAFLD scoring system. J Hepatobiliary Pancreat Sci. 2010;17(3):296–304.

36. Francque SM, Verrijken A, Mertens I, et al. Noninvasive assessment of nonalcoholic fatty liver disease in obese or overweight patients. Clin Gastroenterol Hepatol. 2012; 10(10):1162–8; quiz e87.

37. Festi D, Schiumerini R, Marzi L, et al. Review article: the diagnosis of non-alcoholic fatty liver disease – availability and accuracy of non-invasive methods. Aliment Pharmacol Ther. 2013;37(4):392–400.

38. Prati D, Taioli E, Zanella A, et al. Updated definitions of healthy ranges for serum alanine aminotransferase levels. Ann Intern Med. 2002;137(1):1–10.

39. Miyake T, Kumagi T, Hirooka M, et al. Metabolic markers and ALT cutoff level for diagnosing nonalcoholic fatty liver disease: a community-based cross-sectional study. J Gastroenterol. 2012;47(6):696–703.

40. Bedogni G, Bellentani S, Miglioli L, et al. The Fatty Liver Index: a simple and accurate predictor of hepatic steatosis in the general population. BMC Gastroenterol 2006;6:33.

41. Lee JH, Kim D, Kim HJ, et al. Hepatic steatosis index: a simple screening tool reflecting nonalcoholic fatty liver disease. Dig Liver Dis. 2010;42(7):503–8.

42. Miyasato M, Murase-Mishiba Y, Bessho M, et al. The cytokeratin-18 fragment level as a biomarker of nonalcoholic fatty liver disease in patients with type 2 diabetes mellitus. Clin Chim Acta 2014;433:184–9.

43. Matteoni CA, Younossi ZM, Gramlich T, et al. Nonalcoholic fatty liver disease: a spectrum of clinical and pathological severity. Gastroenterology. 1999;116(6):1413–9.

44. Tsutsui M, Tanaka N, Kawakubo M, et al. Serum fragmented cytokeratin 18 levels reflect the histologic activity score of nonalcoholic fatty liver disease more accurately than serum alanine aminotransferase levels. J Clin Gastroenterol. 2010;44(6):440–7.

45. Clark JM, Brancati FL, Diehl AM. The prevalence and etiology of elevated aminotransferase levels in the United States. Am J Gastroenterol. 2003;98(5):960–7.

46. Yu AS, Keeffe EB. Elevated AST or ALT to nonalcoholic fatty liver disease: accurate predictor of disease prevalence? Am J Gastroenterol. 2003;98(5):955–6.

47. Husain N, Blais P, Kramer J, et al. Nonalcoholic fatty liver disease (NAFLD) in the Veterans Administration population: development and validation of an algorithm for NAFLD using automated data. Aliment Pharmacol Ther. 2014;40(8):949–54.

48. Zheng MH, Shi KQ, Fan YC, et al. Upper limits of normal for serum alanine aminotransferase levels in Chinese Han population. PLoS One. 2012;7(9):e43736.

49. Prati D, Colli A, Conte D, et al. Spectrum of NAFLD and diagnostic implications of the proposed new normal range for serum ALT in obese women. Hepatology. 2005;42(6):1460–1; author reply 1.

50. Kariv R, Leshno M, Beth-Or A, et al. Re-evaluation of serum alanine aminotransferase upper normal limit and its modulating factors in a large-scale population study. Liver Int. 2006;26(4):445–50.

51. Wu WC, Wu CY, Wang YJ, et al. Updated thresholds for serum alanine aminotransferase level in a large-scale population study composed of 34 346 subjects. Aliment Pharmacol Ther. 2012;36(6):560–8.

52. Kang W, Kim SU. Chasing after novel non-invasive markers to identify advanced fibrosis in NAFLD. Clin Mol Hepatol. 2013;19(3):255–7.

53. Dowman JK, Tomlinson JW, Newsome PN. Systematic review: the diagnosis and staging of non-alcoholic fatty liver disease and non-alcoholic steatohepatitis. Aliment Pharmacol Ther. 2011;33(5):525–40.

54. Tomizawa M, Kawanabe Y, Shinozaki F, et al. Elevated levels of alanine transaminase and triglycerides within normal limits are associated with fatty liver. Exp Ther Med. 2014;8(3):759–62.

55. Schwenzer NF, Springer F, Schraml C, et al. Non-invasive assessment and quantification of liver steatosis by ultrasound, computed tomography and magnetic resonance. J Hepatol. 2009;51(3):433–45.

56. Strauss S, Gavish E, Gottlieb P, et al. Interobserver and intraobserver variability in the sonographic assessment of fatty liver. AJR Am J Roentgenol. 2007;189(6):W320–3.

# PART IV
## Value of Treatment Measures

# 19 Defining the role of metabolic physician

**Nicholas Finer**

Centre for Weight Loss, Metabolic and Endocrine Surgery, University College London Hospitals, London, UK
National Centre for Cardiovascular Prevention and Outcomes, UCL Institute of Cardiovascular Science, London, UK

## LEARNING POINTS

- There are a growing role and need for physicians specialising in obesity and obesity-related disorders, and this has been recognised in the United States with the establishment of the American Board of Obesity Medicine and Specialist Certification of Obesity Professional Education (SCOPE) accreditation from the World Obesity Federation.

- The Edmonton Obesity Staging System is increasingly used to clinically stage patients by risk/disease severity and better predicts prognosis than BMI.

- Obesity is strongly heritable, with many risk genes identified, but specific genetic causes are uncommon and tend to present in childhood.

- The metabolic physician's role is to comprehensively evaluate the patient to diagnose and assess diseases implicated in or resulting from obesity and to co-ordinate management as part of a multidisciplinary team.

- The increasing adoption of bariatric surgery worldwide is placing ever greater demands for metabolic physicians.

The obesity, metabolic or bariatric physician (terms used interchangeably in this chapter) who focuses on caring for people with obesity is a rare breed. Obesity is historically a recent disease and its status as a disease is still disputed [1–3]. Treatment for overweight and obesity primarily focuses on weight loss and is managed outside of formal medical care. Patients self-select and initiate diets that are often faddish and nutritionally unsound, elect to join commercial slimming clubs or self-medicate with dubious or ineffective medications increasingly bought over the Internet. Even when medicalised, much care is delivered through 'slimming clinics', which sit more comfortably in the field of cosmetics. To a large extent these facts reflect an underappreciation of the health implications of overweight and obesity, a lack of appropriate training of specialists in obesity and obesity-related disease and also limited provision of medical services and treatment by healthcare systems. The growth in obesity prevalence, the recognition of obesity as a risk for an ever-increasing number of diseases and illnesses as well as a cause of ill health in its own right and the increasing availability of medically supervised diet and lifestyle programmes, pharmacotherapy and surgical treatment suggest a role and need for the metabolic or bariatric physician (Figure 19.1). This person will also be better placed to understand how obesity may modify the relationship between common symptoms (such as headache or breathlessness) to specific diseases [4] (Table 19.1).

As yet there is little explicit accreditation for the metabolic physician in most countries. However, in 2011, the American Board of Obesity Medicine (ABOM) was established in the United States, and this official body has established a credentialing protocol and serves to maintain standards for assessment and certification of candidate physicians. Certification as a diplomate of ABOM recognises 'excellence in the practice of obesity medicine and distinguishes a physician as having achieved a high level of competency and understanding in obesity care'. ABOM collaborates with the National Board of Medical Examiners to administer the annual credentialing exam. ABOM has defined an obesity physician as:

- A physician with expertise in the subspecialty of obesity medicine requiring competency in, and a thorough understanding of, the treatment of obesity and the genetic, biologic, environmental, social and behavioural factors that contribute to obesity

*Clinical Dilemmas in Non-Alcoholic Fatty Liver Disease*, First Edition. Edited by Roger Williams and Simon D. Taylor-Robinson.
© 2016 John Wiley & Sons, Ltd. Published 2016 by John Wiley & Sons, Ltd.

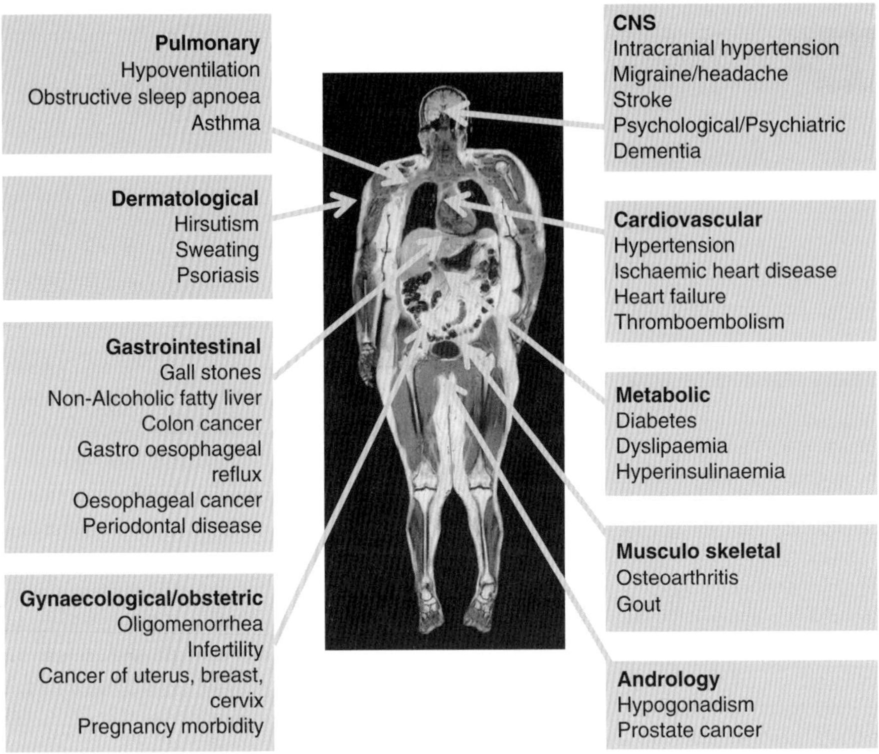

**FIG 19.1** The spectrum of disease linked to overweight and obesity (*Source*: Science Photo Library C007/2245 (Obese woman, MRI scan). Reproduced with permission from Science Photo Library). (*See insert for color representation of the figure.*)

**TABLE 19.1** Genetic syndromes linked to obesity

| Developmental delay and/or dysmorphic features | Without developmental delay | Variably associated with obesity |
| --- | --- | --- |
| Prader–Willi syndrome or fragile X syndrome | Leptin deficiency | Down's syndrome |
| Bardet–Biedl Syndrome | Leptin receptor deficiency | Polycystic ovary syndrome |
| Cohen syndrome | POMC disorders | |
| Albright's hereditary osteodystrophy | PCSK1 deficiency | |
| SIM1 deficiency | MC4R deficiency | |
| BDNF deficiency | | |
| TrkB deficiency | | |

BDNF, brain-derived neurotrophic factor; MC4R, melanocortin 4 receptor; PCSK1, proprotein convertase subtilisin/kexin; POMC, pro-opiomelanocortin; SIM1, single-minded 1; TrkB, tyrosine kinase receptor tropomyosin-related kinase B.

- Employing therapeutic interventions including diet, physical activity, behavioural change and pharmacotherapy
- Utilising a comprehensive approach that may include further resources such as nutritionists, exercise physiologists, mental health professionals and bariatric surgeons as indicated to achieve optimal results

Additionally, the obesity medicine physician maintains competency in providing pre-, peri- and post-surgical care of bariatric surgery patients, promotes the prevention of obesity and advocates for those who suffer from obesity [5]. The World Obesity Federation (formerly the International Association for the Study of

Obesity) also has an accreditation programme Specialist Certification of Obesity Professional Education (SCOPE) that is an internationally recognised standard of obesity management expertise, which acknowledges excellence in obesity prevention and treatment awarded to healthcare practitioners who have completed the SCOPE training programme [6].

While obesity may present in its own right, it is more usually the obesity-related disease or risk factor that prompts referral. Although obesity has become the dominant underlying cause for the very diseases specialist physicians are specialised in (e.g. respiratory physicians and obstructive sleep apnoea, endocrinologists and type 2 diabetes, hepatologists and non-alcoholic fatty liver disease), few such specialities engage in treating it. In the United States where an estimated 13 million adults are severely obese, a survey of 298 physicians carried out by STOP Obesity Alliance revealed that while 89% believed it was their responsibility to help overweight or obese patients lose weight, 72% acknowledged that no one in their practice has been trained to deal with weight-related issues [7]. This may reflect poor training within the medical curriculum. In the Netherlands a study of GP trainees found that 'First-year trainees lack a positive attitude towards and knowledge of the treatment of obese patients; they feel helpless. Third-year trainees complain about attitude problems, even after having been trained in motivational interviewing techniques. Both groups are afraid to offend a patient when addressing his/her weight and lack support of their despondent trainers. Trainees do not feel more competent in treating overweight patients successfully over the course of their GP specialty training' [8]. Practice nurses in the United Kingdom question their adequacy (sense of self-efficacy in responding to patients' problems) and legitimacy (their perceived boundaries of professional responsibility and right to intervene) when it comes to managing the obese patient [9]. The lack of metabolic physicians makes referral from primary care for specialist advice difficult or impossible in most cases, and even teams undertaking bariatric surgery may struggle to find a suitable physician either trained or funded to join a multidisciplinary team (MDT). This deficiency was recognised in the United Kingdom by the Royal College of Physicians (RCP) in 2010 [10] and later in their 2013 report 'Action on Obesity: Comprehensive Care for All' [11]. Among its recommendations were:

- A need to develop and integrate weight management services with those healthcare services that manage the complications and conditions that arise from obesity such as coronary heart disease (CHD), diabetes, arthritis, sleep disorders and gynaecological disorders.
- There should be a physician, ideally in due course a bariatric physician, within each hospital trust to lead on obesity.
- A need to establish a subspecialty of obesity medicine for physicians. The terms 'bariatric medicine' and 'bariatric physician' are proposed.
- The subspecialty should be within the umbrella of diabetes and endocrinology, although this does not preclude physicians with other primary specialties from developing subspecialty recognition in bariatric medicine.
- Physicians specialised in bariatric medicine will provide local leadership in the planning, provision and delivery of obesity treatments, within secondary care and in collaboration and partnership with primary care.

While the role of the metabolic physician will in part be determined by the clinical pathways that determine how patients enter specialist obesity care, the development of this specialty might be considered akin to the development of geriatric medicine in the 1960s, in response to the need of ageing populations for specialist care. In many instances, elderly patients were transformed from ignored, medically neglected and dependent individuals to fully mobile, self-sufficient and rational individuals by specialist MDT, including nutritionists, physiotherapists, occupational therapists, physicians and nurses [12].

## Diagnosis and assessment of the obese patient

While the diagnosis of obesity is all too easy being based upon body mass index (BMI), this classification was derived for population and epidemiological purposes rather than the individual. The recently developed Edmonton Obesity Staging System (Table 19.2) is increasingly being adopted as it links a clinical staging of risk/disease severity to the anthropometric measure of BMI and has been shown to be a better predictor of outcome than BMI, even within any BMI band [13, 14]. The underlying pathophysiology of obesity is the presence not only of excess adipose tissue but also its distribution, especially

**TABLE 19.2** Edmonton obesity staging system

| Stage | Features |
|---|---|
| 0 | NO sign of obesity-related risk factors<br>NO physical symptoms<br>NO psychological symptoms<br>NO functional limitations |
| 1 | SUBCLINICAL obesity-related risk factors – or<br>MILD physical symptoms not requiring medical treatment – or<br>MILD obesity-related psychology and/or impairment of well-being |
| 2 | ESTABLISHED co-morbidity requiring intervention – or<br>MODERATE obesity-related psychological symptoms – or<br>MODERATE functional limitations on daily activities |
| 3 | SIGNIFICANT obesity-related end-organ damage – or<br>SIGNIFICANT obesity-related psychological symptoms – or<br>SIGNIFCANT functional limitations – or<br>SIGNIFICANT impairment of well-being |
| 4 | SEVERE (potentially end-stage) obesity-related chronic disease – or<br>SEVERE disabling psychological symptoms – or<br>SEVERE functional limitations |

*Source*: Data from Ref. [13].

visceral or 'ectopic' within tissue such as liver and muscle. Measuring waist circumference, or sagittal abdominal diameter, can make an estimate of visceral fat distribution, but more detailed characterisation of the amount and distribution of body fat require imaging techniques (CT, MRI or DXA) not routinely used. Such measures may however be important in the obese elderly in whom the coexistence of a low body lean mass with excess fat (sarcopaenic obesity) may be a particular risk for mortality and could contraindicate therapeutic weight loss [15, 16].

While obesity is strongly heritable, and many risk genes have been identified, specific genetic causes are uncommon and tend to present in childhood. Most present either as syndromes related to chromosomal abnormalities (such as Prader–Willi syndrome) or more rarely as homozygous gene mutations (such as leptin hormone or receptor deficiency) and have a phenotype that includes hyperphagia (Table 19.2). The most common gene mutation linked to obesity is of the melanocortin receptor 4 with a prevalence of about 1% in those with a BMI > 30 kg.m². Heterozygotes have a variable phenotype that may have mild features of hyperphagia. Polymorphisms of the fat mass and

obesity-associated protein (FTO) gene are also linked to obesity, metabolic syndrome, insulin resistance (IR) and type 2 diabetes mellitus and recently also to a lower likelihood of achieving successful virologic response to HCV therapy in HIV/HCV-co-infected patients [17]. In the POUNDS LOST trial of diet-induced weight loss, carriers of the FTO risk allele had a greater reduction in weight, body composition and fat distribution in response to a high-protein diet, whereas an opposite genetic effect was observed on changes in fat distribution in response to a low-protein diet [18]. Genotype may also influence the response to bariatric surgery [19] and weight loss drugs [20]. While pharmaco-, nutri- and surgico-genetics have not yet influenced treatment decisions in the form of personalising medical care, it seems likely that the future metabolic physician will need to increasingly consider these aspects.

Another key role for the metabolic physician is to undertake a comprehensive evaluation of the patient to diagnose and assess diseases implicated in or resulting from obesity [21]. Hypercortisolaemia in Cushing's syndrome, while rare, is an easily overlooked diagnosis as its features overlap with obesity (weight gain, hypertension, depression, diabetes). If suspected, formal endocrine investigation is required. Polycystic ovary syndrome also strongly overlaps with obesity in having common features of IR, hyper-androgenaemia and menstrual irregularity. Thyroid disease, while rarely a cause of obesity, is often thought to be by patients and non-specialists. An increasing number of medications are linked to weight gain including corticosteroids, β-blockers, psychotropic medications, anticonvulsants such as valproate, amitriptyline, sulphonylureas and insulin.

Clinical assessment of the obese patient by a metabolic physician should start with taking a comprehensive history to cover the onset of obesity and its progression and life events connected with increases in weight. A psychosocial history is important, as there is a strong association between childhood abuse and deprivation and later weight gain. Patient expectations need evaluating and their beliefs about the causes and treatment of their obesity need to be explored, and this is best done using techniques of motivational interviewing. Assessment of diet and physical activity (and patient attitudes and beliefs around these) is important – this may be delegated to a dietitian and/or exercise specialist where they form part of the metabolic physician's team. Where patients already have established obesity-related co-morbidity, a careful evaluation of their management and control is needed in order to allow opti-misation of treatment in the light of the coexisting obesity. Specific questioning to explore the undiagnosed presence of co-morbidities or risks such as gastro-oesophageal reflux, obstructive sleep apnoea, eating disorders and anovulatory amenorrhea is also needed.

Examination will entail accurate determination of height, weight, waist circumference with scales and meas-ures appropriate to the size of the patient. Blood pressure measurement requires a large cuff size, and pulse oxime-try may reveal hypoxia suggesting hypoventilation syn-drome. The presence of acanthosis nigricans and skin tags in the neck and axilla will suggest the presence of IR. Other specific features related to the obese state include intertrigo, varicose veins and lympho- or lipo-oedema. However in the severely obese patient, examination by palpation and auscultation may prove difficult. The phy-sician needs to be alert to the increased incidence of many cancers in the obese such as breast, uterus and colon.

Investigations will be primarily focused on assessing the consequences of obesity. Metabolic profiling (fasting blood glucose and possibly insulin, glycated haemoglobin, lipids, urate) will help confirm, or exclude diabetes, prediabetes or the metabolic syndrome. Specific parameters related to excess adiposity can be evaluated with liver function tests, renal function, androgen status and in women (especially if oligo- or amenorrheic) gonadotrophins and oestradiol. Despite caloric over-nutrition, many obese have poor qual-ity diets, and this may be linked to deficiencies of vitamins D, B12 and B1, folate and iron. A blood count may reveal some of these deficiencies or polycythemia – a feature of hypoventilation syndrome. Lastly assessment of high-sensitivity C-reactive protein may indicate the degree of obesity-related chronic inflammation – an increasingly recognised component of the metabolic syndrome. Pulmonary and cardiac function requires more formal assessment and questionnaires to assess mood, sleep, eat-ing disorders and readiness to change useful.

## Medical management of obesity

The metabolic physician is ideally place within secondary care to co-ordinate the management of the obese patient – be it medical or surgical. Many evidence-based guidelines now exist to guide management [22–25]. The recent National Institute for Health and Care Excellence (NICE)

guidelines, for example, recommend referral of patients to a specialist service if:

- The underlying causes of being overweight or obese need to be assessed.
- The person has complex disease states or needs that cannot be managed adequately in community-based services (e.g. the additional support needs of people with learning disabilities).
- Conventional treatment has been unsuccessful.
- Specialist interventions (such as a very-low-calorie diet) may be needed or surgery is being considered.

It is likely, and desirable, that the metabolic physician is part of an MDT including dietitian, exercise therapist or physiotherapist, clinical psychologist, nurse specialist and bariatric or metabolic surgeons. The MDT and specifically the metabolic physician will need close links with hepatol-ogists and renal, respiratory, cardiology and diabetes physi-cians. Initial optimisation of obesity-related co-morbidities (control of blood pressure, achieving glycaemic control in those with diabetes, treatment of obstructive sleep apnoea) is a priority but will need to be achieved in relation to the management of the obesity itself; this will involve colla-borative working with the patient's other specialists. Treatment may involve changes in medications (e.g. the switching from weight-gaining drugs such as sulphonylu-reas for diabetes to weight-neutral or weight-losing hypo-glycaemic medications such as DPP4 inhibitors, SGLT2 inhibitors or GLP-1 agonists, or the use of antipsychotic medications with less potent effects on weight). These changes will need to be agreed with other specialists, who may also need to sanction changes in medications needed as a result of weight loss (e.g. reductions of hypotensive agents or diuretics).

The physician should also involve the patient in making decisions about their treatment. Thus patients referred for consideration of bariatric surgery may be unsuited or out with commissioning and national guidelines, may themselves not wish to undergo surgery, or vice versa those referred for medi-cal management may need to be directed towards surgical treatment. In practice such considerations are more likely addressed by the physician rather than the surgeon.

Dietary management falls into two broad categories: those aiming at initial rapid and major loss driven by an urgent clinical need and those directed towards long-term weight loss and weight loss maintenance. The latter are likely to be provided within primary care, with the metabolic physician and secondary care MDT providing more intensive management programmes. Dietary approaches include assessing the energy needs of the individual and advising and supporting the patient on achieving a 600 kcal/day energy deficit, so predicting initially a rate of weight loss of 0.5 kg/week. More intensive regimens may include low- or very-low-energy diets, often composed partially of fully of liquid meal 'replacements'. NICE recently updated their guidance to recommend that very-low-calorie diets should only be prescribed as part of a multicomponent weight management strategy for people who are obese and who have a clinically assessed need to rapidly lose weight (e.g. people who need joint replacement surgery or who are seeking fertility services). The guidance also recommends that such diets are nutritionally complete, followed for a maximum of 12 weeks (continuously or intermittently), and that the person following the diet is given ongoing clinical support, so placing such interventions firmly within the roles and responsibilities of a metabolic physician. Weight loss in such programmes may be rapid and require various considerations: total protein intake in those with chronic renal impairment and adjustment (often including withdrawal of insulin) of concomitant medications for diabetes, heart failure and hypertension. While such programmes can induce rapid and substantial weight loss in the short term (6 months–1 year), weight regain is common even when ongoing support with behavioural and exercise counselling is provided.

The last few years have seen the approval and introduction of new pharmacological treatments for obesity to join the lipase inhibitor orlistat. These new drugs target central nervous systems involved in appetite regulation: central serotonin (lorcaserin), dopamine and GABAergic (phentermine + topiramate) and pro-opiomelanocortin and opioid (bupropion + naltrexone). High-dose GLP-1 agonist (liraglutide) also has direct central effects to enhance satiety and decrease appetite. Weight loss with these drugs ranges from about 7 to 12% when combined with comprehensive lifestyle management. Improvements in cardiometabolic status are seen, largely driven not only by weight loss but also by specific pharmacological actions of the drugs themselves (e.g. glycaemic improvement with liraglutide and lipid lowering with orlistat). The use of anti-obesity pharmacotherapy in combination or more accurately following the induction of weight loss with a low-energy diet has proven highly effective with a total weight loss at 1 year of 13% in the case of liraglutide [26] and may be the most effective way of using these drugs [27]. Clinical experience with these drugs is limited, and the metabolic physician is probably best placed to help develop the integration of pharmacotherapy into the routine care of obese subjects.

## Management of bariatric surgical patients

The increasing adoption of bariatric surgery worldwide is placing ever greater demands for metabolic physicians, who should be an integral part of the MDT. Surgery is increasingly being considered as metabolic surgery, in that independent of weight loss, procedures such as gastric bypass and sleeve gastrectomy have profound beneficial effects on 'metabolic' diseases such as diabetes, dyslipidaemia, non-alcoholic fatty liver disease as well as all other obesity-related morbidity [28–31].

The metabolic physician will have a key role in optimising the patient pre-surgery [32] often in collaboration with the bariatric anaesthetist. Pre-operative weight loss may be indicated in patients with severe central obesity in the face of an extreme BMI or where it is felt that a conventional 'liver shrinkage' diet may be inadequate to ensure sufficient regression of hepatomegaly to allow laparoscopic access. Guidelines suggest that glycaemic control should be achieved before elective surgery [33] based on much evidence that poor glycaemic control increases risks of infection and anastomosis leak [34, 35], and some data suggest that tight pre-operative glycaemic control improves the outcomes of diabetes remission after surgery [36]. Optimising other medications may also be important, for example, withdrawal of non-steroidal anti-inflammatory drugs [37]. Along with controlling blood pressure, ensuring that patients are optimised in relation to concomitant ischaemic heart disease or renal failure will also be the remit of the metabolic physician, in collaboration with the patient's other specialists (who may themselves have little experience of bariatric surgery). Many bariatric patients will have nutritional deficiencies that may require investigation (e.g. iron deficiency) or at the least correction (e.g. vitamin D). Where vitamin D deficiency does occur, awareness of secondary hyperparathyroidism and its appropriate treatment and ensuring that a diagnosis of primary hyperparathyroidism is not missed also come within the remit of the metabolic physician.

At the same time there are increasing recognition and emergence of iatrogenic and nosohypokatastatic disease (disease substitution) [38, 39]. Malabsorption (an integral part of gastric bypass surgery) may compound mineral, vitamin and trace element deficiencies that also result from poor nutrition that can be worsened by the restricted intake imposed by weight loss surgery. Thiamine deficiency (especially in those who have frequent vomiting) can present acutely as Wernicke encephalopathy. The effect of extreme weight loss (with or without micronutrient deficiencies) on bone mineral density (BMD) and bone mass, both of which serve as indirect measures of osteoporosis and fracture risk remains controversial. Technical limitations of screening measures of BMD with DXA also exist.

While one of the major benefits of bariatric surgery is to improve glycaemic control in patients with diabetes, with marked reductions in A1c even after withdrawal of hypoglycaemic therapy, it does not normalise blood glucose profiles. The significance of the (inevitable) excessive rises in postprandial glucose levels to long-term micro- and macrovascular disease is unclear. However, an increasingly recognised metabolic consequence is 'reactive' or postprandial hypoglycaemia (PPH) [40, 41] that appears to result from the hyper-responsiveness of incretin response to meals [42]. There continues to be debate as to whether nesidioblastosis or insulinoma can result from the continued exposure of the β-cell to incretins, but if this does occur, it is rare [43–45]. Some evidence points to an acquired hypothalamic unresponsiveness to hypoglycaemia as a contributory factor. PPH is, however, producing increasing demands on the metabolic physician. Exclusion of insulinoma may require detailed endocrine investigation [46, 47]. Once excluded, management of PPH will require intensive advice to help the patient adhere to a low glycaemic index diet, but medical therapy with drugs such as acarbose [48, 49] or even somatostatin analogues [50] or GLP-1 antagonists [51] is needed.

## Conclusions

The metabolic physician is becoming an increasingly valuable specialist as the prevalence of obesity increases and as an ever-growing number of diseases linked to, caused by or exacerbated in obesity becomes apparent. The physician is likely to be integrated into secondary care endocrine or metabolic services or as part of a bariatric surgery team.

The physician will be both a generalist with skills spanning specialties across the whole of internal medicine and a specialist in managing the ever-increasing metabolic consequences of obesity and its treatments. Many will or should take on the role of co-ordinating care of the obese patient within hospital and participate in providing comprehensive weight management services in both primary and secondary care. The development in the United States of board certification is a step forward that needs developing worldwide.

## References

1. Kopelman PG, Finer N. Reply: Is obesity a disease? Int J Obes Relat Metab Disord [Internet]. 2001 Oct;25(10):1405–6.
2. Jensen MD, Ryan DH, Apovian CM, Ard JD, Comuzzie AG, Donato KA, et al. 2013 AHA/ACC/TOS guideline for the management of overweight and obesity in adults: A report of the American college of cardiology/american heart association task force on practice guidelines and the obesity society. J Am Coll Cardiol. 2014 Jul 1;63(25 Pt B): 2985–3023.
3. Katz DL. Perspective: Obesity is not a disease. Nature [Internet]. 2014 Apr 17;508(7496):S57.
4. Pucci A, Finer N. In: Matfin G, editor. Acute Medical Aspects Related to Obesity A Clinician's Guide: Endocrine and Metabolic Medical Emergencies. Washington, DC: Endocrine Press, Endocrine Society; 2014. p. 377–80.
5. American Board of Obesity Medicine (ABOM) [Internet]. Available from: http://abom.org (accessed on 26 October 2015).
6. World Obesity Federation. Get obesity certification online with SCOPE! [Internet]. Available from: http://www.worldobesity.org/scope/certification/ (accessed on 26 October 2015).
7. EurekAlert! Science News. STOP Obesity Alliance surveys show doctors, patients share role in weight loss, but ask, now what? [Internet]. Available from: http://www.eurekalert.org/pub_releases/2010-03/cca-soa031510.php (accessed on 26 October 2015).
8. Jochemsen-van der Leeuw HGA, van Dijk N, Wieringa-de Waard M. Attitudes towards obesity treatment in GP training practices: A focus group study. Fam Pract 2011;28(4):422–9.
9. Nolan C, Deehan A, Wylie A, Jones R. Practice nurses and obesity: Professional and practice-based factors affecting role adequacy and role legitimacy. Prim Health Care Res Dev [Internet]. 2012 Oct;13(4):353–63.
10. Royal College. The training of health professionals for the prevention and treatment of overweight and obesity Report

prepared for Foresight by the Royal College of Physicians. Evaluation. 2010 (March).

11. Wass J, Finer N. Action on Obesity: Comprehensive Care for All. Report of a Working Party. Royal College of Physicians, London; 2013 p. 1–64.

12. Finer N. Clinical Obesity – A new journal for a new clinical era. Clin Obes [Internet]. 2011 Feb 22;1(1):1–2.

13. Kuk JL, Ardern CI, Church TS, Sharma AM, Padwal R, Sui X, et al. Edmonton obesity staging system: Association with weight history and mortality risk. Appl Physiol Nutr Metab [Internet]. 2011 Aug;36(4):570–6.

14. Sharma AM, Kushner RF. A proposed clinical staging system for obesity. Int J Obes (Lond) [Internet]. 2009 Mar;33(3):289–95.

15. Prado CMM, Heymsfield SB. Lean tissue imaging: A new era for nutritional assessment and intervention. JPEN J Parenter Enteral Nutr. 2014 Nov;38:940–53.

16. Mathus-Vliegen EMH, Basdevant A, Finer N, Hainer V, Hauner H, Micic D, et al. Prevalence, pathophysiology, health consequences and treatment options of obesity in the elderly: A guideline. Obes Facts [Internet]. 2012;5(3): 460–83.

17. Pineda-Tenor D, Berenguer J, Jiménez-Sousa MA, García-Alvarez M, Aldámiz-Echevarria T, Carrero A, et al. FTO rs9939609 polymorphism is associated with metabolic disturbances and response to HCV therapy in HIV/HCV-coinfected patients. BMC Med [Internet]. 2014 Jan;12:198.

18. Zhang X, Qi Q, Zhang C, Smith SR, Hu FB, Sacks FM, et al. FTO genotype and 2-year change in body composition and fat distribution in response to weight-loss diets: The POUNDS LOST Trial. Diabetes [Internet]. 2012 Nov;61(11): 3005–11.

19. Liou T-H, Chen H-H, Wang W, Wu S-F, Lee Y-C, Yang W-S, et al. ESR1, FTO, and UCP2 genes interact with bariatric surgery affecting weight loss and glycemic control in severely obese patients. Obes Surg [Internet]. 2011 Nov;21(11):1758–65.

20. Finer N. Predicting therapeutic weight loss. Am J Clin Nutr. 2015;101(3):419–20.

21. Kushner RF. Clinical assessment and management of adult obesity. Circulation [Internet]. 2012 Dec 11;126(24): 2870–7.

22. Apovian CM, Aronne LJ, Bessesen DH, Mcdonnell ME, Murad MH, Pagotto U, et al. Pharmacological management of obesity: An endocrine society clinical practice guideline. J Clin Endocrinol Metab. 2015 Feb;100:342–62.

23. Scottish Intercollegiate Guidelines Network (SIGN). Management of obesity, a national clinical guideline [Internet]. 2010. p. 1–87.

24. National Clinical Guideline Centre (UK). Obesity: Identification, assessment and management of overweight

and obesity in children, young people and adults: Partial update of CG43. 2014. p. 1–154.

25. Document C. Joint statement of the European Association for the Study of Obesity and the European Society of Hypertension: Obesity and difficult to treat arterial hypertension. 2012. p. 1047–55.

26. Wadden TA, Hollander P, Klein S, Niswender K, Woo V, Hale PM, et al. Weight maintenance and additional weight loss with liraglutide after low-calorie-diet-induced weight loss: The SCALE Maintenance randomized study. Int J Obes (Lond) [Internet]. 2013 Nov;37(11):1443–51.

27. Johansson K, Neovius M, Hemmingsson E. Effects of anti-obesity drugs, diet, and exercise on weight-loss maintenance after a very-low-calorie diet or low-calorie diet: A systematic review and meta-analysis of randomized controlled trials. Am J Clin Nutr. 2013;99(1):14–23.

28. Rubino F, Cummings DE. Surgery: The coming of age of metabolic surgery. Nat Rev Endocrinol [Internet]. 2012 Dec;8(12):702–4.

29. Rubino F, Shukla A, Pomp A, Moreira M, Ahn SM, Dakin G. Bariatric, metabolic, and diabetes surgery: What's in a name?. Ann Surg [Internet]. 2014 Jan;259(1):117–22.

30. Geiker NRW, Swe Myint K, Heck PM, Dhatariya K, Larsen SH, Andersen MR, et al. Intentional weight loss improved performance in obese ischaemic heart patients: A two centre intervention trial. Jacobs J Food Nutr. 2014;1(1):1–9.

31. Rubino F, Shukla A, Pomp A, Moreira M, Ahn SM, Dakin G. Bariatric, metabolic, and diabetes surgery: What's in a name?. Ann Surg [Internet]. 2014 Jan;259(1):117–22.

32. Mechanick JI, Youdim A, Jones DB, Garvey WT, Hurley DL, McMahon MM, et al. Clinical practice guidelines for the perioperative nutritional, metabolic, and nonsurgical support of the bariatric surgery patient-2013 update: Cosponsored by American association of clinical endocrinologists, the obesity society, and American society for Metabolic & Bariatric Surgery. Endocr Pract [Internet]. 2013;19(2):337–72.

33. Diabetes. Management of adults with diabetes undergoing surgery and elective procedures: Improving standards. 2011 April.

34. King JT, Goulet JL, Perkal MF, Rosenthal RA. Glycemic control and infections in patients with diabetes undergoing noncardiac surgery. Ann Surg [Internet]. 2011 Jan;253(1):158–65.

35. Noordzij PG, Boersma E, Schreiner F, Kertai MD, Feringa HHH, Dunkelgrun M, et al. Increased preoperative glucose levels are associated with perioperative mortality in patients undergoing noncardiac, nonvascular surgery. Eur J Endocrinol [Internet]. 2007 Jan;156(1):137–42.

36. English TM, Malkani S, Kinney RL, Omer A, Dziewietin MB, Perugini R. Predicting remission of diabetes after RYGB surgery following intensive management to optimize

preoperative glucose control. Obes Surg [Internet]. 2015 Jan;25(1):1–6.

37. Hakkarainen TW, Steele SR, Bastaworous A, Dellinger EP, Farrokhi E, Farjah F, et al. Nonsteroidal anti-inflammatory drugs and the risk for anastomotic failure: A report from Washington State's Surgical Care and Outcomes Assessment Program (SCOAP). JAMA Surg [Internet]. 2015 Jan 21;150(3):223–8.

38. Finer N. Endocrine and metabolic complications post-bariatric surgery. Endocr Abstr [Internet]. 2014 Mar 1; Available from: http://www.endocrine-abstracts.org/ea/0034/ea0034 cmw1.3.htm (accessed on 26 October 2015).

39. Heber D, Greenway FL, Kaplan LM, Livingston E, Salvador J, Still C. Endocrine and nutritional management of the post-bariatric surgery patient: An Endocrine Society Clinical Practice Guideline. J Clin Endocrinol Metab. 2010;95(11):4823–43.

40. Brun J, Fedou C, Mercier J. Postprandial reactive hypoglycemia. Diabetes Metab [Internet]. 2000;26(5):337–52.

41. Goldfine AB, Mun E, Patti ME. Hyperinsulinemic hypoglycemia following gastric bypass surgery for obesity. Curr Opin Endocrinol Diabetes [Internet] 2006 Oct;13(5):419–24.

42. Society TE. Editorial: Incretin hypersecretion in post-gastric bypass hypoglycemia – Primary problem or red herring?. J Clin Endocrinol Metab. 2007;92(12):4563–5.

43. Meier JJ, Butler AE, Galasso R, Butler PC. Hyperinsulinemic hypoglycemia after gastric bypass surgery is not accompanied by islet hyperplasia or increased??-cell turnover. Diabetes Care. 2006;29:1554–9.

44. Sarwar H, Chapman WH, Pender JR, Ivanescu A, Drake AJ, Pories WJ, et al. Hypoglycemia after roux-en-Y gastric bypass: The BOLD experience. Obes Surg [Internet]. 2014 Jul;24(7):1120–4.

45. Service GJ, Thompson GB, Service FJ, Andrews JC, Collazo-clavell ML, Lloyd RV. Hyperinsulinemic hypoglycemia with nesidioblastosis after gastric-bypass surgery. Analyzer. 2005;353(3):249–54.

46. De Heide LJM, Glaudemans AWJM, Oomen PHN, Apers JA, Totté ERE, van Beek AP. Functional imaging in hyperinsulinemic hypoglycemia after gastric bypass surgery for morbid obesity. J Clin Endocrinol Metab [Internet]. 2012 Jun;97(6):E963–7.

47. Halperin F, Patti ME, Skow M, Bajwa M, Goldfine AB. Continuous glucose monitoring for evaluation of glycemic excursions after gastric bypass. J Obes [Internet]. 2011 Jan;2011:869536.

48. Ritz P, Vaurs C, Bertrand M, Anduze Y, Guillaume E, Hanaire H. Usefulness of acarbose and dietary modifications to limit glycemic variability following Roux-en-Y gastric bypass as assessed by continuous glucose monitoring. Diabetes Technol Ther [Internet]. 2012 Aug;14(8):736–40.

49. Patti ME, Goldfine AB. Hypoglycaemia following gastric bypass surgery – diabetes remission in the extreme? Diabetologia [Internet]. 2010 Nov;53(11):2276–9.

50. Myint KS, Greenfield JR, Farooqi IS, Henning E, Holst JJ, Finer N. Prolonged successful therapy for hyperinsulinaemic hypoglycaemia after gastric bypass: The pathophysiological role of GLP1 and its response to a somatostatin analogue. Eur J Endocrinol [Internet]. 2012 May;166(5):951–5.

51. Salehi M, Gastaldelli A, D'Alessio DA. Blockade of glucagon-like peptide 1 receptor corrects postprandial hypoglycemia after gastric bypass. Gastroenterology. 2014;146:669–80.

# 20 Should physicians be prescribing or patients self-medicating with orlistat, vitamin E, vitamin D, insulin sensitizers, pentoxifylline, or coffee?

**Haripriya Maddur and Brent A. Neuschwander-Tetri**

Division of Gastroenterology and Hepatology, Saint Louis University, St. Louis, MO, USA

### LEARNING POINTS

- Coffee consumption has been linked to less severe disease in patients with NAFLD, although it has not been examined in any prospective trials.

- Pentoxifylline has shown some benefits in small trials, but its effects in diabetics with NASH remain uncertain.

- Vitamin E was shown to improve NASH in about half of the patients treated in two large randomized trials, but these trials excluded diabetics and cirrhotics, so its role in such patients remains unknown.

- Pioglitazone improved NASH but in less than half the patients who received it in several studies. Pioglitazone can cause weight gain and it has an uncertain safety profile that dampen enthusiasm for its use.

- Lifestyle modification with a focus on healthy eating habits, regular exercise, and weight reduction remains the primary treatment for NASH.

## Introduction

Non-alcoholic steatohepatitis (NASH) is present in ~3–5% of the US population with 10–15% of these patients going on to develop cirrhosis [1–6]. In fact, NASH is the third most common indication for liver transplantation, with the projection that it will surpass hepatitis C in the next decade as the leading cause for liver transplantation [7]. With the increase in metabolic syndrome and insulin resistance, both of which are implicated in the pathogenesis of NASH, the need for therapeutic modalities to halt the progression of this ominous disease is paramount. In this section, we will review the data on available pharmacologic agents as well as the role of coffee consumption on halting NASH progression.

## Coffee consumption

Coffee, one of the most widely consumed beverages worldwide, has been reported to have numerous health benefits including decreased risks of heart disease, stroke, and diabetes [8]. Benefits to the liver have been described that include a decreased risk of hepatocellular carcinoma and reduced histologic activity in patients infected with hepatitis C [9].

In studies of patients with NAFLD, beneficial effects of coffee have been shown in laboratory markers and proinflammatory cytokines, as well as less severe steatosis by ultrasound [10, 11]. A study of liver histology also found that coffee consumption was linked to less fibrosis in patients with NASH [12]. A study in bariatric subjects concluded that coffee consumption was associated with less hepatic fibrosis in severely obese patients, but interestingly, this potential benefit of coffee was not seen in patients who consumed coffee in the form of espresso [13]. It was

*Clinical Dilemmas in Non-Alcoholic Fatty Liver Disease*, First Edition. Edited by Roger Williams and Simon D. Taylor-Robinson.
© 2016 John Wiley & Sons, Ltd. Published 2016 by John Wiley & Sons, Ltd.

hypothesized that the lack of observed benefit may be linked to the addition of sucrose in espresso drinks based on the role of sucrose and fructose in the pathogenesis of NASH. Alternatively, compounds extracted from coffee beans during the emulsification process inherent in espresso preparation may be different from those extracted during standard water filtration. Additional evidence for the benefits of coffee includes a dose effect that has also been observed with greater coffee consumption in patients with bland steatosis compared to those with NASH [14]. The benefits of coffee were further corroborated in a large cross-sectional survey from the Non-alcoholic Steatohepatitis Clinical Research Network (NASH CRN) in which lower histology scores were found in coffee drinkers compared to noncoffee drinkers having the full spectrum of NAFLD, although, in this study, the benefits appeared to be limited to those with less severe insulin resistance [15].

Animal studies of NAFLD models have provided additional insights. Coffee feeding has been associated with decreased serum aspartate aminotransferase (AST), alanine aminotransferase (ALT), as well as proinflammatory markers in animals administered a high-fat diet [16, 17]. The mechanisms responsible for the hepatoprotective benefits of coffee continue to be investigated in animal models. Caffeine is an obvious constituent because of its well-known stimulant properties. However, a study in rats showed that decaffeinated coffee was beneficial and that decaffeinated espresso improved liver histology [18]. In this study, fat-fed rats were randomized to 12 weeks of decaffeinated espresso versus water. The rats randomized to coffee consumption were noted to have milder steatosis, decreased ballooning, and decreased inflammation compared to water-fed rats. The coffee-fed rats also had greater hepatic expression of the endoplasmic reticulum protein chaperones glucose-regulated protein 78 (GRP78) and protein disulfide-isomerase A3.

Coffee is comprised of >100 known compounds, and it is unclear which ones are responsible for its reported health benefits. Different coffee preparations may contain different amounts of important compounds such as diterpene lipids, cafestol, and kahweol, which have anticarcinogenic properties in rats but are absent in filtered coffee [19]. Polyphenols and melanoidins in coffee have been proposed to possess antioxidant properties [20]. In another study of rats fed a high-fat diet, groups were given decaffeinated coffee, water, polyphenols, or melanoidins, the latter two of which were extracted from decaffeinated coffee [17]. This study demonstrated decreased hepatic fat and collagen deposition linked to coffee consumption and decreased evidence of oxidant stress linked to both coffee consumption and its constituents (polyphenols and melanoidins).

Thus it appears based on animal studies and clinical data that coffee has benefits in patients with NAFLD, and it appears that its benefits accrue in the absence of caffeine although the exact components responsible for these effects have yet to be identified. So far, it appears that polyphenols may be one class of agents responsible for its therapeutic benefits, although further study is warranted before widespread implementation of coffee consumption as an effective therapy for NASH. However, based on the available data, it certainly appears safe not to restrict coffee consumption in patients with the spectrum of NAFLD.

## Orlistat

Modest weight loss has been shown to improve aminotransferases and markers of insulin resistance in patients with NASH [21]. Pharmacologic vehicles of weight loss induction have thus been studied as potential treatment adjuncts. Orlistat, an inhibitor of gastric and pancreatic lipase, is available over the counter and has been studied based on its inhibition of intestinal breakdown and fat absorption [22]. Initial data examining the use of orlistat in patients with NASH appeared promising. In a case series of three patients with biopsy-proven NASH treated with low-fat diet and orlistat 120 mg three times daily, a significant reduction in weight and aminotransferase levels was observed in addition to histologic improvement of steatosis and fibrosis [23]. A subsequent pilot study using orlistat for 6 months in patients with histologically confirmed NASH in conjunction with lifestyle modification was notable for 10% weight reduction in half of the patients, of which three had histologic improvement of fibrosis [24]. In this pilot study, histological improvement correlated with weight loss rather than orlistat use.

Data comparing orlistat and placebo was published by Zelber-Sagi et al. [25]. In this trial, 52 patients were randomized to placebo versus orlistat 120 mg three times daily in conjunction with caloric restriction. This study was notable for a statistically significant reduction in ALT levels and sonographic reversal of steatosis in the orlistat group compared to placebo. Additionally, body mass index (BMI) reduction was observed to a greater extent in the orlistat group; however this did not reach statistical significance. Interestingly, although there was a reduction in steatosis and fibrosis in patients treated with orlistat, this too did not achieve statistical significance when compared to placebo, although only a subset of patients underwent follow-up biopsy.

As data has suggested that vitamin E may be beneficial in the treatment of NASH, an additional randomized controlled trial enrolled 50 patients randomized to orlistat 120 mg three times daily along with vitamin E 800 International Units (IU) daily and a hypocaloric diet compared to these interventions without orlistat for 36 weeks. Although treatment with orlistat did result in aminotransferase reductions, weight loss, and improvement in histopathology, these changes were not statistically significant. Analysis of subjects who had at least a 5% weight loss demonstrated improved insulin sensitivity and steatosis compared to those who did not demonstrate such weight reduction [26].

These data suggest that orlistat does not provide significant benefit compared to placebo in regard to histologic regression of fibrosis and steatosis. It is important to note, however, that the implementation of dietary restriction in control groups confirmed available data regarding the benefit of weight reduction as a means for improvement in NASH. These small studies of orlistat in patients with NASH did not demonstrate a benefit in terms of weight loss although larger studies of orlistat as a treatment for obesity have shown that it promotes weight loss. Orlistat can be difficult to tolerate, but for the select few who can tolerate it and achieve weight loss through its use, it may have a role in treating their NASH.

## Pentoxifylline

Pentoxifylline, a nonspecific phosphodiesterase inhibitor, has been shown to reduce proinflammatory cytokine production by reduction of TNFα transcription [27, 28]. Given that elevated TNFα levels have been found to be elevated in both alcoholic hepatitis and NASH, therapy with pentoxifylline has been investigated as a potential therapeutic agent. In patients with alcoholic hepatitis, pentoxifylline has been shown to improve short-term survival [29]. In NASH, varying doses of pentoxifylline were found to reduce TNFα release by lipopolysaccharide-stimulated peripheral blood mononuclear cells [30].

Based on such *in vitro* and early pilot studies, a randomized placebo-controlled trial of 20 patients assessed the effect of pentoxifylline 400 mg three times daily, exercise, and caloric restriction compared to caloric restriction and exercise alone for 3 months. AST reduction was lower in the pentoxifylline group with a trend toward ALT reduction. Although TNFα and IL-6 levels were reduced, this was found to occur in both arms, suggesting that the anti-inflammatory effects were achieved through exercise and dietary changes. Interestingly, no BMI reduction was observed [31].

An additional placebo-controlled randomized trial by Van Wagner et al. comparing pentoxifylline 1200 mg daily for 1 year in subjects with biopsy-proven NASH demonstrated a trend toward histologic improvement of steatosis and reduction in aminotransferase levels; however these changes were not statistically significant when compared to placebo [32]. These results were not commensurate, however, with a subsequent study by Zein et al., in which 55 patients with biopsy-proven NASH randomized to pentoxifylline 400 mg three times daily versus placebo for one year demonstrated improvement in the NAFLD activity score (NAS). A nonsignificant trend toward improvement of fibrosis was also observed. Interestingly, despite improvement in histology, no reduction was appreciated in serum TNFα levels. The authors speculated that the lack of a reduction in serum TNFα was due to a discordance between hepatic and serum TNFα. A limitation of this study was that few patients were diabetic, precluding statistical assessment of the effects of pentoxifylline on diabetics. In addition, the discrepancy between histologic improvement in the two studies may be related to the lack of cirrhotic patients in the study by Zein et al. [33].

Based on available data, it appears that pentoxifylline may show promise as a potentially effective therapy for NASH. Although improvements in aminotransferases and histologic activity scores were found in some studies, these findings were not found to differ from placebo in other studies. The aforementioned studies, however, demonstrated the relative safety of pentoxifylline in NASH patients. Larger, more prolonged studies are required with greater inclusion of cirrhotics and diabetics before its routine implementation as a treatment for NASH.

## Vitamin E

Although animal studies have suggested that oxidant stress plays a role in the pathogenesis of NASH, human studies have not been able to make this causative association. It is not known whether this is because the animal models used such as the methionine–choline-deficient diet model lack clinical relevance, if antioxidants used in human studies lack adequate potency or bioavailability at the location(s) where oxidant stress plays a role, or if oxidant stress occurs but does not play a causal role in NASH. The data with vitamin E has been the most encouraging, but the results have been mixed. Two multicenter placebo-controlled trials of vitamin E, one in adults [34] and one in children [35], demonstrated histological improvement in NASH in about half of the subjects, but in neither trial were any indices of improvement in oxidant stress reported. Both trials used natural vitamin E at a dose of 800 IU daily for 96 weeks in subjects without evidence of diabetes or cirrhosis. Whether the results can be extrapolated to patients with diabetes is unknown.

Importantly, vitamin E may not be completely benign as the available literature has suggested that its use may be associated with significant side effects. One meta-analysis implicated vitamin E as a risk factor for hemorrhagic stroke [36]. In addition to stroke risk, a randomized trial also linked high-dose vitamin E (defined as >400 IU/day) as a risk factor for prostate cancer in men treated for >7 years [37]. Thus a recommendation that patients with NASH take vitamin E must take the risks and benefits into account.

Based on this data, a reasonable approach would be to avoid use of vitamin E in those individuals without histologically confirmed NASH and to avoid its use in those individuals with documented diabetes as the aforementioned trials excluded diabetics. Patients given vitamin E should still be encouraged to lose weight as part of their treatment. An analysis of the adult trial of vitamin E demonstrated that those who took vitamin E and lost weight as well had the greatest histological benefit [38]. The complexities of the vitamin E response were further characterized in another analysis of the adult and pediatric trials that demonstrated no relationship between α-tocopherol levels before or during treatment and histological response [39].

## Insulin sensitizers

Adipose insulin resistance has been implicated in the pathogenesis of NASH, specifically contributing to the accumulation of fat within the liver as well as the development and progression of steatohepatitis [40, 41]. Thiazolidinediones (TZDs) have been studied in patients with NASH as a means of improving adipose tissue insulin sensitivity. TZDs enhance insulin sensitivity by activation of peroxisome proliferator-activated receptors, thus increasing adiponectin release and facilitating the retention of fatty acids within triglyceride in adipocytes [42].

Initial studies evaluating TZDs in NASH were promising. In a pilot study of rosiglitazone, 30 obese patients with biopsy-proven NASH were given rosiglitazone 4 mg daily for 48 weeks. In this study, 45% of patients who had posttreatment biopsies had histologic regression of NASH along with improvement of zone 3 perisinusoidal fibrosis and hepatocellular ballooning. In addition, of the 25 patients who completed therapy, improved insulin sensitivity and aminotransferases were noted. Of note, 67% of patients within the study experienced weight gain, and, within six months of cessation of therapy, aminotransferase levels increased to pretreatment levels [43]. In an additional pilot study by Ratziu et al., another TZD, pioglitazone, was examined in eighteen nondiabetic patients for 48 weeks. In this study, nearly three-quarters of the patients studied had aminotransferase normalization. In addition, there was a statistically significant reduction in hepatic steatosis and fibrosis on biopsy. Similar to previous studies, weight gain was appreciated (an average of 4%) in addition to an increase in total body adiposity [44].

In a subsequent randomized controlled trial by Ratziu et al., 63 patients were randomized to rosiglitazone (4 mg daily for 1 month and then increased to 8 mg daily) versus placebo for 1 year. Compared to placebo, those patients receiving rosiglitazone had a statistically significant improvement in aminotransferases and steatosis but no improvement in fibrosis. Weight gain was observed, with a mean weight gain of 1.5 kg in the rosiglitazone group [45].

In the PIVENS trial, 247 patients were randomized to receive 800 IU of natural vitamin E versus 30 mg pioglitazone daily versus placebo. In this trial, the primary endpoint was histologic improvement of NASH based on a composite score of steatosis, lobular inflammation, hepatocyte ballooning, and fibrosis. Treatment with pioglitazone was associated with resolution of NASH in 50% of subjects compared to 28% receiving placebo ($P < 0.01$). In addition, although there was a statistically significant improvement in aminotransferases, no improvement in fibrosis was observed. As with other TZD studies, weight gain was also seen in the TZD group [34].

It should be noted that in addition to observed side effect of weight gain associated with TZDs, these agents have also been reported to result in bone loss, congestive heart failure, fluid retention, and bladder cancer [46]. Additionally, several studies have shown that the response to TZDs is not sustained following drug cessation. Given the risk associated with use of TZDs and the need for prolonged or indefinite treatment, the risks associated with these agents should be taken into strong consideration prior to drug initiation [43, 47].

## Vitamin D

Vitamin D has been implicated in the development and progression of NASH as well as the progression of other liver diseases such as hepatitis C and the development of hepatocellular carcinoma in alcoholic cirrhosis [48–50]. Animal studies with vitamin D receptor knockout mice have shown spontaneous development of hepatic steatosis [51]. However clinical studies have been mixed. In a recent clinical study controlled for insulin resistance, age, and sex, vitamin D deficiency was linked to imaging evidence of hepatic steatosis [52], but another study found no relationship between NASH and vitamin D levels [53]. Results of ongoing and future treatment trials of vitamin D supplementation should shed light on the role of vitamin D as an adjunct in the treatment of NASH.

## Conclusion

At this time, there remain limited viable therapies for NASH beyond lifestyle modification. Although many of the available agents show promise, their efficacy and scope of implementation are limited to carefully selected patients. In particular, vitamin E appears to be the most effective therapy based on currently available studies in nondiabetic subjects with insulin sensitizers being a suitable option for diabetic patients with careful consideration of side effects. As for the use of coffee consumption, it appears to be safe in patients with NASH although more studies are needed before it can be routinely recommended as a viable treatment option. Further studies with larger treatment groups are needed to determine the effects of readily available therapies in patients with NASH.

## References

1. Williams CD, Stengel J, Asike MI, et al. Prevalence of nonalcoholic fatty liver disease and nonalcoholic steatohepatitis among a largely middle-aged population utilizing ultrasound and liver biopsy: a prospective study. Gastroenterology 2011;140:124–31.

2. Vernon G, Baranova A, Younossi ZM. Systematic review: the epidemiology and natural history of non-alcoholic fatty liver disease and non-alcoholic steatohepatitis in adults. Alimentary Pharmacology & Therapeutics 2011;34: 274–85.

3. Lazo M, Hernaez R, Eberhardt MS, et al. Prevalence of non-alcoholic fatty liver disease in the United States: the Third National Health and Nutrition Examination Survey, 1988–1994. American Journal of Epidemiology 2013;178:38–45.

4. Matteoni CA, Younossi ZM, Gramlich T, Boparai N, Liu YC, McCullough AJ. Nonalcoholic fatty liver disease: a spectrum of clinical and pathological severity. Gastroenterology 1999;116:1413–9.

5. Ekstedt M, Franzen LE, Mathiesen UL, et al. Long-term follow-up of patients with NAFLD and elevated liver enzymes. Hepatology 2006;44:865–73.

6. Adams LA, Lymp JF, St Sauver J, et al. The natural history of nonalcoholic fatty liver disease: a population-based cohort study. Gastroenterology 2005;129:113–21.

7. Charlton MR, Burns JM, Pedersen RA, Watt KD, Heimbach JK, Dierkhising RA. Frequency and outcomes of liver transplantation for nonalcoholic steatohepatitis in the United States. Gastroenterology 2011;141:1249–53.

8. Freedman ND, Park Y, Abnet CC, Hollenbeck AR, Sinha R. Association of coffee drinking with total and cause-specific mortality. The New England Journal of Medicine 2012;366:1891–904.

9. Chen S, Teoh NC, Chitturi S, Farrell GC. Coffee and non-alcoholic fatty liver disease: brewing evidence for hepatoprotection? Journal of Gastroenterology and Hepatology 2014;29:435–41.

10. Catalano D, Martines GF, Tonzuso A, Pirri C, Trovato FM, Trovato GM. Protective role of coffee in non-alcoholic fatty liver disease (NAFLD). Digestive Diseases and Sciences 2010;55:3200–6.

11. Gutierrez-Grobe Y, Chavez-Tapia N, Sanchez-Valle V, et al. High coffee intake is associated with lower grade nonalcoholic fatty liver disease: the role of peripheral antioxidant activity. Annals of Hepatology 2012;11:350–5.

12. Brosson D, Kuhn L, Delbac F, Garin J, Christian PV, Texier C. Proteomic analysis of the eukaryotic parasite *Encephalitozoon cuniculi* (microsporidia): a reference map for proteins expressed in late sporogonial stages. Proteomics 2006;6: 3625–35.

13. Anty R, Marjoux S, Iannelli A, et al. Regular coffee but not espresso drinking is protective against fibrosis in a cohort mainly composed of morbidly obese European women with NAFLD undergoing bariatric surgery. Journal of Hepatology 2012;57:1090–6.

14. Molloy JW, Calcagno CJ, Williams CD, Jones FJ, Torres DM, Harrison SA. Association of coffee and caffeine

consumption with fatty liver disease, nonalcoholic steato-hepatitis, and degree of hepatic fibrosis. Hepatology 2012;55:429–36.

15. Bambha K, Wilson LA, Unalp A, et al. Coffee consumption in NAFLD patients with lower insulin resistance is associated with lower risk of severe fibrosis. Liver International 2014;34:1250–8.

16. Fukushima Y, Kasuga M, Nakao K, Shimomura I, Matsuzawa Y. Effects of coffee on inflammatory cytokine gene expression in mice fed high-fat diets. Journal of Agricultural and Food Chemistry 2009;57:11100–5.

17. Vitaglione P, Morisco F, Mazzone G, et al. Coffee reduces liver damage in a rat model of steatohepatitis: the underlying mechanisms and the role of polyphenols and melanoidins. Hepatology 2010;52:1652–61.

18. Salomone F, Li Volti G, Vitaglione P, et al. Coffee enhances the expression of chaperones and antioxidant proteins in rats with nonalcoholic fatty liver disease. Translational Research 2014;163:593–602.

19. Urgert R, Essed N, van der Weg G, Kosmeijer-Schuil TG, Katan MB. Separate effects of the coffee diterpenes cafestol and kahweol on serum lipids and liver aminotransferases. The American Journal of Clinical Nutrition 1997;65:519–24.

20. Wang Y, Ho CT. Polyphenolic chemistry of tea and coffee: a century of progress. Journal of Agricultural and Food Chemistry 2009;57:8109–14.

21. Harrison SA, Day CP. Benefits of lifestyle modification in NAFLD. Gut 2007;56:1760–9.

22. Padwal R, Li SK, Lau DC. Long-term pharmacotherapy for obesity and overweight. The Cochrane Database of Systematic Reviews 2004;(3):CD004094.

23. Harrison SA, Ramrakhiani S, Brunt EM, Anbari MA, Cortese C, Bacon BR. Orlistat in the treatment of NASH: a case series. The American Journal of Gastroenterology 2003;98:926–30.

24. Harrison SA, Fincke C, Helinski D, Torgerson S, Hayashi P. A pilot study of orlistat treatment in obese, non-alcoholic steatohepatitis patients. Alimentary Pharmacology & Therapeutics 2004;20:623–8.

25. Zelber-Sagi S, Kessler A, Brazowsky E, et al. A double-blind randomized placebo-controlled trial of orlistat for the treatment of nonalcoholic fatty liver disease. Clinical Gastroenterology and Hepatology 2006;4:639–44.

26. Harrison SA, Fecht W, Brunt EM, Neuschwander-Tetri BA. Orlistat for overweight subjects with nonalcoholic steato-hepatitis: a randomized, prospective trial. Hepatology 2009;49:80–6.

27. Windmeier C, Gressner AM. Pharmacological aspects of pentoxifylline with emphasis on its inhibitory actions on hepatic fibrogenesis. General Pharmacology 1997;29:181–96.

28. Du J, Ma YY, Yu CH, Li YM. Effects of pentoxifylline on nonalcoholic fatty liver disease: a meta-analysis. World Journal of Gastroenterology 2014;20:569–77.

29. Akriviadis E, Botla R, Briggs W, Han S, Reynolds T, Shakil O. Pentoxifylline improves short-term survival in severe acute alcoholic hepatitis: a double-blind, placebo-controlled trial. Gastroenterology 2000;119:1637–48.

30. Duman DG, Ozdemir F, Birben E, et al. Effects of pentoxi-fylline on TNF-alpha production by peripheral blood mononuclear cells in patients with nonalcoholic steatohepatitis. Digestive Diseases and Sciences 2007;52:2520–4.

31. Lee YM, Sutedja DS, Wai CT, et al. A randomized controlled pilot study of Pentoxifylline in patients with non-alcoholic steatohepatitis (NASH). Hepatology International 2008;2:196–201.

32. Van Wagner LB, Koppe SW, Brunt EM, et al. Pentoxifylline for the treatment of non-alcoholic steatohepatitis: a randomized controlled trial. Annals of Hepatology 2011;10:277–86.

33. Zein CO, Yerian LM, Gogate P, et al. Pentoxifylline improves nonalcoholic steatohepatitis: a randomized placebo-con-trolled trial. Hepatology 2011;54:1610–9.

34. Sanyal AJ, Chalasani N, Kowdley KV, et al. Pioglitazone, vitamin E, or placebo for nonalcoholic steatohepatitis. The New England Journal of Medicine 2010;362:1675–85.

35. Lavine JE, Schwimmer JB, Van Natta ML, et al. Effect of vita-min E or metformin for treatment of nonalcoholic fatty liver disease in children and adolescents: the TONIC randomized controlled trial. Journal of the American Medical Association 2011;305:1659–68.

36. Schurks M, Glynn RJ, Rist PM, Tzourio C, Kurth T. Effects of vitamin E on stroke subtypes: meta-analysis of ran-domised controlled trials. BMJ 2010;341:c5702.

37. Albanes D, Till C, Klein EA, et al. Plasma tocopherols and risk of prostate cancer in the selenium and vitamin E cancer prevention trial (SELECT). Cancer Prevention Research 2014;7:886–95.

38. Hoofnagle JH, Van Natta ML, Kleiner DE, et al. Vitamin E and changes in serum alanine aminotransferase levels in patients with non-alcoholic steatohepatitis. Alimentary Pharmacology & Therapeutics 2013;38:134–43.

39. Athinarayanan S, Wei R, Zhang M, et al. Genetic polymor-phism of cytochrome P450 4F2, vitamin E level and histo-logical response in adults and children with nonalcoholic fatty liver disease who participated in PIVENS and TONIC clinical trials. PLoS One 2014;9:e95366.

40. Sanyal AJ, Campbell-Sargent C, Mirshahi F, et al. Nonalcoholic steatohepatitis: association of insulin resistance and mitochon-drial abnormalities. Gastroenterology 2001;120:1183–92.

41. Cusi K. Role of obesity and lipotoxicity in the development of nonalcoholic steatohepatitis: pathophysiology and clini-cal implications. Gastroenterology 2012;142:711–25.e6.

42. Younossi ZM, Reyes MJ, Mishra A, Mehta R, Henry L. Systematic review with meta-analysis: non-alcoholic steatohepatitis—a case for personalised treatment based on pathogenic targets. Alimentary Pharmacology & Therapeutics 2014;39:3–14.

43. Neuschwander-Tetri BA, Brunt EM, Wehmeier KR, Oliver D, Bacon BR. Improved nonalcoholic steatohepatitis after 48 weeks of treatment with the PPAR-gamma ligand rosiglitazone. Hepatology 2003;38:1008–17.

44. Promrat K, Lutchman G, Uwaifo GI, et al. A pilot study of pioglitazone treatment for nonalcoholic steatohepatitis. Hepatology 2004;39:188–96.

45. Ratziu V, Giral P, Jacqueminet S, et al. Rosiglitazone for nonalcoholic steatohepatitis: one-year results of the randomized placebo-controlled Fatty Liver Improvement with Rosiglitazone Therapy (FLIRT) Trial. Gastroenterology 2008;135:100–10.

46. Ahmadian M, Suh JM, Hah N, et al. PPARgamma signaling and metabolism: the good, the bad and the future. Nature Medicine 2013;19:557–66.

47. Lutchman G, Modi A, Kleiner DE, et al. The effects of discontinuing pioglitazone in patients with nonalcoholic steatohepatitis. Hepatology 2007;46:424–9.

48. Bechmann LP, Hannivoort RA, Gerken G, Hotamisligil GS, Trauner M, Canbay A. The interaction of hepatic lipid and glucose metabolism in liver diseases. Journal of Hepatology 2012;56:952–64.

49. Nobili V, Reif S. Vitamin D and liver fibrosis: let's start soon before it's too late. Gut 2015;64:698–9.

50. Kwok RM, Torres DM, Harrison SA. Vitamin D and nonalcoholic fatty liver disease (NAFLD): is it more than just an association? Hepatology 2013;58:1166–74.

51. Robertson G, Leclercq I, Farrell GC. Nonalcoholic steatosis and steatohepatitis. II. Cytochrome P-450 enzymes and oxidative stress. American Journal of Physiology. Gastrointestinal and Liver Physiology 2001;281:G1135–9.

52. Barchetta I, De Bernardinis M, Capoccia D, et al. Hypovitaminosis D is independently associated with metabolic syndrome in obese patients. PLoS One 2013;8:e68689.

53. Bril F, Maximos M, Portillo-Sanchez P, et al. Relationship of vitamin D with insulin resistance and disease severity in nonalcoholic steatohepatitis. Journal of Hepatology 2014;62:405–11.

# 21 Effects of treatment of NAFLD on the metabolic syndrome

**Hannele Yki-Järvinen**

Department of Medicine, University of Helsinki, Helsinki, Finland

---

### LEARNING POINTS

- The liver is the site of production of two key components of the metabolic/insulin resistance syndrome, glucose and triglycerides.

- Treatment of NAFLD with lifestyle modification ameliorates features of the metabolic syndrome.

- Vitamin E and obeticholic acid are effective treatments of NAFLD but not the metabolic syndrome.

- Amelioration of insulin resistance is not necessary for the treatment of NASH but is important for the prevention of cardiovascular disease and type 2 diabetes.

## Introduction

The metabolic syndrome (MetS) represents a cluster of actors that identifies subjects at risk for type 2 diabetes and cardiovascular disease (CVD). Each component of the MetS is either a cause or a consequence of insulin resistance. The most recent version defines the MetS as a condition that includes any three of the following five: increased fasting glucose or type 2 diabetes, hypertriglyceridemia, low HDL cholesterol, increased waist circumference (ethnicity dependent), and hypertension. It thus allows diagnosis of the syndrome in 10 ways [1]. Although the extent to which various definitions of the MetS increase the risk of type 2 diabetes and CVD is unknown, it is well established that each component predisposes to these complications.

NAFLD and the MetS share common pathophysiology. The liver is the site of production of two of the key components of the MetS, fasting serum glucose and very-low-density lipoprotein (VLDL), which contains most of the triglycerides present in serum. In subjects with NAFLD, the ability of insulin to normally suppress production of glucose and VLDL is impaired, resulting in hyperglycemia and hypertriglyceridemia. The liver, once fatty, also overproduces many other markers of cardiovascular risk such as C-reactive protein, fibrinogen, and coagulation factors [1]. One might therefore predict that treatment of NAFLD ameliorates features of the MetS. On the other hand, while mild hyperglycemia, hyperinsulinemia, and hypertriglyceridemia/low HDL cholesterol seem consequences of insulin resistance in the liver, there is no clear mechanistic link between NAFLD and hypertension. Also, NAFLD and insulin resistance frequently dissociate as subjects with NAFLD carrying the common I148M variant in PNPLA3 or those carrying the TM6SF2 gene variant at rs58542926 are not insulin resistant [2–5] (see Chapters 6 and 11). Furthermore, the pathophysiology of NASH involves features such as increased oxidative stress, which treatment cannot be predicted to reverse insulin resistance or type 2 diabetes. The ensuing discussion reviews effects of treatment of NAFLD on features of insulin resistance and the MetS. This is of clinical interest as insulin resistance is essential in the pathogenesis of CVD, which, rather than liver disease, is the major cause of death in NAFLD [6].

---

*Clinical Dilemmas in Non-Alcoholic Fatty Liver Disease*, First Edition. Edited by Roger Williams and Simon D. Taylor-Robinson.
© 2016 John Wiley & Sons, Ltd. Published 2016 by John Wiley & Sons, Ltd.

## Effect of insulin-sensitizing antidiabetic treatments on NAFLD and the MetS (Table 8.1)

### Lifestyle

#### Weight loss induced by hypocaloric diets

Weight loss induced by hypocaloric diets rapidly decreases liver fat content. For example, merely a 48-h low-carbohydrate (<50 g/day) energy-deficit diet decreases liver fat content by 30% [7]. This decrease occurred in the face of a 2% change in body weight [7]. In the same study, liver fat content decreased by 9% by a high-carbohydrate, low-fat, energy-deficit diet. Fasting plasma glucose and insulin and free fatty acids decreased significantly more with the low- than the high-carbohydrate diet [7]. However, as discussed in the following, the magnitude of changes in features of the MetS is very modest even with 10% of weight loss.

The largest of studies examining the effects of lifestyle intervention on liver fat content and features of the MetS is the Fatty Liver Ancillary Study in the Look AHEAD trial. Overweight or obese patients with type 2 diabetes (BMI ~35 kg/m², baseline liver fat ~4%, serum triglycerides 1.3 mmol/L, $HbA_{1c}$ 7.1%) were randomized into intensive lifestyle intervention or a control group receiving diabetes support and education [8]. Liver fat content was measured with proton magnetic resonance spectroscopy in 96 subjects with type 2 diabetes. Weight loss averaged 8.5 kg in the group receiving intensive lifestyle education and 0.05 kg in the control group. Liver fat content decreased significantly by 51% in the intensive lifestyle intervention group [8]. Glycemic control improved significantly more in the intervention than the control group. No significant differences were observed in the changes in serum lipids between groups. Meta-analysis of effects of weight reduction on lipids has also supported the view that such effects are very modest despite substantial weight loss [9]. Serum triglycerides decrease by 0.15 mmol/L, while HDL cholesterol increases by 0.09 mmol/L for every 10 kg of weight loss. More importantly, the Look AHEAD trial proper did not find that the intensive lifestyle intervention that promoted weight loss of 8.6% and increased fitness decreased cardiovascular morbidity in overweight or obese adults with type 2 diabetes [10]. This implies that the 3–5% reduction in body weight recommended by the AASLD [11] may not have significant benefits with respect to the MetS or CVD. Weight loss also lowers blood pressure, but this effect is unlikely to be mediated via changes in liver fat content.

**TABLE 21.1** Examples of dissociation of effects of pharmacotherapy of NAFLD on liver fat content, insulin sensitivity, glycemia, and body weight

| Treatment | Liver fat | Insulin sensitivity | Glycaemia | Body weight |
|---|---|---|---|---|
| *Glucose-lowering* | | | | |
| Pioglitazone | −40 to 50% | ↑ | +++ | ↑ |
| Metformin | No change | ↑ | +++ | ↓ |
| Insulin | −20 to −45% | ↑ | ++++ | ↑[a] |
| *Anti-obesity* | | | | |
| Orlistat | −40%[b] | ↑[b] | +[b] | ↓↓[b] |
| CB-1 blockade | −70%[b] | ↑[b] | +[b] | ↓↓[b] |
| *Lipid lowering* | | | | |
| Fibrates | No change | No change | No change | No change |
| Nicotinic acid | No change | ↓ | − | No change |
| Omega-3 fatty acids | ~30% (*p* = 0.1) | No change | No change | No change |
| Statins | No change | No change | − | ↑ |
| Ezetimibe | No change | No change | − | No change |
| *Drugs targeting NAFLD* | | | | |
| Vitamin E | Decrease | No change | No change | No change |
| Pentoxifylline | Decrease | No change | No change | No change |
| FXR agonist | Decrease | ↓ | No change | No change |

↑, increase; ↓, decrease; +, improvement; −, deterioration.
[a] Proportional to improvement in glycaemic control.
[b] Effects on liver fat, insulin sensitivity, and glycemia secondary to effect on body weight.

*Weight loss by bariatric surgery*

During the 15 years of follow-up in the Swedish Obese Subjects study, bariatric surgery decreased the incidence of type 2 diabetes by 93% [12]. Weight loss averaged 20 kg more in the surgically than conventionally treated group. Although no histologic data are available from this study, changes in ALT and AST during follow-up were proportional to weight loss [13]. These data support the view that the more weight loss, the greater the long-term benefit both with respect to the incidence of type 2 diabetes and frequency of abnormal liver chemistries. Effects of lifestyle treatment on NAFLD have been discussed more extensively in Chapter 19 and bariatric surgery in Chapter 22.

## Antidiabetic pharmacotherapies
### Glitazones

Early small mechanistic studies measuring liver fat content with proton magnetic resonance spectroscopy and hepatic insulin sensitivity in type 2 diabetic patients treated for 16 weeks showed that rosiglitazone but not metformin decreases liver fat content, although both agents increase hepatic insulin sensitivity and similarly improve glycemic control [14]. Pioglitazone compared to placebo was shown to decrease liver fat by 50% and enhance hepatic insulin sensitivity within 16 weeks compared to placebo in patients with type 2 diabetes [15]. The concentration of plasma adiponectin increases remarkably by two- to threefold during glitazone but not metformin treatment and is likely to be one of the key mediators of the beneficial effects of glitazones on insulin sensitivity. The increase in insulin sensitivity is observed despite weight gain [16].

Randomized controlled trials and a meta-analysis have shown that pioglitazone decreases not only steatosis but also hepatocellular ballooning, lobular inflammation, and possibly fibrosis in patients with and without type 2 diabetes [17]. It also enhances insulin sensitivity measured using a glucose tolerance test combined with glucose tracers [18], C-peptide concentrations [19] and homeostasis model assessment insulin resistance (HOMA-IR) [20, 21]. The histologic benefits have been attributed at least in part to changes in circulating adiponectin concentrations [22].

### Metformin

Metformin enhances hepatic insulin sensitivity but does not change liver fat content [14] or liver histology [11].

*Subcutaneous insulin therapy*

There are no randomized controlled trials addressing the effects of insulin therapy on liver fat content or hepatic insulin sensitivity or liver histology. In an open trial, seven months of insulin therapy decreased liver fat content by 20% and increased hepatic insulin sensitivity as measured using the euglycemic insulin clamp technique combined with a glucose tracer [23]. Serum adiponectin did not change, but free fatty acids, which are quantitatively the most important sources of intrahepatocellular triglycerides [24], decreased significantly. In another open study, 3 months of insulin therapy decreased liver fat content by 45% [25].

### GLP-1 agonists and DPP-4 inhibitors

GLP-1 agonists such as exenatide, liraglutide, lixisenatide, and albiglutide are synthetic agonists of the gut-derived GLP-1 peptide. All these drugs are currently approved for the treatment of type 2 diabetes and liraglutide also for the treatment of obesity. As an example of effects on body weight, exenatide compared to insulin in the face of similar improvement in glycemic control induced a ~8 kg decrease in body weight over 3 years of treatment in type 2 diabetic patients [26]. Randomized controlled trials examining the effects of GLP-1 agonists and DPP-4 inhibitors on NAFLD are currently ongoing.

## Antiobesity drugs
### Orlistat

Orlistat is an intestinal lipase inhibitor that prevents fat absorption. It does promote weight loss and also because of its mechanism of action lowers LDL cholesterol more than placebo for the same amount of weight loss [27]. Orlistat improves insulin sensitivity and decreases liver fat content in proportion to weight loss.

### Cannabinoid receptor blockade

CB-1 receptor blockers have shown promise in rodent models for the treatment of NASH [28]. In humans, the CB-1 receptor blocker rimonabant was effective in promoting weight loss but was withdrawn because of psychiatric side effects. Rimonabant decreased liver fat content and features of the MetS in proportion to weight loss [29].

## Lipid-lowering therapies
### Fibrates

Recent evidence from a meta-analysis suggested that fibrate therapy on a background of statin treatment provides clinical benefits with respect to cardiovascular events in subgroups of patients with the dyslipidemia characterizing the MetS, that is, high triglycerides (≥1.7 mmol/L or 150 mg/dL) and low HDL cholesterol (<1.0 mmol/L or 40 mg/dL) [30]. The mechanism of such benefit does not seem to involve a decrease in liver fat content or insulin sensitivity [31].

*Nicotinic acid*

The AIM-HIGH trial randomized 3414 subjects with high triglycerides (1.7–4.5 mmol/L), low HDL cholesterol (<1 mmol/L in men, <1.3 mmol/L in women), and LDL cholesterol <4.6 mmol/L to receive nicotinic acid or placebo in addition to statin therapy. Nicotinic acid lowered serum triglycerides from 1.8 to 1.4 mmol/L and increased HDL cholesterol from 0.91 to 1.08 mmol/L but had no effect on cardiovascular events [32]. Similar data were reported in the HPS2-THRIVE study with extended-release niacin [33]. The incidence of type 2 diabetes increased and glycemic control deteriorated in this trial [33]. Nicotinic acid does not change liver fat content and may cause a deterioration in insulin sensitivity [31].

*Omega-3 fatty acids*

In the first randomized, double-blind, placebo-controlled trial testing the efficacy of omega-3 fatty acids on liver fat content, 104 patients with NAFLD received either omega-3 fatty acids (docosahexaenoic and eicosapentaenoic acids 4 g/day) of placebo for 15–18 months [34]. Liver fat content decreased marginally significantly by 29% in the omega-3 compared to the placebo group. Serum triglycerides decreased and HDL cholesterol increased in the omega-3 fatty acid compared to the placebo group, but glycosylated hemoglobin concentrations remained unchanged. In the ORIGIN study including 12,536 patients with impaired fasting glucose, impaired glucose tolerance, or type 2 diabetes, 1 g of n-3 fatty acids daily for 6.2 years did not reduce the incidence of cardiovascular events and had no effect on glycemia [35]. Serum triglyceride concentrations decreased significantly by 0.16 mmol/L from a baseline concentration of 1.6 mmol/L. Taken together these studies suggest that omega-3 fatty acids may favorably influence NAFLD and the lipid abnormalities of the MetS but not glycemia or CVD.

*Statins and ezetimibe*

Only two placebo-controlled randomized clinical trials have examined the effects of statins on liver function tests or liver histology. Nelson et al. took liver biopsies from 16 subjects before and after 12 months of simvastatin or placebo treatment and found no differences in liver histology between the groups [36]. A larger study with 204 subjects found no differences in liver function tests between pravastatin and placebo-treated patients [37]. Statins do not change insulin sensitivity [38]. However, a recent Mendelian randomization analysis showed that statin use is associated with increased obesity and risk of type 2 diabetes [39]. The mechanism underlying this association is unknown. One open-label randomized clinical trial has been performed to compare the effects of the cholesterol synthesis inhibitor ezetimibe and placebo on insulin sensitivity and liver histology in patients with NAFLD. The plan was to enroll 80 patients, but the trial was stopped early because ezetimibe treatment significantly increased glycosylated hemoglobin concentrations. The fibrosis stage and ballooning score were, however, significantly improved with ezetimibe [40].

## Drugs primarily targeting NAFLD/NASH
*Vitamin E*

Vitamin E is a fat-soluble antioxidant vitamin that has in several randomized controlled trials in adults been shown to improve liver histology in NASH [20, 41–43]. In the PIVENS trial, vitamin E did not change insulin sensitivity of glucose metabolism or lipolysis as determined from products of fasting glucose and insulin (HOMA-IR) [20, 42] and fasting free fatty acids and insulin [41].

*Pentoxifylline*

Pentoxifylline is an methyl xanthine derivative that inhibits production of proinflammatory cytokine such as tumor necrosis factor alpha. It has been shown to reduce steatosis, lobular inflammation, and fibrosis but not ballooning in noncirrhotic patients with NASH [44]. Pentoxifylline did not change serum concentrations of tumor necrosis factor alpha or adiponectin or insulin sensitivity as assessed by the frequently sampled intravenous glucose tolerance test and HOMA-IR [44]. Another study including patients with NASH and cirrhosis did not report improvements with pentoxifylline [45].

*Farnesoid X receptor agonists*

The farnesoid X receptor (FXR) ligand obeticholic acid is a synthetic variant of the natural bile acid chenodeoxycholic acid. This agent was recently tested versus placebo in a multicenter randomized trial (FLINT) of 72 weeks in 200 patients with biopsy-proven NASH [46]. *In vitro*, FXR agonism leads to repression of the key lipogenic transcription factor SREBP$_{1c}$ in addition to preventing cellular accumulation of bile acids to toxic levels [47]. Liver fibrosis, hepatocellular ballooning, steatosis, and lobular inflammation improved significantly in obeticholic acid as compared to placebo-treated patients. Body weight decreased slightly more in the obeticholic acid than the placebo group. Despite weight loss, metabolic parameters such as fasting insulin and HOMA-IR increased significantly more in the obeticholic acid than the placebo-treated patients. HDL cholesterol and triglycerides decreased, while LDL cholesterol, perhaps because of the inhibition of bile acid synthesis, increased significantly in the obeticholic acid-treated patients [46]. These data demonstrate that reversal of insulin resistance is not necessary for the treatment of NASH.

### Other treatments

Four small (total number of patients 20–66) randomized controlled trials have examined the effects of probiotic treatments (lactobacillus, bifidobacterium, streptococcus) on NAFLD. The duration of treatment ranged from 8 weeks to 6 months. In a meta-analysis of these trials, probiotics had no effect on BMI, lipids, glucose, or HOMA-IR but decreased ALT and AST [48]. Data on liver histology were too sparse to allow conclusions.

In a phase 1B placebo-controlled trial with 82 patients treated for 12 weeks, a decrease in local cortisol production via inhibition of the enzyme 11β-hydroxysteroid dehydrogenase type 1 slightly decreased body weight and liver fat content (−15%) [49]. Insulin sensitivity remained unchanged.

### Conclusions

NAFLD alone is not considered an indication for pharmacotherapy at present. However, NAFLD is often, although not uniformly, associated with obesity and features of the MetS, which increase the risk of CVD and diabetes. Lifestyle intervention is advised in all patients with NAFLD and the MetS to prevent these complications. Weight loss combined with exercise is effective in decreasing liver fat content as well as all aspects of the MetS, although the magnitude of weight loss necessary to observe metabolic benefits is substantial, at least around 10%.

Pharmacologic therapies aim at preventing progression and reversing NASH. Such therapies have variable effects on components of the MetS. Pioglitazone induces weight gain despite improving NASH histology and insulin sensitivity. Insulin therapy lowers liver fat content and enhances insulin sensitivity, but there are no randomized controlled trials or data on its effects on liver histology. The currently two perhaps most promising pharmacotherapies for NASH, vitamin E and obeticholic acid, have neutral or even deleterious effects on insulin sensitivity. This suggests that lifestyle and other insulin-sensitizing therapies should perhaps be combined with drugs specifically targeting NASH.

### References

1. Yki-Jarvinen H. Non-alcoholic fatty liver disease as a cause and a consequence of metabolic syndrome. The Lancet Diabetes & Endocrinology 2014; 2(11): 901–10.
2. Romeo S, Kozlitina J, Xing C, et al. Genetic variation in PNPLA3 confers susceptibility to nonalcoholic fatty liver disease. Nature Genetics 2008; 40(12): 1461–5.
3. Kozlitina J, Smagris E, Stender S, et al. Exome-wide association study identifies a TM6SF2 variant that confers susceptibility to nonalcoholic fatty liver disease. Nature Genetics 2014; 46(4): 352–6.
4. Liu YL, Reeves HL, Burt AD, et al. TM6SF2 rs58542926 influences hepatic fibrosis progression in patients with non-alcoholic fatty liver disease. Nature Communications 2014; 5: 4309.
5. Zhou Y, Llaurado G, Oresic M, Hyotylainen T, Orho-Melander M, Yki-Jarvinen H. Circulating triacylglycerol signatures and insulin sensitivity in NAFLD associated with the E167K variant in TM6SF2. Journal of Hepatology 2015; 62: 657–63.
6. Anstee QM, Targher G, Day CP. Progression of NAFLD to diabetes mellitus, cardiovascular disease or cirrhosis. Nature Reviews Gastroenterology & Hepatology 2013; 10(6): 330–44.
7. Kirk E, Reeds DN, Finck BN, Mayurranjan SM, Patterson BW, Klein S. Dietary fat and carbohydrates differentially alter insulin sensitivity during caloric restriction. Gastroenterology 2009; 136(5): 1552–60.
8. Lazo M, Solga SF, Horska A, et al. Effect of a 12-month intensive lifestyle intervention on hepatic steatosis in adults with type 2 diabetes. Diabetes Care 2010; 33(10): 2156–63.
9. Dattilo AM, Kris-Etherton PM. Effects of weight reduction on blood lipids and lipoproteins: a meta-analysis. The American Journal of Clinical Nutrition 1992; 56(2): 320–8.
10. Look ARG, Wing RR, Bolin P, et al. Cardiovascular effects of intensive lifestyle intervention in type 2 diabetes. The New England Journal of Medicine 2013; 369(2): 145–54.
11. Chalasani N, Younossi Z, Lavine JE, et al. The diagnosis and management of non-alcoholic fatty liver disease: practice guideline by the American Gastroenterological Association,

American Association for the Study of Liver Diseases, and American College of Gastroenterology. Gastroenterology 2012; 142(7): 1592–609.

12. Carlsson LM, Peltonen M, Ahlin S, et al. Bariatric surgery and prevention of type 2 diabetes in Swedish obese subjects. The New England Journal of Medicine 2012; 367(8): 695–704.

13. Burza MA, Romeo S, Kotronen A, et al. Long-term effect of bariatric surgery on liver enzymes in the Swedish Obese Subjects (SOS) study. PLoS One 2013; 8(3): e60495.

14. Tiikkainen M, Hakkinen AM, Korsheninnikova E, Nyman T, Makimattila S, Yki-Jarvinen H. Effects of rosiglitazone and metformin on liver fat content, hepatic insulin resistance, insulin clearance, and gene expression in adipose tissue in patients with type 2 diabetes. Diabetes 2004; 53(8): 2169–76.

15. Bajaj M, Suraamornkul S, Piper P, et al. Decreased plasma adiponectin concentrations are closely related to hepatic fat content and hepatic insulin resistance in pioglitazone-treated type 2 diabetic patients. The Journal of Clinical Endocrinology and Metabolism 2004; 89(1): 200–6.

16. Yki-Jarvinen H. Thiazolidinediones. The New England Journal of Medicine 2004; 351(11): 1106–18.

17. Boettcher E, Csako G, Pucino F, Wesley R, Loomba R. Meta-analysis: pioglitazone improves liver histology and fibrosis in patients with non-alcoholic steatohepatitis. Alimentary Pharmacology & Therapeutics 2012; 35(1): 66–75.

18. Belfort R, Harrison SA, Brown K, et al. A placebo-controlled trial of pioglitazone in subjects with nonalcoholic steatohepatitis. The New England Journal of Medicine 2006; 355(22): 2297–307.

19. Aithal GP, Thomas JA, Kaye PV, et al. Randomized, placebo-controlled trial of pioglitazone in nondiabetic subjects with nonalcoholic steatohepatitis. Gastroenterology 2008; 135(4): 1176–84.

20. Sanyal AJ, Chalasani N, Kowdley KV, et al. Pioglitazone, vitamin E, or placebo for nonalcoholic steatohepatitis. The New England Journal of Medicine 2010; 362(18): 1675–85.

21. Ratziu V, Giral P, Jacqueminet S, et al. Rosiglitazone for non-alcoholic steatohepatitis: one-year results of the randomized placebo-controlled Fatty Liver Improvement with Rosiglitazone Therapy (FLIRT) trial. Gastroenterology 2008; 135(1): 100–10.

22. Gastaldelli A, Harrison S, Belfort-Aguiar R, et al. Pioglitazone in the treatment of NASH: the role of adiponectin. Alimentary Pharmacology & Therapeutics 2010; 32(6): 769–75.

23. Juurinen L, Tiikkainen M, Hakkinen AM, Hakkarainen A, Yki-Jarvinen H. Effects of insulin therapy on liver fat content and hepatic insulin sensitivity in patients with type 2 diabetes. American Journal of Physiology, Endocrinology and Metabolism 2007; 292(3): E829–35.

24. Lambert JE, Ramos-Roman MA, Browning JD, Parks EJ. Increased de novo lipogenesis is a distinct characteristic of individuals with nonalcoholic fatty liver disease. Gastroenterology 2014; 146: 726–35.

25. Lingvay I, Roe ED, Duong J, Leonard D, Szczepaniak LS. Effect of insulin versus triple oral therapy on the progression of hepatic steatosis in type 2 diabetes. Journal of Investigative Medicine 2012; 60(7): 1059–63.

26. Bunck MC, Corner A, Eliasson B, et al. Effects of exenatide on measures of beta-cell function after 3 years in metformin-treated patients with type 2 diabetes. Diabetes Care 2011; 34(9): 2041–7.

27. Tiikkainen M, Bergholm R, Rissanen A, et al. Effects of equal weight loss with orlistat and placebo on body fat and serum fatty acid composition and insulin resistance in obese women. The American Journal of Clinical Nutrition 2004; 79(1): 22–30.

28. Osei-Hyiaman D, Liu J, Zhou L, et al. Hepatic CB1 receptor is required for development of diet-induced steatosis, dyslipidemia, and insulin and leptin resistance in mice. The Journal of Clinical Investigation 2008; 118(9): 3160–9.

29. Bergholm R, Sevastianova K, Santos A, et al. CB(1) blockade-induced weight loss over 48 weeks decreases liver fat in proportion to weight loss in humans. International Journal of Obesity 2013; 37(5): 699–703.

30. Chapman MJ, Ginsberg HN, Amarenco P, et al. Triglyceride-rich lipoproteins and high-density lipoprotein cholesterol in patients at high risk of cardiovascular disease: evidence and guidance for management. European Heart Journal 2011; 32(11): 1345–61.

31. Fabbrini E, Mohammed BS, Korenblat KM, et al. Effect of fenofibrate and niacin on intrahepatic triglyceride content, very low-density lipoprotein kinetics, and insulin action in obese subjects with nonalcoholic fatty liver disease. The Journal of Clinical Endocrinology and Metabolism 2010; 95(6): 2727–35.

32. Investigators A-H, Boden WE, Probstfield JL, et al. Niacin in patients with low HDL cholesterol levels receiving intensive statin therapy. The New England Journal of Medicine 2011; 365(24): 2255–67.

33. Group HTC, Landray MJ, Haynes R, et al. Effects of extended-release niacin with laropiprant in high-risk patients. The New England Journal of Medicine 2014; 371(3): 203–12.

34. Scorletti E, Bhatia L, McCormick KG, et al. Effects of purified eicosapentaenoic and docosahexaenoic acids in non-alcoholic fatty liver disease: results from the *WELCOME study. Hepatology 2014; 60: 1211–21.

35. ORIGIN Trial Investigators; Bosch J, Gerstein HC, et al. n-3 fatty acids and cardiovascular outcomes in patients with dysglycemia. The New England Journal of Medicine 2012; 367(4): 309–18.

36. Nelson A, Torres DM, Morgan AE, Fincke C, Harrison SA. A pilot study using simvastatin in the treatment of nonalcoholic steatohepatitis: A randomized placebo-controlled trial. Journal of clinical gastroenterology 2009; 43(10): 990–4.

37. Eslami L, Merat S, Malekzadeh R, Nasseri-Moghaddam S, Aramin H. Statins for non-alcoholic fatty liver disease and non-alcoholic steatohepatitis. The Cochrane database of systematic reviews 2013; 12: CD008623.

38. Sheu WH, Shieh SM, Shen DD, et al. Effect of pravastatin treatment on glucose, insulin, and lipoprotein metabolism in patients with hypercholesterolemia. American Heart Journal 1994; 127(2): 331–6.

39. Swerdlow DI, Preiss D, Kuchenbaecker KB, et al. HMG-coenzyme A reductase inhibition, type 2 diabetes, and body-weight: evidence from genetic analysis and randomised trials. Lancet 2015; 385: 351–61.

40. Takeshita Y, Takamura T, Honda M, et al. The effects of ezetimibe on non-alcoholic fatty liver disease and glucose metabolism: a randomised controlled trial. Diabetologia 2014; 57(5): 878–90.

41. Bell LN, Wang J, Muralidharan S, et al. Relationship between adipose tissue insulin resistance and liver histology in non-alcoholic steatohepatitis: a pioglitazone versus vitamin E versus placebo for the treatment of nondiabetic patients with nonalcoholic steatohepatitis trial follow-up study. Hepatology 2012; 56(4): 1311–8.

42. Lavine JE, Schwimmer JB, Van Natta ML, et al. Effect of vitamin E or metformin for treatment of nonalcoholic fatty liver disease in children and adolescents: the TONIC randomized controlled trial. JAMA 2011; 305(16): 1659–68.

43. Hoofnagle JH, Van Natta ML, Kleiner DE, et al. Vitamin E and changes in serum alanine aminotransferase levels in patients with non-alcoholic steatohepatitis. Alimentary Pharmacology & Therapeutics 2013; 38(2): 134–43.

44. Zein CO, Yerian LM, Gogate P, et al. Pentoxifylline improves nonalcoholic steatohepatitis: a randomized placebo-controlled trial. Hepatology 2011; 54(5): 1610–9.

45. Van Wagner LB, Koppe SW, Brunt EM, et al. Pentoxifylline for the treatment of non-alcoholic steatohepatitis: a randomized controlled trial. Annals of Hepatology 2011; 10(3): 277–86.

46. Neuschwander-Tetri BA, Loomba R, Sanyal AJ, et al. Farnesoid X nuclear receptor ligand obeticholic acid for non-cirrhotic, non-alcoholic steatohepatitis (FLINT): a multicentre, randomised, placebo-controlled trial. Lancet 2015; 385: 956–65.

47. de Aguiar Vallim TQ, Tarling EJ, Edwards PA. Pleiotropic roles of bile acids in metabolism. Cell Metabolism 2013; 17(5): 657–69.

48. Ma YY, Li L, Yu CH, Shen Z, Chen LH, Li YM. Effects of probiotics on nonalcoholic fatty liver disease: a meta-analysis. World journal of gastroenterology 2013; 19(40): 6911–8.

49. Stefan N, Ramsauer M, Jordan P, et al. Inhibition of 11beta-HSD1 with RO5093151 for non-alcoholic fatty liver disease: a multicentre, randomised, double-blind, placebo-controlled trial. The Lancet Diabetes & Endocrinology 2014; 2(5): 406–16.

# 22 What are the dangers as well as the true benefits of bariatric surgery?

**Andrew Jenkinson**

Clinical Lead Department of Metabolic and Bariatric Surgery, University College London Hospital, London, UK

> **LEARNING POINTS**
>
> - Understand the genetic aspects of the obesity epidemic
> - Explain the metabolic defence against low-calorie dieting
> - Describe the historical perspective of bariatric surgery
> - Clarify the true risks and benefits of the currently popular procedures

## Introduction

Human evolution has been inexorably linked to our ability to select, prepare and cook food. These skills conferred to early man a significant metabolic advantage. Pre-cooked foods require less digestive effort, and therefore over time a smaller GI tract was evolved, leaving metabolic room for cephalisation and the development of a large brain [1]. Unfortunately the hunter-gatherer humans of 150 000 years ago continued to develop their skills in food preparation, resulting in the advent of agriculture and farming 20 000 years ago to the current explosion in the availability of sugar and highly palatable processed foods. Our relentless fascination and ability to grow and process foods, the very reason we were able to evolve to be humans in the first place, have led us to develop an obesogenic environment that is no longer suited to our health.

Thirty percent of the world's population or 2.1 billion people are now overweight or obese 2.5 times more than the number of malnourished people. If the current rise in obesity rates is continued, then by 2050 half of the population of the United Kingdom will be obese (currently 23% of UK adults are obese). In 2014 the McKinsey Global Institute calculated that the cost of obesity to the UK economy was £47 billion per year. They compared the economic threat of obesity to the world as similar to smoking and armed conflict and more costly than alcoholism and climate change [2].

## Morbid obesity

It is well known that obesity causes a number of medical conditions in addition to non-alcoholic fatty liver disease (NAFLD). The central visceral adiposity characterised by the android fat distribution found particularly in men is a direct risk factor in the development of type 2 diabetes, hypertension and dyslipidaemia. This constellation of disorders, commonly referred to as metabolic syndrome, subsequently drives the future risk of cardiovascular complications.

What is less commonly understood are the physiological changes that drive obesity and make it so hard for patients to lose weight permanently by 'dieting and will power'.

## Obesity, genetics and physiology

Genetic studies have suggested that some people are sensitive to an obesogenic environment and some people seem resistant to it. In fact genetic factors contribute to ~85% of a person's body mass index (BMI) [3]. In an obese person the normal homeostatic factors that should maintain energy balance break down. The development of leptin resistance results in a failure of the hypothalamus to respond appropriately to the signal that energy stores in the form of adipose tissue have exceeded requirements.

*Clinical Dilemmas in Non-Alcoholic Fatty Liver Disease*, First Edition. Edited by Roger Williams and Simon D. Taylor-Robinson.
© 2016 John Wiley & Sons, Ltd. Published 2016 by John Wiley & Sons, Ltd.

The physiological changes that occur when a person diets are also misunderstood. The longer the period of calorific restriction, the more pronounced the rise in ghrelin, a hormone secreted by the stomach driving appetite, and the lower the level of peptide YY, the satiety hormone, secreted by the small bowel. Increasing evidence suggests that in individuals that have tried low-calorie dieting in order to lose weight, the appetite and satiety changes that are experienced during a diet are in fact still present a year after dieting has ceased [4]. This explains the common description of yo-yo weight fluctuation in response to dieting, with a slow and inexorable long-term weight gain. In 2014 the cumulative evidence that ultra-low-calorie dieting is in fact counterproductive in weight regulation led NICE (the UK commissioning advisory body) to warn against this form of intervention for obese persons [5].

In the face of the development of our obesogenic environment and the subsequent obesity pandemic, coupled with the failure of conservative forms of treatment for obesity, it is not surprising that bariatric surgery has risen in popularity. In the United States the number of bariatric procedures now exceeds the number of gallbladder operation with over 200 000 procedures performed annually.

But how effective and how safe is this type of surgery?

## Development of bariatric surgical procedures

Bariatric surgery is new in comparison to most established specialities. Since the start of the rapid rise in obesity rates in the 1980s, different types of surgical procedure have come into and then gone out of fashion to be replaced by newer more effective procedures. The reason that we see more and more patients now requesting this type of surgery is that as the obesity crisis has worsened, so the safety and effectiveness of surgery have improved.

### Jejunoileal bypass

The first type of bariatric surgery to become popular was the jejunoileal bypass. This rapidly gained popularity in the 1960s and 1970s but then rapidly fell out of favour due to long-term complications. The problems with this procedure were twofold. Firstly the degree of malabsorption was too extreme, with the creation of a virtual short bowel syndrome. This led to severe mineral, vitamin and protein deficiency with many reports of liver failure, steatosis and sudden death. Secondly the redundant bypassed bowel was left blind-ended, meaning that over time bacteria overgrowth and translocation from this segment resulted in significant arthralgia and dermatitis. Due to the frequency and severity of these side effects, most of these procedures have now either been reversed or revised to the successor to the jejunoileal bypass: the gastric bypass.

### Gastric bypass

The gastric bypass is still considered to be the 'gold standard' procedure in bariatric surgery (see Figure 22.1). Due to concerns about the malabsorptive complications caused by jejunoileal bypass, the gastric bypass was developed to be a hybrid procedure combining a much lesser degree of malabsorption combined with restriction in the capacity of the stomach. It has only recently become apparent, however, that malabsorption is not the prominent cause of weight loss after bypass. In fact the rerouting of the bowel causes significant changes to the secretion of the appetite and satiety hormones (ghrelin and PYY). The biological signal to eat in response to weight loss is therefore switched off, making weight loss much easier for patients. In addition to this GLP-1, another peptide secreted in excess post-operatively, has a crucial role in glycaemic control and peripheral insulin sensitivity explaining the rapid improvement or resolution of type 2 diabetes following this procedure.

Despite the good results of the gastric bypass in weight loss and improvement in diabetes, it remained a procedure performed by the open technique until recently. Open surgery carries the inherent risk of respiratory complications and DVT/pulmonary embolism (PE). These risks are amplified in obese patients. The procedure was painful and required an extended inpatient stay. These risks remained significant until the advent of laparoscopic surgery in the late 1990s.

### Laparoscopic gastric bypass

The gastric bypass, initially performed as an open operation, was increasingly performed laparoscopically in the early 2000s. Throughout the decade with further developments in training and technology, including high-definition monitors, advanced stapling devices and advances in thermal dissection technology, the safety of the bypass improved. A procedure that we knew to be effective in the long term, with good long-term follow-up data from the open era of surgery, could now be performed with significantly decreased pain and morbidity, leading to a much faster recovery.

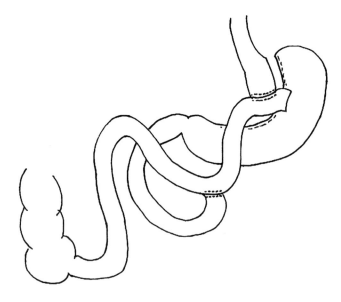

**FIG 22.1** Gastric bypass.

## Vertical banded gastroplasty

The vertical banded gastroplasty (VBG) was the first bariatric procedure to work through purely restriction of the stomach capacity. The procedure involved placement of a non-adjustable restrictive band between the upper stomach pouch and the distal stomach. These procedures were carried out as open operations and thus conferred risks of PE. Long-term outcome was poor as the procedure did not change the patients' desire to eat in response to weight loss leading to weight regain. The procedure was superseded in the 1990s by the advent of the adjustable gastric band (AGB), a procedure that was performed laparoscopically.

## Laparoscopic AGB

The AGB is a silicon ring that is placed around the upper part of the stomach, dividing the stomach into a small 20–30 cc upper part and a large distal part. The band contains an inflatable inner tube that is connected to tubing and an inflation port that sits subcutaneously, usually in the upper abdomen. On inflating the inner tube via percutaneous cannulation of the port in clinic, the bands' inner diameter is reduced, increasing the restrictive effect of the band and forcing the patient to eat slower and chew the food more thoroughly. The tighter the band, the more vigilant a patient has to be with choice of foods and length of chewing. When the band is working, the patient will be forced to chew each mouthful of food 20–30 times before swallowing and then waiting for the food bolus to travel through the restrictive band before a further mouthful of food can be taken. A small meal should take 20–30 min to consume.

The AGB had several significant advantages over the VBG. Firstly it was easy to place laparoscopically, and therefore the risks associated with open VBG surgery were immediately negated. Secondly the procedure did not require stapling and cutting of the stomach; therefore the risk of post-operative bleeding became minimal with the gastric band. Finally the degree of restriction of the band could be adjusted in clinic, a feature that many patients viewed positively. The AGB superseded the VBG as the restrictive procedure of choice by patients and surgeons in the 1990s. Within 10 years of its introduction, the gastric band had become the most popular bariatric procedure performed.

However, the AGB behaved in a similar simple restrictive fashion to the VBG, and just as VBG patients had experienced good initial weight loss followed by significant weight regain, so do AGB patients. In addition to this, as the number of AGBs rose throughout the world, so did its long-term complication rate in relation to the hardware of the gastric band. Complications such as leakage for the band tubing and migration or erosion of the band into stomach became common, and many bands are still being removed today.

Due to the common occurrence of long-term complications requiring band removal plus the weight regain experienced by many patients, the gastric band is now rapidly losing popularity after the introduction of a procedure that promised a restrictive element, a metabolic effect and no malabsorption: the sleeve gastrectomy.

## Laparoscopic sleeve gastrectomy

The sleeve gastrectomy has risen to become currently the most commonly performed bariatric procedure worldwide having recently superseded the laparoscopic gastric bypass in popularity. The sleeve procedure has seen a meteoric rise in popularity considering that it was rarely being performed only 5 years ago (see Figure 22.2).

The procedure is simple to understand and relatively easy to perform compared to the gastric bypass. Both patients and surgeons like this simplicity.

Performed laparoscopically, the stomach is stapled and separated. The division of the stomach begins in the antrum and continues in parallel to the lesser curvature (the right-sided concave border) to the lower oesophageal sphincter area. A new tube-shaped stomach is created to replace the old cavernous stomach, reducing its capacity from ~2000 to 300 cc. The redundant stomach is removed.

The early (2-year) results for sleeve gastrectomy as far as weight loss and resolution of obesity-related co-morbidities are comparable to the gastric bypass. These outcomes may be a surprise if the sleeve is considered to be purely a restrictive procedure, reducing the stomach capacity; however this procedure also works to change appetite and satiety drives. The resection of the body and the fundus of the stomach removes the major ghrelin-secreting area from the GI tract. This is the hormone that leads to a voracious appetite in response to caloric restriction. Removal of this part of the stomach nullifies this appetite response. In addition, the reduced capacity of the stomach encourages faster delivery of nutrients into the small bowel, stimulating an early and exaggerated PYY response from this area and producing an early feeling of satiety. With early delivery of nutrients to the small bowel comes a GLP-1 response similar to that seen in the gastric bypass and explaining the sleeve gastrectomies excellent effect on glycaemic control in type 2 diabetics.

## Other procedures

The *duodenal switch* is rarely practised in the United Kingdom. This is a truly malabsorptive procedure, and although it produces slightly better weight loss and resolution of type 2 diabetes compared to the gastric bypass, it has significant disadvantages. Malabsorption leads to patients complaining of frequent episodes of steatorrhoea. In the long term, vitamin, mineral and protein deficiencies are not unusual, and patients need to be carefully selected to ensure long-term compliance with follow-up.

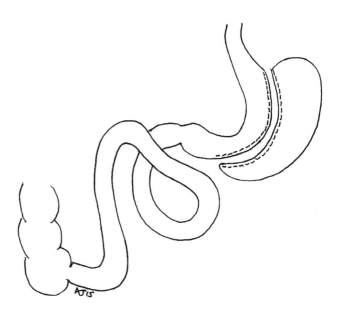

**FIG 22.2** Sleeve gastrectomy.

The *mini-gastric bypass* is a procedure gaining increasing popularity. This procedure was developed by a single unit in the United States but is now performed in multiple centres worldwide. It involves the bypass of a much larger section of the small bowel than the traditional gastric bypass, and therefore the prefix 'mini' is a misnomer. It could be argued that the perception by patients that this is a mini, or lesser, form of gastric bypass has contributed to its current popularity.

The surgery itself employs a single anastomosis of a loop of jejunum onto the stomach pouch. Controversy persists as to whether the surgical shortcut of not diverting biliary secretions away from the stomach, as occurs in the gastric bypass, could cause chronic biliary gastritis or oesophagitis with increased risk of long-term dysplasia and future malignancy [6].

### Current frequently performed procedures

Currently the most common procedures performed in bariatric surgery are the sleeve gastrectomy and the gastric bypass. These are the two most effective procedures with low risk in appropriately selected patients. All procedures are now performed laparoscopically. The gastric band is losing popularity to the sleeve gastrectomy and in many centres is no longer performed. The mini-gastric bypass conversely is increasing in popularity, and some surgeons now prefer this procedure to the gastric bypass, as it is simpler to perform.

## What are the risks of bariatric surgery?

When deciding on any operative intervention, including bariatric surgery, surgeons must use their knowledge and experience to decide whether they are truly benefiting the patient with their intervention. They must calculate the risk (of significant complications) versus the benefit (improvements in health and quality of life). The risks of surgery are dependent on several factors. These include patient factors, the type of procedure performed and the expertise of the unit.

### Acute complications of bariatric surgery

Acute complications following the three common bariatric surgery procedures – the gastric band, gastric bypass and sleeve gastrectomy – are rare. The main significant complication of the bypass and sleeve is either bleeding from the staple line (or a transected vessel) or staple line leakage.

Post-operative bleeding occurs in ~2–4% of patients. In most cases the bleeding will stop spontaneously, and the patient will only require treatment with a blood transfusion. Occasionally the bleeding will be more profuse and will require re-laparoscopy to control it.

Staple line leakage is even less common but can be a more difficult complication to treat. A reasonable bariatric unit will have a staple line leakage rate of 1–2%.

Staple line leakage in the gastric bypass is termed anastomotic leak as it is at the site of one of the anastomoses. In the sleeve gastrectomy leakage occurs in most cases at the top of the staple line, near the gastro-oesophageal junction. Ninety percent of leaks will occur whilst the patient is still an inpatient in the first two post-operative days. The mainstay of treatment is early recognition, re-laparoscopy and placement of drains. The patient is then fed either enterally (nasal tube or feeding jejunostomy) or parenterally. If the drains are placed in the correct position, gastric bypass leaks will heal invariably in 2–4 weeks.

Staple line leakage from the sleeve gastrectomy can sometimes be more troublesome to treat. The intraluminal pressure within the sleeve gastrectomy is high, meaning that leaks can become persistent despite good drain placement and optimal nutrition. Many techniques for the treatment of sleeve gastrectomy leaks have been reported. These include stent placement, fibrin sealant, endoscopic clipping and botox to the pylorus. The success of these techniques is variable. Sleeve leaks are rare and so even large centres have few patients in their series. In rare instances patients can develop a chronic gastro-cutaneous fistula and may need conversion of the sleeve to a gastric bypass in order to reduce the high intraluminal sleeve pressure driving the leak.

### Long-term complications following bariatric surgery

The gastric band, although simple and safe to place, is plagued by high rates of long-term complications. These include damage or malfunction of the band itself resulting in leakage and loss of restriction. The band can also migrate upwards or downwards, or the fundus to the stomach can push through the band causing acute gastric proximal pouch dilation. This complication requires urgent band deflation and laparoscopic band removal in order to prevent gastric perforation. Finally the band can erode or migrate into the gastric wall, causing dysphagia and again requiring laparo-scopic removal.

The incidence of band complications has been variably reported as anywhere between 5 and 40% [7]. This is the major reason that the gastric band is falling out of favour amongst both patients and surgeons.

Following gastric bypass surgery, two main potential long-term complications can occur: internal herniation or vitamin deficiencies. Following surgery patients are requested to take long-term vitamin, iron and calcium sup-plements. In non-compliant patients, or patients who have had poor post-operative advice and are not taking supple-ments, vitamin and mineral deficiency is likely. The most commonly seen deficiencies are iron deficiency anaemia, vitamin B12 deficiency and vitamin D deficiency.

Internal small bowel herniation is a rare but potentially serious long-term complication following gastric bypass. The changes in anatomy following this procedure cause potential internal hernias, or holes, within the small bowel mesentery. Between 2 and 5% of patients may return years after surgery with loops of small bowel herniating through an internal hernia. In most cases this will cause intermit-tent episodes of abdominal colic. However there are rare cases of small bowel strangulation requiring urgent surgery and small bowel resection.

Abdominal wall hernia can occur in any patient after laparoscopic surgery and will be more common in obese subjects. Incisional hernias through the laparoscopic post site can occur in up to 1–2% of patients and usually require elective repair.

Apart from abdominal wall hernias, there are no signifi-cant long-term complications following sleeve gastrec-tomy. No foreign body has been placed and there is no change in the intestinal anatomy apart from a reduction in gastric capacity. The absence of long-term problems fol-lowing sleeve gastrectomy is a factor in its growing popularity.

### Mortality following bariatric surgery

Risk of death following bariatric surgery is very low. The UK National Bariatric Surgery Registry reported that there were seven deaths from bariatric surgery reported since 2012 out of a total of 9642 patients operated on a mortality risk of 0.7% [8]. The same mean mortality risk (0.7%) was found in a cohort of 2075 patients who were split into subgroup depending on their risk as calculated from the obesity surgery mortality risk score. Risk was stratified according to five criteria (male gender, $BMI > 50 kg/m^2$, age >45, presence of hypertension and history of DVT/PE). Scores of 0–1 calculated a low mor-tality rate of 0.2%, scores of 2–3 gave an intermediate risk of 1.1%, and high-risk patients (score = 5) had a mortality rate of 2.4%, or 12 times the higher than low risk [9]. Therefore mortality risk can be controlled by appropriate patient selection and optimisation. In addition it is accepted that mortality rates are lower if surgery is carried out in high-volume centres.

## Benefits of bariatric surgery

Following gastric bypass or sleeve gastrectomy surgery, patients routinely report that their lives have been trans-formed. After decades of struggles with dieting and yo-yo weight fluctuation, their weight loss is maintained. A good estimate of weight loss following either of these proce-dures is at least 70% excess weight lost. For example, a man of average height (1.75 m, 5 ft 9 in.) weighing 120 kg (18 stone 12 lbs) would expect to reset his weight to 89 kg (14 stone 1 lb), or lower, within a year of surgery. This level of weight loss is generally maintained in the long term if patients are give appropriate lifestyle and dietetic education.

As well as good weight loss the sleeve and bypass procedures have an excellent effect on metabolic syndrome. Over 60% of diabetic patients will be off medication following surgery, and the remainder will have better glycaemic control. The majority of patients with hypertension, dyslipidaemia and sleep apnoea will have resolution or significant improvement in their symptoms.

For women of reproductive age, fertility will improve following weight loss through bariatric surgery, pregnancy will be safer, and there will be less chance of emergency caesarean section. In addition to weight loss and better health, quality of life scores improve dramatically following gastric bypass and sleeve gastrectomy.

### Effect on NAFLD

NAFLD is present in between 75 and 100% of patient undergoing bariatric surgery. Small prospective studies have shown that bariatric surgery has positive effects on liver function tests and steatosis. However the long-term effect of bariatric surgery on hepatic inflammation and fibrosis is unclear and requires larger well-designed studies [10].

**TABLE 22.1** Summary of common bariatric surgical procedures

|  | Band | Sleeve | Bypass |
|---|---|---|---|
| Risks | Mortality, <1 in 2000<br>Early complications, 1 in 100<br>Late complications, 1 in 4 | Mortality, 0.7%. Low-risk patient mortality, 0.2%<br>Early complications, 1 in 20<br>Late complications, 1 in 20 | |
| Hospital stay | 1 night | 2 nights | |
| Recovery | 1–2 weeks | 2–3 weeks | |
| Average weight loss | 50% excess weight loss | 70% excess weight loss | 70–80% excess weight loss |
| Resolution or improvement in co-morbidities [11] | T2DM 47%<br>HT 43%<br>Cholesterol 59%<br>OSA 95% | T2DM 70% | T2DM 90%<br>HT 60–73%<br>Cholesterol 96%<br>OSA 94% |

## Conclusion

Obesity, and its associated problems, can now be safely treated by bariatric surgery. The risks of surgery have significantly reduced following the introduction of new procedures, new techniques and new technology (Table 22.1). In appropriately selected patients treated by a specialist team in a large specialist centre, the risks of bariatric surgery can now be equated to the risk of gallbladder surgery. In addition the rapid and sustained benefits of bariatric surgery are now being understood. The metabolic effects of surgery on appetite and satiety driving gut peptides and on metabolism have improved our understanding of obesity as a disease.

If a medical intervention that had such a dramatically beneficial effect on weight, health and quality of life and at such a low risk were discovered, it would be proclaimed the 'trillion-dollar pill' by the pharma industry. For now, whilst we await this discovery, bariatric surgery remains our only effective treatment for obesity.

## References

1. LC Aiello, P Wheeler. The expensive tissue hypothesis – the brain and the digestive system in human and primate evolution. Current Anthropology 1995; 36(2): S199–S221.
2. R Dobbs, C Sawers, F Thompson, J Manyika, JR Woetzel, P Child, S McKenna, A Spatharou; McKinsey Global Institute. Overcoming obesity: an initial economic analysis. The McKinsey Global Institute Washington, DC, November 2014.
3. J Wardle, S Carnell, CMA Haworth, R Plomin. Evidence for a strong genetic influence on childhood adiposity despite the force of the obesogenic environment. Am J Clin Nutr February 2008; 87(2): 398–404.
4. P Sumithrano, LA Prendergast, E Delbridge, K Purcell, A Shulkes, A Kriketos, J Proietto. Long term persistence of hormonal adaptations to weight loss. N Engl J Med 2011; 365(17): 1597–604.
5. National Institute for Health and Care Excellence. Managing overweight and obesity in adults – lifestyle weight management services. NICE guidelines [PH53]. May 2014.
6. KK Mahawar, WR Carr, S Balupuri, PK Small. Controversy surrounding 'mini' gastric bypass. Obes Surg 2014; 24(2): 324–33.
7. M Suter, JM Calmes, A Paroz, V Giusti. A 10-year experience with laparoscopic gastric banding for morbid obesity: high long-term complication and failure rates. Obes Surg 2006; 16(7): 829–35.
8. R Welbourn. National Bariatric Surgery Registry. 2nd Report: 2014.
9. EJ DeMaria, L Wolfe, M Murr, TK Byrne, R Blackstone, JP Grant, A Budak. Validation of the obesity surgery mortality risk score in a multicenter study proves it stratifies mortality risk in patients undergoing gastric bypass for morbid obesity. Ann Surg 2007;246(4): 578–82.
10. KJP Schwenger, JP Allard. Clinical approaches to non-alcoholic fatty liver disease. World J Gastroenterol 2014; 20(7): 1712–23.
11. H Buchwald, Y Avidor, E Braunwald, MD Jensen, W Pories, K Fahrbach, K Schoelles. Bariatric surgery: a systematic review and meta-analysis. JAMA 2004; 292(14): 1724–37.

# 23 Liver transplantation: What can it offer?

## Roger Williams

The Institute of Hepatology, Foundation for Liver Research, London, UK

### LEARNING POINTS

- An increasing number of transplants from non-alcoholic fatty liver disease (NAFLD).
- Careful selection needed.
- Survival figures as high as 75% at 5 years.
- Pre- and post-transplant management of metabolic syndrome is essential.

The simple answer to the question raised in the title to this chapter is yes. Indeed liver transplantation can offer a great deal for NAFLD patients when carefully selected, even though severe liver damage is found in 5–10% only of patients with NAFLD and morbidity/mortality is much more likely to be related to cardiac events than cirrhosis. Obesity rates are so high worldwide that the number of cases with end-stage liver disease will continue to increase and constitute a major burden on health-care systems. Unlike other common causes of cirrhosis such as viral hepatitis B/C and alcohol related, in which other forms of treatment can give benefit, there are no such possibilities once cirrhosis has developed in NAFLD. Once decompensation has occurred, the usual course is one of rapid downhill progression, and liver transplantation becomes the only option for recovery. Furthermore, hepatocellular carcinoma cases associated with NAFLD are rising dramatically according to recent data from a large UK series and accounted for 35% of all cases [1].

In fact, transplant programmes the world over are already reporting an increased number of liver transplants being carried out for NAFLD. In the United Kingdom, an analysis of the NHS Blood and Transplant Agency data for patients undergoing liver transplantation showed that decompensated NASH cirrhosis accounted for a growing proportion of cases – 12% in 2013 compared with 4% in 1995. During the past decade according to a database of the United Network for Organ Sharing (UNOS), the proportion of first-time adult cadaveric liver transplants performed for NASH between 1 January 1997 and 31 October 2010 rose from 1.2 to 7.4% [2]. Also from the United States, data from the Scientific Registry of Transplant Recipients for 2001–2009 showed that NASH was the primary or secondary indication for transplantation in 1 959 of the 35 781 cases who underwent primary liver transplantation and compared with the 1.2% of cases transplanted in 2001, 9.79% were transplanted in 2009 [3]. As a substantial percentage of the cases of cryptogenic cirrhosis transplanted were likely to have been secondary to NASH, figures for NASH plus 50% of cryptogenic cirrhosis cases were also analysed, the proportions of the total number of transplants increasing from 1.2 to 6.7% for 2001 and from 9.79 to 12.5% for 2009. According to Charlton and colleagues, NASH was the third most common indication for liver transplantation in the United States at that time and was on a trajectory to become the most common indication over the next 10–20 years.

In this chapter I will address three main questions:

1. Do transplant survival results for NASH justify the use of donor organs when compared with results obtained for other common disease indications?

2. Is the frequency with which NAFLD recurs in the transplanted liver and the underlying metabolic syndrome of clinical significance?

---

*Clinical Dilemmas in Non-Alcoholic Fatty Liver Disease*, First Edition. Edited by Roger Williams and Simon D. Taylor-Robinson.
© 2016 John Wiley & Sons, Ltd. Published 2016 by John Wiley & Sons, Ltd.

3.  Does obesity pre- and post-transplant have an impact on long-term outcomes after liver transplantation for non-NASH disease indications?

The emphasis throughout will be on current data and of the lessons that need to be taken forward.

## Current results of liver transplantation for NASH

In a 2009 report, the outcomes after transplantation for NASH cirrhosis were compared with those for alcoholic cirrhosis in a single large transplant centre over the period 1997–2007 [4]. Sepsis was the leading cause of post-transplant deaths in both groups with a higher percentage of cardiovascular deaths in the NASH group (26% vs. 7%) and of malignancies in those transplanted for alcoholic cirrhosis (29% vs. 0%). Interestingly, acute rejection was significantly more frequent in the NASH/cirrhosis transplants (41% vs. 23%), but there was no difference in graft failure rate (24% vs. 18%). Survival probabilities were considered to be inferior for NASH but not significantly so with 1-, 3-, 5- and 9-year survival rates for the NASH group of 82, 79, 75 and 62%, respectively, compared with 92, 86, 86 and 76% for alcoholic cirrhosis.

In the 2011 series of Charlton et al., from the database of Scientific Registry of Transplant Recipients, survival rates at 1 and 3 years were 84 and 78%, respectively, for NASH compared with 87 and 78% for all other indications transplanted. Patient and graft survival was similar for NASH and non-NASH patients after adjusting for creatinine, sex, age and BMI in multivariate analysis [3]. This review also refers to a number of papers showing graft loss on longer-term follow-up occurred in 2.5–5% only, as a result of recurrent NASH. Relevant to the excellent early survival rates for NASH as compared with transplants for other indications is the lesser severity of disease recurrence as compared, for instance, with HCV recurrence. Also, the frequency of HCC among NASH-transplanted recipients was lower – 12% compared with 19% for other aetiologies [3]. Nearly half of the liver transplant recipients with HCC had HCV as a primary or secondary indication in which, interestingly, hepatic steatosis is known to be an adverse risk factor in the progression of the disease.

The 2012 publication from the database of UNOS already referred to included survival results for 1810 patients who underwent transplantation for NASH-related cirrhosis [2]. The figures of 87% at 1 year, 82.2% at 3 years and 76.7% at 5 years were superior to those for patients with hepatocellular carcinoma, hepatitis C and alcoholic liver disease and inferior only for four groups of patients, namely, primary biliary cirrhosis, primary sclerosing cholangitis, autoimmune hepatitis and hepatitis B.

A single centre experience (Baylor Medical Centre) of 257 patients transplanted for diagnosis of cytogenesis cirrhosis (239) or NASH (18) showed 1-, 5- and 10-year survivals to be the same for cryptogenic cirrhosis or NASH (86, 71 and 56%) for those undergoing transplantation for other indications (86, 71 and 53%). Death was more often due to cardiovascular disease and less likely to be due to recurrent liver disease [5]. In another single centre experience of 129 NASH and 275 non-NASH transplants, Kennedy et al. found an increased early mortality in the NASH group most commonly caused by infections (38% vs. 26%) and cardiac complications (19 vs. 7%). Overall survivals though were similar with figures of 90, 88 and 85%, respectively, at 1, 3 and 5 years for NASH compared with 92, 86 and 80% in the non-NASH group [6].

## Frequency of NAFLD recurrence and of metabolic syndrome after transplantation and clinical significance

The risk factors for NASH – namely, obesity and the metabolic syndrome particularly diabetes – are likely to persist or become even greater after liver transplantation. Whether recurrent steatosis is clinically silent as it is in the non-transplanted situation at least for the initial years or whether histological changes and the rate of progression to cirrhosis are enhanced post-transplant as a result of immunosuppression as with other recurrent diseases is not known. Furthermore, with the continuing increase in the frequency of obesity and diabetes in the population, the appearance of NAFLD in the transplanted organ could represent de novo rather than recurrent disease. The distinction, however, is largely a semantic one as the histological changes and outcome effects are likely to be the same. Relevant to the interpretation of histological evolution of post-transplant is the possible occurrence of other post-transplant pathology, namely, de novo autoimmune chronic hepatitis and late cellular rejection, which may complicate the histological interpretation of NAFLD/NASH recurrence.

Patil and Yerian in an excellent recent review found that the majority of studies on NASH recurrence following transplantation were retrospective in nature and the absence of a standard biopsy protocol and the wide variation in timing of liver biopsies made comparisons difficult [7]. The frequency of recurrent disease as reported varied considerably. Of seven series in which histological reviews had been performed, the percentages for steatosis ranged from 8.2 to 62.5% over follow-up periods of 4 months to 10 years and for steatohepatitis 4 to 33% over periods of 6 weeks to 20 years. Advanced fibrosis found in the later follow-up periods was reported in a frequency of 0–33%. The finding that those with cryptogenic cirrhosis were more likely to be steatosis free at 1, 2 and 5 years than those transplanted for NASH raises the question as to whether all cases of cryptogenic cirrhosis can be attributed to an earlier NAFLD. Overall it would appear that recurrence or de novo NAFLD in the graft is common but progression to more severe NASH disease is uncommon and, as described earlier, has little adverse effect on survival figures. Included in the series of seven was that of Yalamanchili et al., for whom long-term survival figures were quoted earlier [5]. These workers found that post-transplant steatosis in 31% of their cases was more common when the pre-transplant diagnosis was NASH – 45% at 5 years compared with 23% for cryptogenic cirrhosis. NASH was found in 4% only and bridging fibrosis in 5 and 10%, respectively, after 5 and 10 years. Their findings also suggest that not all cases of cryptogenic cirrhosis are caused by NASH.

All the evidence as also considered later points to the underlying metabolic syndrome as the driving force in the frequency and severity of NASH recurrent disease rather than steatosis alone. Thus, El Atrache et al. in a retrospective study of 83 patients transplanted for NASH/cryptogenic cirrhosis found that 34% of the patients with metabolic syndrome had recurrent disease compared with 13% of those without metabolic syndrome. Disease recurrence was present in 32% of the patients with hypertension versus 12% of those without and similarly in 37% of those on insulin compared to 6% of those not on insulin [8]. Nevertheless, the series reporting the highest BMI had the greatest frequency of steatosis, steatohepatitis and advanced fibrosis. Nearly 85% of the patients in the series of Charlton and colleagues had a BMI > 30 kg/m$^2$ [3], and in two other series, mean BMIs were 28.7 and 29 kg/m$^2$, respectively [5, 9]. The frequency of type 2 diabetes varied from 22.6 to 53.3% in these three series reflecting differences in the patient population pre-transplant in terms of obesity and the metabolic syndrome.

According to O'Leary et al., in a comparison cohort study, NASH/CC patients were almost twice as likely as those with end-stage liver disease from HCV to be denied listing for transplantation because of co-morbid conditions mainly those of the metabolic syndrome [10]. Interestingly in that series, unlike others referred to earlier, the presence of co-morbid conditions did not appear to effect early post-transplant outcomes compared with those who had received a transplant for other diseases although over the longer term NASH/CC transplant recipients were more likely to die of cardiovascular disease while HCV patients were more likely to die of recurrent liver disease. This study also showed that NASH/CC patients with a MELD score of <15 were less likely to progress than the HCV group (1.3 vs. 3.2 MELD points per year) and as a result were less likely to receive a transplant and were more likely to die or be delisted because of co-morbid conditions relating to the metabolic syndrome. With a MELD score of >15 there was no difference in rate of progression or in percentages receiving transplants [10].

### Post-transplant cardiovascular (CVS) events

Although 5- and 10-year survival rates for NASH after transplantation are comparable to those for other disease indications, most of the evidence points to mortality being higher in the early post-transplant stages as a result of infections and CVS complications. Thus in the series of Vanwagner et al., adverse CVS events <1 year after transplant were higher in NASH-transplanted patients in comparison to an alcohol-induced liver disease [11]. Arrhythmias and cardiac arrests accounted for over 50% of all cardiac complications with a 50% overall mortality. The majority (70%) of events occurred in the perioperative period. A prolonged QTc interval in the pre-operative ECG was noted in 77% of the cases, and it is known that insulin resistance and the metabolic syndrome are independent risk factors for QTc prolongation. A prolonged QTc is also the electrophysiological hallmark of cirrhotic cardiomyopathy, which may be the cause of at least some of the increases in CVS events during the early post-operative period. Further studies are needed to evaluate the potential benefit of intensified pre-transplant CVS management including the pre-operative use of beta blockers, which have been shown to be protective for combined cardiac outcomes in a liver transplant population [12]. Statins also may be of benefit in the pre-operative period irrespective of the patients' cholesterol levels [13].

## Occurrence of chronic kidney injury

Obesity is known to be an independent predictor for the development of chronic kidney injury (CKI) in diabetic patients with NAFLD, and the further effects of transplantation were looked at by Houlihan et al. in a single centre comparison study of 48 NASH patients and a non-NASH group [14]. Strictly matched for variables including MELD score, the estimated GFR was significantly lower in the NASH group at 3, 6, 12 and 24 months after transplantation. Within 2 years, 31.2% of NASH patients had evidence of CKI stage III disease compared with 8.3% of the non-NASH group. Renal dysfunction early in the post-operative period is known to be a predictor of CKI in the longer term, and delayed introduction/low dose of calcineurin inhibitors together with the use of the renal-sparing agent sirolimus will reduce the likelihood of developing CKI.

## Impact of obesity on long-term outcome after liver transplantation for non-NASH indications

Morbid obesity was considered to be a contraindication to transplantation in the guidelines of AASLD although several reports have shown acceptable outcomes in obese patients transplanted for a variety of liver disease indications. As the presence of hepatic steatosis from obesity is known to increase the severity of liver disease from other aetiologies including alcohol, HCV/HBV and even genetic disorders such as haemochromatosis, its presence might be expected to have an impact on the results of liver transplantation for those indications.

Relevant to the assessment of obesity pre-transplant is the confounding influence of fluid accumulation from liver decompensation on measurements of the BMI. Modification of the BMI by multiplying its value with that of the serum albumin level to compensate for ascites and more general fluid accumulation was used in a study of a cohort of 507 patients mainly transplanted for HCV, PBC or HCC in a single Canadian centre [15]. The recipients at the extremes of modified BMI – namely, >40 kg/m$^2$ and <18.5 kg/m$^2$ – were found to have significantly lower patient and graft survival. At these extremes, however, the poorer results are more likely to be related to generally poor health states, with high MELD scores and ITU stays at the time of the transplantation rather than directly due to obesity or malnutrition. For the overall series no significant difference was found in patient survival across the modified BMI categories.

Whatever the disease indication, hepatic steatosis inevitably is common post-transplant as result of increases in weight of the patients. Dumortier and colleagues in a series of 599 adult liver transplants for a range of non-NASH disease indications found steatosis to be present on histological examination in 31% of those who did not have a recurrence of their original disease. On multivariate analysis, seven factors were shown to be risk factors for post-transplant steatosis, namely, obesity, tacrolimus-based immunosuppression, diabetes mellitus, hyperlipidaemia, arterial hypertension, cirrhosis as primary indication and pre-transplant donor graft steatosis [16].

In a 2014 recent review, the impact of type 2 diabetes and obesity on long-term outcomes was analysed in a series of more than 85 000 liver transplant recipients of whom 11.2% had diabetes pre-transplant and 7.9% of the donors had a history of diabetes [17]. Multivariate analysis showed that the presence of pre-transplant diabetes and the development of diabetes post-transplant and diabetes in the donor (presumably as a result of associated graft steatosis) were accompanied by an increased risk of liver graft failure and were independently associated with higher recipient mortality. Almost 65% of liver transplant recipients and 53% of the donors were in the overweight or obese categories. The standard BMI that does not take into account ascites and fluid retention as already referred to was not predictive of a poor long-term outcome. One benefit from the high prevalence of diabetes post-transplant is an increased bone mineral density and a lower incidence of osteoporosis and osteopenia as a result of a complex interaction of insulin resistance and high BMI on bone physiology [18].

Another 2014 published study looked at the additional effect of pre-transplant obesity and diabetes on CVS risk factors and outcomes after transplantation. The cohort comprised 202 consecutive patients transplanted at the National Centre in New Zealand [19]. Obesity together with concomitant diabetes was the strongest predictor of post-operative events rate and longer hospital stay. Although early post-transplant morbidity may be affected, no influence on long-term survival was noted with similar survival rates up to 5 years after for obese, diabetic patients versus non-obese, non-diabetic cases. According to Sarno et al., new-onset diabetes mellitus (NODM) after transplantation for non-NASH disease indications is one of the strongest predictive factors for lower survival and increased co-morbidities. The main factor contributing to NODM is likely to be the immunosuppression. Cyclosporine, tacrolimus particularly and steroids are all diabetogenic, and the other currently used immunosuppressive agent sirolimus gives hypertriglyceridaemia exacerbating metabolic changes that may already have developed as part of the metabolic syndrome [20].

## Conclusion

1. Liver transplantation has much to offer to the patient with NAFLD who has progressed to end-stage liver disease. Five-year survivals of 70–80% are as good as for other disease indications, and NAFLD patients should have similar improvements in quality of life indices as have been demonstrated for other transplanted conditions.
2. Recurrence of NAFLD in association with continued obesity or de novo development is frequent in the grafted organ but unlike recurrent disease from other disease indications appears to have little effect on survival rates with 2 and 5% only of transplanted NAFLD cases developing steatofibrosis and cirrhosis after 5 years. Furthermore, unlike recurrent disease following transplantation for HCV/HBV end-stage liver disease or primary hepatocellular carcinoma, there is no evidence that immunosuppression therapy accelerates the progression of NAFLD in the graft.
3. In contrast, the persistence and various consequences of the underlying metabolic syndrome are of clinical significance with NASH-transplanted patients remaining prone to cardiovascular events and hypertensive and diabetic complications, including renal failure that can lead to an increase in morbidity/mortality in the perioperative and early transplant periods.
4. After transplantation for non-NASH disease indications, the persistence of the metabolic syndrome in association with obesity is not only frequent but a significant cause of early and late post-transplant complications with NODM being one of the strongest predictors for a reduction in survival and increase in co-morbidities.

From these conclusions, it is apparent that post-transplant management for NAFLD recipients should be concerned more with manifestations of the metabolic syndrome, particularly diabetes, than with possible progression of recurrent liver disease. The increased physical activity that has been enabled by the transplant may help with weight reduction although more often body weight increases with a successful transplant, whatever the disease indication, rather than the reverse. A continuing area of uncertainly is the level of acceptable co-morbidity from the metabolic syndrome in terms of listing patients for liver transplantation, and aggressive management pre-transplant through restrictions on high-fat and sugar-containing food and beverages, close diabetic control and anti-hypertension measures is essential to the obtaining of excellent transplant survival and quality of life results.

## Acknowledgement

The author thanks Enda O'Sullivan for much editorial support.

## References

1. Dyson J, Jaques B, Chattopadyhay D, et al. Hepatocellular cancer: the impact of obesity, type 2 diabetes and a multi-disciplinary team. J Hepatol 2014; 60: 110–7.
2. Afzali A, Berry K, Ioannou GN. Excellent posttransplant survival for patients with nonalcoholic steatohepatitis in the United States. Liver Transpl 2012; 18: 29–37.
3. Charlton MR, Burns JM, Pedersen RA, et al. Frequency and outcomes of liver transplantation for nonalcoholic steatohepatitis in the United States. Gastroenterology 2011; 141: 1249–53.
4. Bhagat V, Mindikoglu AL, Nudo CG, et al. Outcomes of liver transplantation in patients with cirrhosis due to nonalcoholic steatohepatitis versus patients with cirrhosis due to alcoholic liver disease. Liver Transpl 2009; 15: 1814–20.
5. Yalamanchili K, Saadeh S, Klintmalm GB, et al. Nonalcoholic fatty liver disease after liver transplantation for cryptogenic cirrhosis or nonalcoholic fatty liver disease. Liver Transpl 2010; 16: 431–9.
6. Kennedy C, Redden D, Gray S, et al. Equivalent survival following liver transplantation in patients with non-alcoholic steatohepatitis compared with patients with other liver diseases. HPB (Oxford). 2012; 14: 625–34.
7. Patil DT, Yerian LM. Evolution of nonalcoholic fatty liver disease recurrence after liver transplantation. Liver Transpl 2012; 18: 1147–53.
8. El Atrache MM, Abouljoud MS, Divine G, et al. Recurrence of non-alcoholic steatohepatitis and cryptogenic cirrhosis following orthotopic liver transplantation in the context of the metabolic syndrome. Clin Transpl 2012; 26: E505–12.
9. Contos MJ, Cales W, Sterling RK, et al. Development of non-alcoholic fatty liver disease after orthotopic liver transplantation for cryptogenic cirrhosis. Liver Transpl 2001; 7: 363–73.

10. O'Leary JG, Landaverde C, Jennings L, et al. Patients with NASH and cryptogenic cirrhosis are less likely than those with hepatitis C to receive liver transplants. Clin Gastroenterol Hepatol. 2011; 9: 700–704.e1.

11. Vanwagner LB, Bhave M, Te HS, et al. Patients transplanted for nonalcoholic steatohepatitis are at increased risk for post-operative cardiovascular events. Hepatology 2012; 56: 1741–50.

12. Safadi A, Homsi M, Maskoun W, et al. Perioperative risk predictors of cardiac outcomes in patients undergoing liver transplantation surgery. Circulation 2009; 120: 1189–94.

13. Lander JS, Coplan NL. Statin therapy in the perioperative period. Rev Cardiovasc Med 2011; 12: 30–7.

14. Houlihan DD, Armstrong MJ, Davidov Y, et al. Renal function in patients undergoing transplantation for nonalcoholic steatohepatitis cirrhosis: time to reconsider immunosup-pression regimens? Liver Transpl 2011; 17: 1292–8.

15. Tanaka T, Renner EL, Selzner N, et al. The impact of obesity as determined by modified body mass index on long-term outcome after liver transplantation: Canadian single-center experience. Transplant Proc 2013; 45: 2288–94.

16. Dumortier J, Giostra E, Belbouab S, et al. Non-alcoholic fatty liver disease in liver transplant recipients: another story of 'seed and soil'. Am J Gastroenterol 2010; 105: 613–20.

17. Younossi ZM, Stepanova M, Saab S, et al. The impact of type 2 diabetes and obesity on the long-term outcomes of more than 85 000 liver transplant recipients in the US. Aliment Pharmacol Ther 2014; 40: 686–94.

18. Boonchaya-anant P, Hardy E, Borg BB, et al. Bone mineral density in patients with nonalcoholic steatohepatitis among end-stage liver disease patients awaiting liver transplanta-tion. Endocr Pract 2013; 19: 414–9.

19. Dare AJ, Plank LD, Phillips AR, et al. Additive effect of pretransplant obesity, diabetes, and cardiovascular risk factors on outcomes after liver transplantation. Liver Transpl 2014; 20: 281–90.

20. Sarno G, Mehta RJ, Guardado-Mendoza R, et al. New-onset diabetes mellitus: predictive factors and impact on the outcome of patients undergoing liver transplantation. Curr Diabetes Rev 2013; 9: 78–85.

**PART V**

# What Does the Future Hold?

# 24 Molecular antagonists, leptin or other hormones in supplementing environmental factors?

**Jonathan M. Hazlehurst[1] and Jeremy W. Tomlinson[2]**

[1] Centre for Diabetes, Endocrinology and Metabolism, School of Clinical and Experimental Medicine, University of Birmingham, Birmingham, UK

[2] Oxford Centre for Diabetes, Endocrinology and Metabolism, University of Oxford, Churchill Hospital, Headington, UK
**Conflict of interest**: Professor Jeremy W. Tomlinson is an investigator on the ongoing LEAN study (Clinical trials.gov identifier: NCT01237119) to which Dr Jonathan M. Hazlehurst has also contributed to although neither have received financial support as part of this study.

---

## LEARNING POINTS

- The pathogenesis of NAFLD is multifactorial, and progression to fibrosis is uncommon and unpredictable.

- Simple steatosis, steatohepatitis and fibrosis represent different points on a disease spectrum and may require different treatments.

- Current studies are heterogeneous in design with some enrolling only those with steatosis and with variable duration and end points.

- Small incremental improvements in steatosis are unlikely to be clinically relevant, and effective treatments must treat more advanced disease.

## Introduction

NAFLD is a spectrum of disease extending from steatosis through to steatohepatitis and then fibrosis. Currently there are no licensed disease-modifying treatments, and medical management is principally aimed at controlling cardiovascular risk [1]. NAFLD is a complex condition with a multifactorial aetiology, which is reflected by the diversity in treatment strategies in development. Given this complexity it is likely that treatment strategies may differ between those with simple steatosis and those with steatohepatitis.

## Strategies to promote 'healthier' adipose tissue function

### Leptin

Leptin is principally released from white adipose and has beneficial effects on satiety and the control of fat mass. However, there is emergent animal data suggesting that it contributes to progression of hepatic oxidative stress and fibrosis. While leptin is an effective obesity treatment in congenital leptin deficiency [2], levels are increased in obese compared to non-obese controls and correlate with percentage fat mass.

The data on leptin levels and NAFLD are conflicting. Leptin levels were not different between those with progressive fibrosis and stable disease [3]. However, other published data have shown leptin levels to be higher in patients with NASH compared to matched controls and correlated with steatosis rather than fibrosis [4] and may contribute to hepatocyte oxidative stress [5]. Furthermore, leptin-deficient mice are protected from diet-induced hepatic fibrosis, an effect that is reversed by leptin replacement [6].

Leptin has been considered as a novel treatment for NAFLD. Leptin administration alongside a calorie-restricted diet in simple obesity resulted in a modest reduction in weight and fat mass [7]. This was not seen when compared to placebo [8]. Depot, 2-weekly leptin

---

preparations achieve modest weight loss alongside calorie restriction [9]. Significant improvements in lipid profiles or measures of insulin resistance have not been shown.

Leptin has been used to treat patients with lipodystrophy with and without NASH with significant improvements in lipid profile, HbA1c and transaminases, grade of steatosis, ballooning injury and overall NAFLD activity score [10]. However, lipodystrophy represents an extreme example of adipose tissue dysfunction, often with low circulating leptin and any extrapolations to patients with NAFLD must be made with caution. There is an ongoing phase II study in patients with NASH without lipodystrophy (Clinical Trails.gov Identifier: NCT00596934) using daily subcutaneous recombinant human Methionyl leptin and results are awaited.

### Metadoxine

Metadoxine (pyridoxine–L-2-pyrrolidone-5-carboxylate) has also been trialled in patients with NAFLD. As well as limiting adipocyte differentiation [11], it also has direct beneficial effects upon the liver, reducing oxidative stress [12] and lipid partitioning. Furthermore, it reduces the deposition of procollagen and fibronectin in animal models of liver fibrosis [13]. In the only published randomised placebo-controlled study, patients in the metadoxine group had a reduction in steatosis on ultrasound, but there was no improvement in either transaminases or histology [14].

## Beyond diabetes and insulin signalling

### Peroxisome proliferator-activated receptor agonists

Improving insulin sensitivity is a potential treatment strategy. Metformin has been used due to its favourable effect on hepatic insulin sensitivity, but in a recent meta-analysis, despite a reduction in weight and transaminases, there has shown to be no histological improvement [15]. Thiazolidinediones (TZDs) activate peroxisome proliferator-activated receptors (PPARs) with the greatest specificity for PPARγ improving insulin sensitivity and lipid metabolism. Although several studies have shown a favourable impact of TZDs upon histology [15], because of safety concerns for long-term use regarding heart failure, bladder cancer and bone loss, clinical use is limited [1]. Therefore, the modulation of insulin signalling remains an attractive therapeutic target, but further agents may be required that target PPARs or even TZDs that work independently of

PPAR activation such as Blx-1002. In combination with metformin, Blx-1002 reduced hepatic steatosis, dyslipidaemia and glucose in animal models [16].

Fenofibrate is a PPARα agonist used in the management of hypertriglyceridaemia. Preclinical data suggests improvements in hepatic insulin resistance and steatosis, increased fatty acid oxidation and reduced hepatic inflammation. Clinical studies have been limited by small sample size and the lack of well-designed RCTs with histological end points [17].

Other selective PPAR modulators (SPPARM) have also been developed including the dual PPARα/δ agonist GFT-505. In animal models of NAFLD, GFT-505 had a protective effect on hepatic steatosis, inflammation and fibrosis. In a combined analysis of phase II studies of patients with metabolic syndrome, GFT-505 improved transaminases [18] and is now the subject of an ongoing phase IIb 52 week study in patients with NASH using histology as the primary end point (Clinical Trails.gov Identifier: NCT01694849).

### Dipeptidyl peptidase-4 inhibition

Dipeptidyl peptidase-4 (DPPIV) is widely expressed and has several roles including the degradation of the incretin molecules notably glucagon-like peptide-1 (GLP-1) [19]. Hepatic and serum expression of DPPIV correlates with hepatic steatosis, and severity of NASH [20]- and DPPIV-deficient rats has reduced lipogenesis, increased β-oxidation and reduced pro-inflammatory and profibrotic cytokines [21]. DPPIV inhibitors are already licensed for patients with type 2 diabetes and in diabetic mice reduce adipose infiltration by inflammatory cells and hepatic steatosis [22]. DPPIV inhibition is efficacious for the control of diabetes in patients with NAFLD [23] and has been shown to improve AST, ALT and gamma-GT although not in the context of a placebo-controlled study [24]. There is an ongoing placebo-controlled randomised double-blind study comparing sitagliptin 100 mg to placebo in patients with NAFLD (Clinical Trails.gov Identifier: NCT01963845).

### GLP-1

GLP-1 is secreted from L-cells of the small intestine and has wide-ranging effects including increasing insulin release and sensitivity, delaying gastric emptying and increasing satiety. In a study of non-diabetic patients with NAFLD, GLP-1 secretion was significantly reduced after an oral glucose tolerance test [25]. GLP-1 agonist is hepatoprotective in mice fed with a HFD with effects independent of weight loss and mediated *via* the GLP-1 receptor [26]. In a large meta-analysis of liraglutide use in patients with type 2 diabetes, 1.8 mg was well tolerated and reduced ALT at 26 weeks; however, this effect was lost when corrected for weight loss and HbA1c improvement [27]. In a non-placebo-controlled study, the administration of 0.9 mg of liraglutide was associated with improvements in transaminases, glycaemic control and visceral fat. 6/10 patients who underwent a liver biopsy at 96 weeks had histological improvements [28]. The LEAN study (Clinical Trails.gov Identifier: NCT01237119) is a randomised double-blind placebo-controlled study investigating both the safety and efficacy of liraglutide 1.8 mg daily for 12 months in patients with NASH [29]. Recruitment is completed and published data are awaited.

## Lipid and dietary modification

### Omega-3 polyunsaturated fatty acids

Polyunsaturated fatty acids can activate PPAR, suppress hepatic lipogenesis and may have anti-inflammatory effects. Dietary administration of PUFA in animal models of NAFLD improves insulin sensitivity and suppresses hepatic lipogenesis [30].

A meta-analysis has shown a beneficial effect of PUFA on liver fat and AST, but not ALT, although there was significant heterogeneity between the studies [31]. Docosahexaenoic acid (DHA) administered to 20 children (250 mg) with NAFLD for 18 months resulted in histological improvement thought in part mediated by the anti-inflammatory action of increased GPR120 expression [32]. However, in a double-blind randomised placebo-controlled trial of DHA (1440 mg) and eicosapentaenoic acid (EPA) (2160 mg) for 48 weeks in patients with NASH and diabetes, there was no improvement in histology and a deterioration in insulin resistance in the intervention arm [33]. In a separate study, 103 patients with NAFLD were randomised to receive either Omacor 4 g ((DHA (1520 mg) and EPA (1840 mg)) or placebo (olive oil 4 g) for up to 18 months [34]. There was a trend towards improvement in liver fat measured by MRS in the Omacor group.

### Bile acids

Bile acids are synthesised in the liver from the oxidation of cholesterol and are further modified by partial dehydroxylation by intestinal bacteria. Secretion is stimulated by cholecystokinin in response to a meal and serves to solubilise dietary lipids promoting absorption via the intrahepatic circulation [35]. Additionally bile acids are important signalling molecules acting on several receptors including the farnesoid X receptor (FXR) and the G protein-coupled receptor TGR5.

FXR is a nuclear receptor that modulates bile acid, lipid and glucose homeostasis and is widely expressed including the liver [35]. FXR knockout mice develop NASH and impaired cholesterol and triglyceride clearance in an LDL receptor knockout model of hypercholesterolaemia [36]. Furthermore, FXR activation improves lipid metabolism and suppresses hepatic gluconeogenesis in diabetic mice [37]. TGR5 is expressed in tissues including the liver, brown adipose and intestines. TGR5 activation within the intestine induces the release of GLP-1 with a resultant improvement in glucose tolerance and hepatic steatosis in mice fed with a HFD [38].

Bile acid sequestrants form insoluble conjugates that are lost in the faeces with a resultant improvement in dyslipidaemia. There are additional improvements in glucose metabolism in patients with type 2 diabetes although whether the effect is mediated in part by GLP-1 secretion is debated [39, 40]. The bile acid sequestrant, Colesevelam, has been trialled in patients with NASH. While LDL cholesterol improved, there was no effect on measures of insulin resistance, anthropometric indices or liver biopsy, and liver fat as measured by magnetic resonance spectroscopy increased [41].

Ursodeoxycholic acid is a secondary bile acid and is used in the management of primary biliary cirrhosis and gallstones. Its use as either monotherapy or in combination with other treatments in patients with NAFLD has been the subject of a recent systematic review. Eight studies examined monotherapy at doses of 13–15 mg/kg/day up to 28–35 mg/kg/day with durations of between 2 and 24 months. Transaminases improved in five studies while steatosis and fibrosis improved in two studies [42].

Aramchol is a fatty acid–bile acid conjugate. A dose of 300 mg when taken for 3 months was well tolerated and resulted in a significant reduction in liver fat measured by MRS with a non-significant trend towards improvement in transaminases [43].

Several FXR receptor agonists have been developed including INT-747. INT-747 (obeticholic acid) has been compared to placebo over 6 weeks with a significant improvement in insulin sensitivity. 25 mg of INT-747 resulted in a significant reduction in non-invasive measures of liver fibrosis and ALT and resulted in a reduction in body weight [44]. There is an ongoing phase IIb study in NASH patients for 72 weeks with histology as the primary outcome (Clinical Trials.gov Identifier: NCT01265498).

### Statins and beyond

Statins are 3-hydroxy-3-methylglutaryl-CoA (HMG-CoA) reductase inhibitors and catalyse the rate-limiting step in cholesterol synthesis. Despite reservations, statins are safe in patients with NAFLD [1], and their use in NAFLD has been the subject of a Cochrane review [45]. There was no improvement in transaminases or histology [45]. In a retrospective study, statin use was associated with a reduction in hepatic steatosis on paired biopsy [46]. There is an ongoing phase II study comparing atorvastatin with metformin (Clinical Trails.gov Identifier: NCT01544751) and a study comparing atorvastatin and vitamin E (Clinical Trails.gov Identifier: NCT01720719) both looking at the effect on hepatic steatosis.

Ezetimibe inhibits cholesterol absorption in the gastrointestinal tract and is licensed for dyslipidaemia in patients intolerant to statins or as an add-on to statins where control is inadequate [47]. A recent, open-label RCT ezetimibe (10 mg/day) for 6 months was associated with an improvement in cholesterol, but not triglycerides, and in those that underwent paired biopsy, there was an improvement in the fibrosis stage and ballooning score. However, hepatic gene expression was indicative of increased oxidative stress. This study was terminated due to increased HbA1c in the ezetimibe-treated group [48].

Diacylglycerol acyltransferase (DGAT) has two isoforms, which catalyse the final step in triglyceride synthesis. In animals fed with a HFD, DGAT2 knockdown reduced intrahepatic lipid, promoted fatty acid oxidation and improved hepatic insulin sensitivity [49]. However, there are concerns from animal models that the inhibition of triglyceride synthesis by DGAT knockdown may increase oxidative stress, inflammation and fibrosis suggesting that triglyceride accumulation may in part be a protective mechanism [50]. Despite these concerns, a phase II study examining the safety and efficacy of LCQ-908, a DGAT1 inhibitor in patients with NAFLD (Clinical Trails.gov Identifier: NCT01811472), is ongoing.

### Hepatic oxidative stress

Vitamin E, an antioxidant, is discussed extensively elsewhere. Pentoxyphylline has wide-ranging effects including hemorrheologic properties, enhanced aerobic glycolysis and oxygen consumption and non-specific inhibition of phosphodiesterase [51]. In a recent meta-analysis of five heterogeneous studies that included a total of 147 patients with NAFLD, pentoxyphylline decreased weight, improved transaminases as well as the histological parameters of lobular inflammation and the NAFLD activity score.

There is emerging data investigating the effect of silymarin, a plant extract, as a potential treatment in patients with NAFLD. Animal data have shown an improvement in the activation of hepatocyte stellate cells that are involved in fibrosis as well as reductions in TNFα [52]. However, clinical studies to date have demonstrated improvements in transaminases with no available data from liver biopsies [53]. There is an ongoing study using histology at 12 months as the primary outcome (Clinical Trails.gov Identifier: NCT00680407).

Cysteamine, a degradation product of the amino acid cysteine, has antioxidant properties. In one non-placebo-controlled paediatric study, patients had an improvement in transaminases at 24 weeks [54]. It is now the subject of a placebo-controlled RCT in paediatric patients with NAFLD with histology as the primary end point (Clinical trials.gov Identifier: NCT01529268).

Nuclear erythroid 2-related factor (Nrf2) is another antioxidant, and Nrf2 knockout mice fed with a HFD developed increased NASH as compared to the simple steatosis seen in control animals [55]. Nrf2 activators, including oltipraz, attenuate histological progression to NASH in animals models [56]. However the available human data have not demonstrated histological improvement following 24 weeks of treatment [57].

### Conclusion

Faced with the diabetes and obesity epidemic fuelling the increase in the prevalence of NAFLD, it is clear that targeted, safe and efficacious therapies are needed urgently. The complexity and chronicity of NAFLD make this a challenge. Several different disease-modifying strategies may need to be applied simultaneously in order to address the different pathological processes that contribute to the different stages of the disease. The treatments that have been outlined here remain at the earliest stages of development. Further detailed clinical studies are clearly warranted, and these must include patients across the whole spectrum of disease, rather than focusing on those patients with simple steatosis, in whom the long-term clinical consequence of their condition is debatable. Studies must be well designed with meaningful clinical end points, and until such time as non-invasive markers can accurately and predictably stage disease, there is still a need for liver biopsy data. In the meantime, the best available management involves aggressive reduction of cardiovascular risk. However, the breadth of the studies discussed and those in development should afford a degree of optimism for the future.

## Acknowledgement

This work has been supported by the Medical Research Council (senior clinical fellowship ref. G0802765, J. W. Tomlinson).

## References

1. Chalasani N, Younossi Z, Lavine JE, et al. The diagnosis and management of non-alcoholic fatty liver disease: practice Guideline by the American Association for the Study of Liver Diseases, American College of Gastroenterology, and the American Gastroenterological Association. Hepatology 2012;55:2005–23.
2. Farooqi IS, Matarese G, Lord GM, et al. Beneficial effects of leptin on obesity, T cell hyporesponsiveness, and neuroendocrine/metabolic dysfunction of human congenital leptin deficiency. J Clin Invest 2002;110:1093–103.
3. Angulo P, Alba LM, Petrovic LM, et al. Leptin, insulin resistance, and liver fibrosis in human nonalcoholic fatty liver disease. J Hepatol 2004;41:943–9.
4. Chitturi S, Farrell G, Frost L, et al. Serum leptin in NASH correlates with hepatic steatosis but not fibrosis: a manifestation of lipotoxicity? Hepatology 2002;36:403–9.
5. Chatterjee S, Ganini D, Tokar EJ, et al. Leptin is key to peroxynitrite-mediated oxidative stress and Kupffer cell activation in experimental non-alcoholic steatohepatitis. J Hepatol 2013;58:778–84.
6. Leclercq IA, Farrell GC, Schriemer R, et al. Leptin is essential for the hepatic fibrogenic response to chronic liver injury. J Hepatol 2002;37:206–13.
7. Heymsfield SB, Greenberg AS, Fujioka K, et al. Recombinant leptin for weight loss in obese and lean adults: a randomized, controlled, dose-escalation trial. JAMA 1999;282:1568–75.
8. Zelissen PM, Stenlof K, Lean ME, et al. Effect of three treatment schedules of recombinant methionyl human leptin on body weight in obese adults: a randomized, placebo-controlled trial. Diabetes Obes Metab 2005;7:755–61.
9. DePaoli A. Leptin in common obesity and associated disorders of metabolism. J Endocrinol 2014;223:T71–81.
10. Safar Zadeh E, Lungu AO, Cochran EK, et al. The liver diseases of lipodystrophy: the long-term effect of leptin treatment. J Hepatol 2013;59:131–7.
11. Yang YM, Kim HE, Ki SH, et al. Metadoxine, an ion-pair of pyridoxine and L-2-pyrrolidone-5-carboxylate, blocks adipocyte differentiation in association with inhibition of the PKA-CREB pathway. Arch Biochem Biophys 2009;488:91–9.
12. Calabrese V, Calderone A, Ragusa N, et al. Effects of Metadoxine on cellular status of glutathione and of enzymatic defence system following acute ethanol intoxication in rats. Drugs Exp Clin Res 1996;22:17–24.
13. Arosio B, Santambrogio D, Gagliano N, et al. Changes in expression of the albumin, fibronectin and type I procollagen genes in CCl4-induced liver fibrosis: effect of pyridoxol L,2-pyrrolidon-5 carboxylate. Pharmacol Toxicol 1993;73:301–4.
14. Shenoy KT, Balakumaran LK, Mathew P, et al. Metadoxine versus placebo for the treatment of non-alcoholic steatohepatitis: a randomized controlled trial. J Clin Exp Hepatol 2014;4:94–100.
15. Musso G, Gambino R, Cassader M, et al. A meta-analysis of randomized trials for the treatment of nonalcoholic fatty liver disease. Hepatology 2010;52:79–104.
16. Narayanan S, Vijayaraj D, Kulkarni NM, et al. 1272 Efficacy of BLX 1002 in animal models of non-alcoholic fatty liver disease and dyslipidaemia. J Hepatol 2014;54:S502.
17. Kostapanos MS, Kei A, Elisaf MS. Current role of fenofibrate in the prevention and management of non-alcoholic fatty liver disease. World J Hepatol 2013;5:470–78.
18. Staels B, Rubenstrunk A, Noel B, et al. Hepatoprotective effects of the dual peroxisome proliferator-activated receptor alpha/delta agonist, GFT505, in rodent models of nonalcoholic fatty liver disease/nonalcoholic steatohepatitis. Hepatology 2013;58:1941–52.
19. Itou M, Kawaguchi T, Taniguchi E, et al. Dipeptidyl peptidase-4: a key player in chronic liver disease. World J Gastroenterol 2013;19:2298–306.
20. Balaban YH, Korkusuz P, Simsek H, et al. Dipeptidyl peptidase IV (DDP IV) in NASH patients. Ann Hepatol 2007;6:242–50.
21. Ben-Shlomo S, Zvibel I, Shnell M, et al. Glucagon-like peptide-1 reduces hepatic lipogenesis via activation of AMP-activated protein kinase. J Hepatol 2011;54:1214–23.
22. Shirakawa J, Fujii H, Ohnuma K, et al. Diet-induced adipose tissue inflammation and liver steatosis are prevented by DPP-4 inhibition in diabetic mice. Diabetes 2011;60:1246–57.

23. Arase Y, Kawamura Y, Seko Y, et al. Efficacy and safety in sitagliptin therapy for diabetes complicated by non-alcoholic fatty liver disease. Hepatol Res 2013;43:1163–8.

24. Fukuhara T, Hyogo H, Ochi H, et al. Efficacy and safety of sitagliptin for the treatment of nonalcoholic fatty liver disease with type 2 diabetes mellitus. Hepatogastroenterology 2014;61:323–8.

25. Bernsmeier C, Meyer-Gerspach AC, Blaser LS, et al. Glucose-induced glucagon-like Peptide 1 secretion is deficient in patients with non-alcoholic fatty liver disease. PLoS One 2014;9:e87488.

26. Trevaskis JL, Griffin PS, Wittmer C, et al. Glucagon-like peptide-1 receptor agonism improves metabolic, biochemical, and histopathological indices of nonalcoholic steatohepatitis in mice. Am J Physiol Gastrointest Liver Physiol 2012;302:G762–72.

27. Armstrong MJ, Houlihan DD, Rowe IA, et al. Safety and efficacy of liraglutide in patients with type 2 diabetes and elevated liver enzymes: individual patient data meta-analysis of the LEAD program. Aliment Pharmacol Ther 2013;37:234–42.

28. Eguchi Y, Kitajima Y, Hyogo H, et al. Pilot study of liraglutide effects in non-alcoholic steatohepatitis and non-alcoholic fatty liver disease with glucose intolerance in Japanese patients (LEAN-J). Hepatol Res 2015;45:269–78.

29. Armstrong MJ, Barton D, Gaunt P, et al. Liraglutide efficacy and action in non-alcoholic steatohepatitis (LEAN): study protocol for a phase II multicentre, double-blinded, randomised, controlled trial. BMJ Open 2013;3:e003995.

30. Sekiya M, Yahagi N, Matsuzaka T, et al. Polyunsaturated fatty acids ameliorate hepatic steatosis in obese mice by SREBP-1 suppression. Hepatology 2003;38:1529–39.

31. Parker HM, Johnson NA, Burdon CA, et al. Omega-3 supplementation and non-alcoholic fatty liver disease: a systematic review and meta-analysis. J Hepatol 2012;56:944–51.

32. Nobili V, Carpino G, Alisi A, et al. Role of docosahexaenoic acid treatment in improving liver histology in pediatric non-alcoholic fatty liver disease. PLoS One 2014;9:e88005.

33. Dasarathy S, Dasarathy J, Khiyami A, et al. Double-blind randomized placebo-controlled clinical trial of omega 3 fatty acids for the treatment of diabetic patients with nonalcoholic steatohepatitis. J Clin Gastroenterol 2015;49:137–44.

34. Scorletti E, Bhatia L, McCormick KG, et al. Effects of purified eicosapentaenoic and docosahexaenoic acids in non-alcoholic fatty liver disease: results from the *WELCOME study. Hepatology 2014;60:1211–21.

35. Li Y, Jadhav K, Zhang Y. Bile acid receptors in non-alcoholic fatty liver disease. Biochem Pharmacol 2013;86:1517–24.

36. Kong B, Luyendyk JP, Tawfik O, et al. Farnesoid X receptor deficiency induces nonalcoholic steatohepatitis in low-density lipoprotein receptor-knockout mice fed a high-fat diet. J Pharmacol Exp Ther 2009;328:116–22.

37. Zhang Y, Lee FY, Barrera G, et al. Activation of the nuclear receptor FXR improves hyperglycemia and hyperlipidemia in diabetic mice. Proc Natl Acad Sci U S A 2006;103:1006–11.

38. Thomas C, Gioiello A, Noriega L, et al. TGR5-mediated bile acid sensing controls glucose homeostasis. Cell Metab 2009;10:167–77.

39. Smushkin G, Sathananthan M, Piccinini F, et al. The effect of a bile acid sequestrant on glucose metabolism in subjects with type 2 diabetes. Diabetes 2013;62:1094–101.

40. Hofmann AF. Bile acid sequestrants improve glycemic control in type 2 diabetes: a proposed mechanism implicating glucagon-like peptide 1 release. Hepatology 2011;53:1784.

41. Le TA, Chen J, Changchien C, et al. Effect of colesevelam on liver fat quantified by magnetic resonance in nonalcoholic steatohepatitis: a randomized controlled trial. Hepatology 2012;56:922–32.

42. Xiang Z, Chen YP, Ma KF, et al. The role of ursodeoxycholic acid in non-alcoholic steatohepatitis: a systematic review. BMC Gastroenterol 2013;13:140.

43. Safadi R, Konikoff FM, Mahamid M, et al. The fatty acid-bile acid conjugate aramchol reduces liver fat content in patients with nonalcoholic fatty liver disease. Clin Gastroenterol Hepatol 2014;12:2085–91.e1.

44. Mudaliar S, Henry RR, Sanyal AJ, et al. Efficacy and safety of the farnesoid X receptor agonist obeticholic acid in patients with type 2 diabetes and nonalcoholic fatty liver disease. Gastroenterology 2013;145:574–82.

45. Eslami L, Merat S, Malekzadeh R, et al. Statins for non-alcoholic fatty liver disease and non-alcoholic steatohepatitis. Cochrane Database Syst Rev 2013;12:CD008623.

46. Ekstedt M, Franzen LE, Mathiesen UL, et al. Statins in non-alcoholic fatty liver disease and chronically elevated liver enzymes: a histopathological follow-up study. J Hepatol 2007;47:135–41.

47. Charles Z, Pugh E, Barnett D. Ezetimibe for the treatment of primary (heterozygous-familial and non-familial) hyper-cholesterolaemia: NICE technology appraisal guidance. Heart 2008;94:642–3.

48. Takeshita Y, Takamura T, Honda M, et al. The effects of ezetimibe on non-alcoholic fatty liver disease and glucose metabolism: a randomised controlled trial. Diabetologia 2014;57:878–90.

49. Choi CS, Savage DB, Kulkarni A, et al. Suppression of diacylglycerol acyltransferase-2 (DGAT2), but not DGAT1, with antisense oligonucleotides reverses diet-induced hepatic steatosis and insulin resistance. J Biol Chem 2007;282:22678–88.

50. Yamaguchi K, Yang L, McCall S, et al. Inhibiting triglyceride synthesis improves hepatic steatosis but exacerbates liver

damage and fibrosis in obese mice with nonalcoholic steato-hepatitis. Hepatology 2007;45:1366–74.

51. Du J, Ma YY, Yu CH, et al. Effects of pentoxifylline on non-alcoholic fatty liver disease: a meta-analysis. World J Gastroenterol 2014;20:569–77.

52. Kim M, Yang SG, Kim JM, et al. Silymarin suppresses hepatic stellate cell activation in a dietary rat model of non-alcoholic steatohepatitis: analysis of isolated hepatic stellate cells. Int J Mol Med 2012;30:473–9.

53. Solhi H, Ghahremani R, Kazemifar AM, et al. Silymarin in treatment of non-alcoholic steatohepatitis: a randomized clinical trial. Caspian J Intern Med 2014;5:9–12.

54. Dohil R, Schmeltzer S, Cabrera BL, et al. Enteric-coated cysteamine for the treatment of paediatric non-alcoholic fatty liver disease. Aliment Pharmacol Ther 2011;33:1036–44.

55. Wang C, Cui Y, Li C, et al. Nrf2 deletion causes "benign" simple steatosis to develop into nonalcoholic steatohepatitis in mice fed a high-fat diet. Lipids Health Dis 2013;12:165.

56. Shimozono R, Asaoka Y, Yoshizawa Y, et al. Nrf2 activators attenuate the progression of nonalcoholic steatohepatitis-related fibrosis in a dietary rat model. Mol Pharmacol 2013;84:62–70.

57. Kim SG, Kim YM, Choi JY, et al. Oltipraz therapy in patients with liver fibrosis or cirrhosis: a randomized, double-blind, placebo-controlled phase II trial. J Pharm Pharmacol 2011;63:627–35.

# What is the role of antifibrotic therapies in the current and future management of NAFLD?

25

**Natasha McDonald and Jonathan Fallowfield**

MRC/University of Edinburgh Centre for Inflammation Research, Queen's Medical Research Institute, University of Edinburgh, Edinburgh, UK

LEARNING POINTS

- The overall aim of antifibrotic therapy in NAFLD is to prevent or reduce progression to cirrhosis and, therefore, decrease liver-related outcomes and death.

- Currently, there are no effective antifibrotic agents in clinical use. Trials focusing on the use of existing medication and/or vitamin supplementation have been disappointing.

- Clinical trial design in NAFLD faces many challenges such as lack of knowledge of natural history of disease, difficulties with patient selection and non-invasive monitoring of disease progression, as well as defining suitable trial end points.

- Broadly speaking, emerging antifibrotic approaches either target the drivers of NASH or specific components of the fibrotic cascade, and several new agents are being investigated in phase 1 and 2 clinical trials.

- It is possible that integrated approaches, targeting two or more distinct inflammatory/fibrogenic pathways, will be required to combat steatohepatitis and resolve accumulated fibrosis.

Due to obesity epidemic, non-alcoholic fatty liver disease (NAFLD) is becoming the most common cause of chronic liver disease worldwide. The overall goal of antifibrotic therapy is to prevent or reduce progression to cirrhosis and, therefore, decrease liver-related outcomes and death. The most important group to treat are patients with non-alcoholic steatohepatitis (NASH) and significant fibrosis or patients with mild fibrosis and severe NASH phenotype/strong risk factors for fibrosis progression. Despite a large number of human trials over the past two decades, there are no effective antifibrotic agents in current clinical use. In this chapter, we will revise the potential therapeutic targets in liver fibrosis, review the challenges of trial design in NAFLD, summarise the results of antifibrotic trials to date, and look at the most likely future therapeutic candidates in the NAFLD fibrosis field.

## Antifibrotic targets in NAFLD

A number of potential antifibrotic targets have been identified in preclinical studies, and many are now being evaluated in clinical trials (Figure 25.1). In some cases (e.g. PDE4 inhibitors), promising preclinical data have not translated to clinical efficacy, at least in part, because animal models used for proof of concept do not accurately reproduce the pathobiological milieu of human NASH [1]. Broadly, drug approaches either target drivers of NASH (insulin resistance, lipotoxicity and cell injury) or specific components of the fibrotic cascade (hepatic stellate cell (HSC) behaviour and matrix degradation). This distinction is important as different trial designs, study populations and end points will be required depending on the choice of therapeutic target.

*Clinical Dilemmas in Non-Alcoholic Fatty Liver Disease*, First Edition. Edited by Roger Williams and Simon D. Taylor-Robinson.
© 2016 John Wiley & Sons, Ltd. Published 2016 by John Wiley & Sons, Ltd.

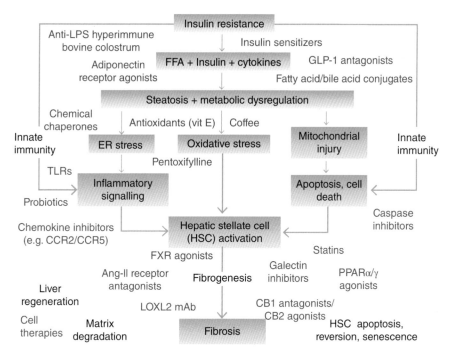

**FIG 25.1** Potential pharmacological targets in NASH. Ang-2, angiotensin 2; CB, cannabinoid receptor; CCR, CC chemokine receptors; ER, endoplasmic reticulum; FFA, free fatty acids; FXR, farnesoid X receptor; GLP, glucagon-like peptide; LOX, lysyl oxidase; LPS, lipopolysaccharide; PPAR, peroxisome proliferator-activated receptor; TLR, toll-like receptor; vit E, vitamin E.

## Challenges of clinical trial design in NAFLD

### Lack of knowledge of natural history of disease

Despite rising prevalence and clinical significance, NAFLD remains a disease that lacks robust natural history data, mainly due to its long and typically asymptomatic course that often begins in adolescence or even childhood. In the absence of non-invasive biomarkers that correlate with disease stage, longitudinal follow-up of patients with liver biopsies is required to assess changes in disease severity and characterisation of disease on a histological and molecular level. Moreover, NAFLD course is not linear with both deterioration and improvement between all categories and severity of disease and lack of the full knowledge of factors that are predictive of disease regression or progression.

### Difficulties with patient selection

In NASH patients, advanced fibrosis (but not grades of steatosis, lobular inflammation or ballooning degeneration) predicts increased risk of liver-related mortality. Lack of non-invasive markers to stratify disease often necessitates liver biopsy to assess NAFLD Activity Score (NAS) prior to trial entry and often on trial exit, with all its associated costs and risks. The often complex past medical and medication history of each NAFLD patient needs to be carefully considered at the trial entry, as these factors may interact with the trial medication or preclude patients from entering into trials. Since a number of gene variants associated with accelerated course of NAFLD (e.g. PNPLA3, TM6SF2) have been identified, future therapeutic trials may need to stratify the patients on enrolment based on their genetic risk profile.

### Difficulties with non-invasive monitoring of disease progression/regression

The need for a non-invasive biomarker or biomarker panel that will align with the histological grade of disease is the most important unmet need in the field of NAFLD. Currently available biochemical tests lack sufficient sensitivity and specificity to gain widespread implementation, and imaging is unable to identify NASH in the setting of NAFLD, as apoptosis, ballooning and cell injury are not detectable by available techniques [2].

Equally, the accurate non-invasive assessment of fibrosis stage remains an elusive target, not least owing to the poor performance of liver biopsy as the gold standard comparison [3]. Elastography techniques have limited ability to discriminate low or intermediate stages of fibrosis, their reproducibility in NAFLD has not been fully verified, and their performance in monitoring longitudinal changes in liver fibrosis in clinical trials has not been evaluated.

Promising results have been obtained with a novel magnetic resonance protocol for liver tissue characterisation, quantifying liver fibrosis, steatosis and siderosis in unselected adult patients requiring liver biopsy as part of their routine care [4]. As a truly quantitative, non-invasive technique, this methodology has the potential for the safe longitudinal assessment and prediction of disease progression and/or response to therapy, and further studies are ongoing.

### The challenge of defining suitable trial end points in NAFLD

The indolent progression of NAFLD, often over decades, poses a major challenge because clinical events are uncommon in non-cirrhotic patients, and none of the existing non-invasive biochemical or imaging tests has been validated to support the 'reasonably likely to predict clinical benefit' standard of a surrogate trial end point. Currently, reduction in NAS combined with either improvement or lack of progression in fibrosis score is the suggested end point for trials of 12–24-month duration.

### What have we learnt from NAFLD antifibrotic trials to date?

To date, interventional trials in NASH have been disappointing. Although lifestyle interventions are recommended in NAFLD, there are very few randomised controlled trials of adequate size to support their efficacy; in particular there is no convincing evidence of histological improvement in fibrosis, and motivation and adherence remain significant barriers [5]. Moreover, there is a relative paucity of published clinical trials in NAFLD where hepatic fibrosis is a primary or secondary end point (summarised in Table 25.1). These trials focused on the use of existing medication and/or vitamin supplementation in the hope that they will beneficially affect liver fibrosis.

### What are the most promising emerging antifibrotic therapies in NAFLD?

Insulin resistance is probably the main driver in NAFLD but also has an important role in the initiation and perpetuation of NASH, including fibrosis progression [25]. However, correcting insulin resistance alone is not sufficient to effectively treat NASH in the majority of patients [26], suggesting the need for a broader hepatoprotective approach, which also targets fibrogenic pathways.

### Obeticholic acid (INT747, 6α-ethyl-chenodeoxycholic acid)

Obeticholic acid (OCA) is a semi-synthetic derivative of the primary human bile acid, chenodeoxycholic acid, the natural agonist of the farnesoid X receptor (FXR), a nuclear hormone receptor involved in the regulation of glucose and lipid metabolism and immune responses. FXR activation in HSCs promotes resolution of fibrosis in animal models [27, 28]. OCA also avidly binds to the TGR5 receptor on L cells of the enterochromaffin system and may exert its beneficial effects via increased production of glucagon-like peptides (GLP) (see in the following text). In a proof of concept phase 2 placebo-controlled study that included type 2 diabetes patients with NAFLD and mild-to-moderate or moderate liver fibrosis, there was a modest but significant reduction in the mean enhanced liver fibrosis (ELF) score in the 25 mg OCA group compared with placebo [29]. Based on the efficacy and safety shown in this study and on the emerging preclinical evidence for potential beneficial effects of OCA in NAFLD/NASH [30], a phase 2b double-blind trial of OCA versus placebo for 72 weeks of treatment in biopsy-proven NASH patients was initiated (FLINT; NCT01265498). In fact, the FLINT study was stopped early for efficacy as primary end point of the trial was met at the interim analysis. In addition, recently published data from animal studies point to the role of OCA in reducing portal pressure [31].

### Dual peroxisome proliferator-activated receptor α/δ agonist (GFT505)

Peroxisome proliferator-activated receptors (PPARs) are nuclear receptors that play key roles in the regulation of metabolic homeostasis, inflammation, cellular growth and differentiation. In the liver, PPAR-α is expressed at high level in hepatocytes and plays a major role in regulating fatty acid transport and β-oxidation and modulating

**TABLE 25.1** Summary of antifibrotic trials in NAFLD

| Treatment | Study design | Phase | Patient population | Number of patients | Results | Reference |
|---|---|---|---|---|---|---|
| *Insulin-sensitising agents* | | | | | | |
| Metformin | 48 wks;ol,nr | – | NAFLD | 15 | No effect on fibrosis | [6] |
| | 48 wks;ol,nr | – | NASH | 28 | No effect on fibrosis | [7] |
| | 6 mo;r,db | – | NAFLD | 48 | No effect | [8] |
| | 12 mo; r, ol | – | NASH and IR | 19 | No effect | [9] |
| | 96 wks;r,db | – | Children aged 8–17; NAFLD | 173 | No effect | [10] |
| Pioglitazone | 6 mo;r,db | 4 | NASH; TIIDM or IR | 55 | No effect | [11] |
| | 12 mo; r,db | – | NASH, non-diabetic | 74 | Decreased fibrosis with Pio (=0.05) | [12] |
| | 96 wks; r,db | 3 | NASH, non-diabetic | 247 | No effect | [13] |
| *Antioxidants/cytoprotectants* | | | | | | |
| Vitamin E | 6 mo;r,db | – | NASH | 49 | No effect | [14] |
| | 2 yr;r,db | | NASH, non-diabetic | 247 | No effect | [13] |
| | 96 wks;r,db | – | Children aged 8–17; NAFLD | 173 | No effect | [10] |
| Pentoxifylline | 1 yr;r,db | 2 | NASH | 55 | No effect on fibrosis but improvement in NAS | [15] |
| | 12 mo;r | | NASH | 30 | No effect | [16] |
| Ursodeoxycholic acid | 2 yrs;r,db | | NASH | 166 | No effect | [17] |
| | 2 yrs;r,db | | NASH | 48 | No effect | [18] |
| | 12 mo;r,db | 3 | NASH | 126 | Reduction in FibroTest score | [19] |
| *Orlistat* | | | | | | |
| Orlistat | 36 wks;r,ol | 4 | NAFLD | 52 | No effect | [20] |
| | 36 wks;r | 4 | NASH | 50 | No effect | [21] |
| *Polyunsaturated fatty acids* | | | | | | |
| Ethyl-eicosapentaenoic acid | 12 mo;r,db | 2b | NASH | 243 | No effect | [22] |
| *Angiotensin receptor blockers* | | | | | | |
| Telmisartan versus losartan | 20 mo;r,db, no placebo | | NASH and hypertension | 54 | Reduced fibrosis in telmisartan arm | [23] |
| Losartan + rosiglitazone | 48 wks;r,db | | NASH | 137 | No additional effect | [24] |

db, double blind; IR, insulin resistance; nr, non-randomised; ol, open label; r, randomised; TIIDM, type 2 diabetes mellitus.

gluconeogenesis and inflammatory responses [32, 33]. Similar to PPAR-α, PPAR-δ also governs hepatic glucose utilisation and lipoprotein metabolism and has an important anti-inflammatory activity in the liver through actions in parenchymal and non-parenchymal cells [34]. GFT505 is a novel PPAR modulator with preferential activity on PPAR-α and concomitant activity on PPAR-δ. In animal models of NASH, treatment with GFT505 resulted in a more favourable lipid profile, reduced expression of pro-inflammatory and pro-fibrotic genes [35]. Although the (modest) hepatic fibrosis in NASH models was not significantly reduced by GFT505, it did show both a prophylactic and therapeutic effect in a rat carbon tetrachloride ($CCl_4$) liver fibrosis model [35]. Following on from these encouraging preclinical studies, a phase 2b trial of GFT505 in biopsy-proven NASH patients is currently ongoing (NCT01694849).

### Anti-LOXL2 monoclonal antibody

Lysyl oxidase (LOX) L2 is an enzyme that promotes cross-linking of fibrillar collagen I, a major component of fibrotic stroma and has been proposed as a potential 'core pathway', being critical for the development of fibrosis in the liver and other tissues. Treatment with a LOXL2-specific monoclonal antibody significantly reduced liver fibrosis and increased survival in a mouse $CCl_4$ model [36]. Two phase 2 placebo-controlled trials are currently evaluating the effect of 96 weeks treatment with simtuzumab (GS-6624, a LOXL2 specific monoclonal antibody) on liver collagen content in the setting of compensated NASH cirrhosis (NCT01672879) and advanced NASH fibrosis (NCT01672866).

### Modulating the gut microbiome

Altered interactions between gut microbiota and the host may exacerbate progression of NAFLD and other metabolic syndrome-associated abnormalities, including glucose intolerance and obesity. In a methionine- and choline-deficient diet-induced mouse model of NASH, administration of VSL#3 (a mixture of eight probiotic strains) reduced the progression of liver fibrosis but without significant attenuation of steatosis or inflammation [37]. Unfortunately, to date, there have been no clinical studies demonstrating the efficacy of probiotic treatment in hepatic fibrosis. A recently published trial of VSL#3 in paediatric NAFLD patients demonstrated a reduction in fatty liver on ultrasound after 4 months of treatment, associated with reduction

in BMI and increase in total and activated plasma GLP-1 levels [38]. A small placebo-controlled trial of the effects of synbiotics (combination of pre- and probiotics) in NASH has been completed, and publication of results is awaited (NCT01791959).

### Adiponectin agonists

Adiponectin is an anti-inflammatory cytokine that reduces body fat, ameliorates insulin resistance and has a hepatoprotective action [39]. Evidence from human studies suggests that, when adjusted for age, gender and BMI, the levels of adiponectin are decreased in NASH compared to chronic viral hepatitis [40]. Moreover, NASH patients have significantly lower adiponectin levels than those with simple steatosis or obese controls without NAFLD [41]. Adiponectin receptors (ARs) are abundantly expressed in HSCs, and a recently published study suggests a novel mechanism for its antifibrotic effect via disruption of focal adhesion complexes, preventing crosstalk between activated HSCs and the extracellular matrix [42]. Although the cost of using synthetic adiponectin in clinical trials would be prohibitive, efforts are under way to utilise small peptides that mimic the effects of adiponectin or to use small-molecule AR agonists [43].

### GLP-1 analogues

Glucagon-like peptide 1 (GLP-1) is an incretin hormone secreted by the L cells of the distal small intestine and proximal colon and is degraded by dipeptidyl peptidase IV (DPPIV) preventing the peptide from stimulating pancreatic insulin secretion following feeding. Therapeutic GLP-1 analogues (liraglutide and exenatide) are resistant to DPPIV enzyme cleavage, whereas DPPIV inhibitors (gliptins) prolong the half-life of endogenous GLP-1. As well as enhancing insulin secretion from β-cells, GLP-1 has an anorectic effect through modulation of brain activity in appetite centres and delays gastric emptying. It is also thought to be directly involved, via binding to hepatocyte GLP-1 receptors, in reducing hepatic free fatty acid and triglyceride stores and thereby directly improving hepatocyte insulin resistance and reducing lipotoxicity, both critical factors in NAFLD progression [44]. Liraglutide efficacy and action in NASH (LEAN) is a phase 2 randomised, double-blind, placebo-controlled trial to assess the effect of 48 weeks treatment on liver histological improvement in obese patients with NASH, with or without type 2 diabetes (NCT01237119).

## Galectin inhibitors

Galectin-3 protein appears to play a crucial role in organ fibrosis as galectin-3 knockout mice are resistant to experimental liver, lung and kidney fibrosis [45–47]. Treatment with galectin inhibitor GR-MD-02 significantly improved NASH activity and markedly reduced fibrosis in a mouse model of NASH [48], and a phase 1 trial of intravenous galectin-3 antagonist is currently recruiting (NCT01899859).

## CC Chemokine receptor 2 and 5 antagonists

CC chemokine receptor (CCR) 2 and CCR5 are expressed on monocytes, macrophages and HSCs, promoting their recruitment and migration during liver injury. CCR2/5 signalling promotes hepatic fibrosis in mouse models [49]. Cenicriviroc is an oral dual CCR2/5 antagonist that showed significant antifibrotic activity in the mouse model of NASH [50], and the phase 2 trial of its safety and efficacy in adult subjects with NASH fibrosis (CENTAUR) has recently opened (NCT02217475).

## Other emerging therapies

Finally, other potential antifibrotic therapies in the early stages of development are worthy of mention. Oral administration of anti-LPS hyperimmune bovine colostrum (Imm124-E) led to improvement in insulin resistance and rise in serum GLP-1 and adiponectin levels in a small open-label study in 10 patients with biopsy-proven NASH [51]. In addition, a phase 1b trial evaluating the effect of blocking glucocorticoid action by inhibition of 11β-hydroxysteroid dehydrogenase type 1 (11β-HSD1), an enzyme highly expressed in the liver, resulted in a reduction in liver fat content measured by MR spectroscopy [52].

In recent years, an important role for the hepatic endocannabinoid system in the pathogenesis of liver disease has been demonstrated in animal and human studies. CB1 receptor antagonism is antifibrotic even at advanced stages of chronic liver injury, through anti-proliferative and pro-apoptotic effects on hepatic myofibroblasts, whereas CB2 receptor agonism leads to reduced inflammation and fibrosis [53, 54]. Rimonabant, a promising CB1 receptor antagonist with anorectic properties, was withdrawn as it increased depression and suicidal tendencies. Research efforts are now focused on the development of peripherally restricted CB1 receptor antagonists (or CB2 receptor agonists) to harness the antifibrotic properties of endocannabinoid signalling without unwanted central effects.

## Conclusions

Due to the growing worldwide epidemic of NAFLD, efforts to explain the underlying causes of NASH fibrosis have taken on a new urgency, yielding a number of promising translational targets. Whilst there currently remains no treatment for NAFLD, short of diet and lifestyle modification, multiple clinical trials of potential anti-inflammatory/antifibrotic agents are ongoing. Interestingly, many novel therapeutic strategies converge on the increased production of GLP-1 as a final regulator of hepatic insulin resistance and fatty acid metabolism. It is quite possible that integrated approaches, targeting two or more distinct inflammatory/fibrogenic pathways, will be required to combat steatohepatitis and resolve accumulated fibrosis.

## Acknowledgement

The authors would like to acknowledge the help of Dr Arun Sanyal in the design of Figure 25.1.

## References

1. Ratziu V, Bedossa P, Francque SM, et al. Lack of efficacy of an inhibitor of PDE4 in phase 1 and 2 trials of patients with nonalcoholic steatohepatitis. Clin Gastroenterol Hepatol 2014; 12(10):1724–30.e5.
2. Castera L, Vilgrain V, Angulo P. Noninvasive evaluation of NAFLD. Nat Rev Gastroenterol Hepatol 2013;10(11):666–75.
3. Ratziu V, Charlotte F, Heurtier A, et al. Sampling variability of liver biopsy in nonalcoholic fatty liver disease. Gastroenterology 2005;128(7):1898–906.
4. Banerjee R, Pavlides M, Tunnicliffe EM, et al. Multiparametric magnetic resonance for the non-invasive diagnosis of liver disease. J Hepatol 2014;60(1):69–77.
5. Promrat K, Kleiner DE, Niemeier HM, et al. Randomized controlled trial testing the effects of weight loss on nonalcoholic steatohepatitis. Hepatology 2010;51(1):121–9.
6. Nair S, Diehl AM, Wiseman M, et al. Metformin in the treatment of non-alcoholic steatohepatitis: a pilot open label trial. Aliment Pharmacol Ther 2004;20(1):23–8.
7. Loomba R, Lutchman G, Kleiner DE, et al. Clinical trial: pilot study of metformin for the treatment of non-alcoholic steatohepatitis. Aliment Pharmacol Ther 2009;29(2):172–82.
8. Haukeland JW, Konopski Z, Eggesbo HB, et al. Metformin in patients with non-alcoholic fatty liver disease: a randomized, controlled trial. Scand J Gastroenterol 2009;44(7):853–60.

9. Shields WW, Thompson KE, Grice GA, et al. The effect of metformin and standard therapy versus standard therapy alone in nondiabetic patients with insulin resistance and nonalcoholic steatohepatitis (NASH): a pilot trial. Therap Adv Gastroenterol 2009;2(3):157–63.

10. Lavine JE, Schwimmer JB, Van Natta ML, et al. Effect of vitamin E or metformin for treatment of nonalcoholic fatty liver disease in children and adolescents: the TONIC randomized controlled trial. JAMA 2011;305(16):1659–68.

11. Belfort R, Harrison SA, Brown K, et al. A placebo-controlled trial of pioglitazone in subjects with nonalcoholic steatohepatitis. N Engl J Med 2006;355(22):2297–307.

12. Aithal GP, Thomas JA, Kaye PV, et al. Randomized, placebo-controlled trial of pioglitazone in nondiabetic subjects with nonalcoholic steatohepatitis. Gastroenterology 2008;135(4): 1176–84.

13. Sanyal AJ, Chalasani N, Kowdley KV, et al. Pioglitazone, vitamin E, or placebo for nonalcoholic steatohepatitis. N Engl J Med 2010;362(18):1675–85.

14. Harrison SA, Torgerson S, Hayashi P, et al. Vitamin E and vitamin C treatment improves fibrosis in patients with nonalcoholic steatohepatitis. Am J Gastroenterol 2003; 98(11):2485–90.

15. Zein CO, Yerian LM, Gogate P, et al. Pentoxifylline improves nonalcoholic steatohepatitis: a randomized placebo-controlled trial. Hepatology 2011;54(5):1610–9.

16. Van Wagner LB, Koppe SW, Brunt EM, et al. Pentoxifylline for the treatment of non-alcoholic steatohepatitis: a randomized controlled trial. Ann Hepatol 2011;10(3):277–86.

17. Lindor KD, Kowdley KV, Heathcote EJ, et al. Ursodeoxycholic acid for treatment of nonalcoholic steatohepatitis: results of a randomized trial. Hepatology 2004;39(3):770–8.

18. Dufour JF, Oneta CM, Gonvers JJ, et al. Randomized placebo-controlled trial of ursodeoxycholic acid with vitamin e in nonalcoholic steatohepatitis. Clin Gastroenterol Hepatol 2006;4(12):1537–43.

19. Ratziu V, de Ledinghen V, Oberti F, et al. A randomized controlled trial of high-dose ursodeoxycholic acid for non-alcoholic steatohepatitis. J Hepatol 2011;54(5):1011–9.

20. Zelber-Sagi S, Kessler A, Brazowsky E, et al. A double-blind randomized placebo-controlled trial of orlistat for the treatment of nonalcoholic fatty liver disease. Clin Gastroenterol Hepatol 2006;4(5):639–44.

21. Harrison SA, Fecht W, Brunt EM, et al. Orlistat for overweight subjects with nonalcoholic steatohepatitis: a randomized, prospective trial. Hepatology 2009;49(1): 80–6.

22. Sanyal AJ, Abdelmalek MF, Suzuki A, et al. No significant effects of ethyl-eicosapentanoic acid on histologic features of nonalcoholic steatohepatitis in a phase 2 trial. Gastroenterology 2014;147(2):377–84.e1.

23. Georgescu EF, Ionescu R, Niculescu M, et al. Angiotensin-receptor blockers as therapy for mild-to-moderate hypertension-associated non-alcoholic steatohepatitis. World J Gastroenterol 2009;15(8):942–54.

24. Torres DM, Jones FJ, Shaw JC, et al. Rosiglitazone versus rosiglitazone and metformin versus rosiglitazone and losartan in the treatment of nonalcoholic steatohepatitis in humans: a 12-month randomized, prospective, open-label trial. Hepatology 2011;54(5):1631–9.

25. Fracanzani AL, Valenti L, Bugianesi E, et al. Risk of severe liver disease in nonalcoholic fatty liver disease with normal aminotransferase levels: a role for insulin resistance and diabetes. Hepatology 2008;48(3):792–8.

26. Ratziu V, Pienar L. Pharmacological therapy for non-alcoholic steatohepatitis: how efficient are thiazolidinediones? Hepatol Res 2011;41(7):687–95.

27. Fiorucci S, Antonelli E, Rizzo G, et al. The nuclear receptor SHP mediates inhibition of hepatic stellate cells by FXR and protects against liver fibrosis. Gastroenterology 2004;127(5):1497–512.

28. Fickert P, Fuchsbichler A, Moustafa T, et al. Farnesoid X receptor critically determines the fibrotic response in mice but is expressed to a low extent in human hepatic stellate cells and periductal myofibroblasts. Am J Pathol 2009;175(6):2392–405.

29. Mudaliar S, Henry RR, Sanyal AJ, et al. Efficacy and safety of the farnesoid X receptor agonist obeticholic acid in patients with type 2 diabetes and nonalcoholic fatty liver disease. Gastroenterology 2013;145(3):574–82.e1.

30. Adorini L, Pruzanski M, Shapiro D. Farnesoid X receptor targeting to treat nonalcoholic steatohepatitis. Drug Discov Today 2012;17(17–18):988–97.

31. Mookerjee RP, Mehta G, Balasubramaniyan V, et al. Hepatic dimethylarginine-dimethylaminohydrolase1 is reduced in cirrhosis and is a target for therapy in portal hypertension. J Hepatol 2015;62:325–31.

32. Lefebvre P, Chinetti G, Fruchart JC, et al. Sorting out the roles of PPAR alpha in energy metabolism and vascular homeostasis. J Clin Invest 2006;116(3):571–80.

33. Zambon A, Gervois P, Pauletto P, et al. Modulation of hepatic inflammatory risk markers of cardiovascular diseases by PPAR-alpha activators: clinical and experimental evidence. Arterioscler Thromb Vasc Biol 2006;26(5): 977–86.

34. Odegaard JI, Ricardo-Gonzalez RR, Red Eagle A, et al. Alternative M2 activation of Kupffer cells by PPARdelta ameliorates obesity-induced insulin resistance. Cell Metab 2008;7(6):496–507.

35. Staels B, Rubenstrunk A, Noel B, et al. Hepatoprotective effects of the dual peroxisome proliferator-activated receptor alpha/delta agonist, GFT505, in rodent models of

nonalcoholic fatty liver disease/nonalcoholic steatohepatitis. Hepatology 2013;58(6):1941–52.

36. Barry-Hamilton V, Spangler R, Marshall D, et al. Allosteric inhibition of lysyl oxidase-like-2 impedes the development of a pathologic microenvironment. Nat Med 2010;16(9): 1009–17.

37. Velayudham A, Dolganiuc A, Ellis M, et al. VSL#3 probiotic treatment attenuates fibrosis without changes in steatohepatitis in a diet-induced nonalcoholic steatohepatitis model in mice. Hepatology 2009;49(3):989–97.

38. Alisi A, Bedogni G, Baviera G, et al. Randomised clinical trial: the beneficial effects of VSL#3 in obese children with non-alcoholic steatohepatitis. Aliment Pharmacol Ther 2014;39(11):1276–85.

39. Tsochatzis E, Papatheodoridis GV, Archimandritis AJ. The evolving role of leptin and adiponectin in chronic liver diseases. Am J Gastroenterol 2006;101(11):2629–40.

40. Tsochatzis E, Papatheodoridis GV, Hadziyannis E, et al. Serum adipokine levels in chronic liver diseases: association of resistin levels with fibrosis severity. Scand J Gastroenterol 2008;43(9):1128–36.

41. Jarrar MH, Baranova A, Collantes R, et al. Adipokines and cytokines in non-alcoholic fatty liver disease. Aliment Pharmacol Ther 2008;27(5):412–21.

42. Kumar P, Smith T, Rahman K, et al. Adiponectin modulates focal adhesion disassembly in activated hepatic stellate cells: implication for reversing hepatic fibrosis. FASEB J 2014;28(12):5172–83.

43. Okada-Iwabu M, Yamauchi T, Iwabu M, et al. A small-molecule AdipoR agonist for type 2 diabetes and short life in obesity. Nature 2013;503(7477):493–9.

44. Mells JE, Anania FA. The role of gastrointestinal hormones in hepatic lipid metabolism. Semin Liver Dis 2013;33(4): 343–57.

45. Henderson NC, Mackinnon AC, Farnworth SL, et al. Galectin-3 expression and secretion links macrophages to the promotion of renal fibrosis. Am J Pathol 2008;172(2):288–98.

46. Henderson NC, Mackinnon AC, Farnworth SL, et al. Galectin-3 regulates myofibroblast activation and hepatic fibrosis. Proc Natl Acad Sci U S A 2006;103(13):5060–5.

47. Mackinnon AC, Gibbons MA, Farnworth SL, et al. Regulation of transforming growth factor-beta1-driven lung fibrosis by galectin-3. Am J Respir Crit Care Med 2012; 185(5):537–46.

48. Traber PG, Zomer E. Therapy of experimental NASH and fibrosis with galectin inhibitors. PLoS One 2013; 8(12):e83481.

49. Seki E, de Minicis S, Inokuchi S, et al. CCR2 promotes hepatic fibrosis in mice. Hepatology 2009;50(1):185–97.

50. Oral Presentations. Hepatology 2013;58(S1):36A–91A. doi:10.1002/hep.2672.

51. Mizrahi M, Shabat Y, Ben Ya'acov A, et al. Alleviation of insulin resistance and liver damage by oral administration of Imm124-E is mediated by increased Tregs and associated with increased serum GLP-1 and adiponectin: results of a phase I/II clinical trial in NASH. J Inflamm Res 2012;5:141–50.

52. Stefan N, Ramsauer M, Jordan P, et al. Inhibition of 11beta-HSD1 with RO5093151 for non-alcoholic fatty liver disease: a multicentre, randomised, double-blind, placebo-controlled trial. Lancet Diabetes Endocrinol 2014;2(5):406–16.

53. Teixeira-Clerc F, Julien B, Grenard P, et al. CB1 cannabinoid receptor antagonism: a new strategy for the treatment of liver fibrosis. Nat Med 2006;12(6):671–6.

54. Giannone FA, Baldassarre M, Domenicali M, et al. Reversal of liver fibrosis by the antagonism of endocannabinoid CB1 receptor in a rat model of CCl(4)-induced advanced cirrhosis. Lab Invest 2012;92(3):384–95.

# 26 Developmental programming of non-alcoholic fatty liver disease

**Jiawei Li[1], Paul Cordero[1], and Jude A. Oben[1,2]**

[1] Institute for Liver and Digestive Health, University College London, London, UK
[2] Department of Gastroenterology and Hepatology, Guy's and St Thomas' Hospital, NHS Foundation Trust, London, UK

## LEARNING POINTS

- Developmental programming theory states that nutritional and environmental stimuli during a plastic period of development, such as the perinatal period, may lead to physiological and metabolic changes in descendants, increasing their risk of developing certain diseases later in life.

- There is strong evidence from human studies that maternal obesity predisposes offspring to increased body weight and fat deposition leading to the development of non-alcoholic fatty liver disease (NAFLD).

- Similarly, dietary interventions in animal models have also demonstrated that maternal obesity and perinatal obesogenic diet program the offspring for NAFLD.

- The mechanisms of developmental programming of NAFLD may involve modifications of molecular mechanisms orchestrated by epigenetic modifications of DNA. Recent findings also suggest a role of the innate immune system in the developmental programming of NAFLD.

The early developmental phase is a plastic period in which many factors such as the nutritional milieu and environmental stimuli affect the descendants. During this critical period, permanent structural and physiological changes take place, which can impact on offspring metabolic outcomes and risks of developing diseases later in life [1], a phenomenon termed 'developmental programming'. This concept, also known as Barker's hypothesis, originated from observations by the British epidemiologist David Barker who found that low birth weight in infants is closely associated with higher risks of cardiovascular disease in later life [2]. Barker et al. further proposed the 'thrifty phenotype hypothesis', with the core idea that epigenetic alterations might take place during development as a survival mechanism. The disease condition that develops later in life is due to a mismatch between *in utero* and *ex utero* conditions [3, 4]. Furthermore, cellular differentiation takes place early in fetal development in support of the concept of developmental programming [5].

Non-alcoholic fatty liver disease (NAFLD) is essentially the main hepatic manifestation of the metabolic syndrome, characterised by hepatic steatosis, hepatic inflammation and liver fibrosis and in some cases, hepatocellular carcinoma [6]. The underlying pathogenesis is uncertain, although it is known that obesity and insulin resistance have major roles. The 'two-hit hypothesis' suggests that manifestation of NAFLD involves two stages. The first hit is due to fat deposition in the liver induced by obesity and insulin resistance making the liver vulnerable to a second hit involving endoplasmic reticulum (ER) stress, reactive oxygen species (ROS) or cytokine responses [7–9]. Recently, the idea has expanded to multiple hits suggesting that the pathogenesis might also involve mitochondrial dysfunction, inflammation and gut microbiota [10]. Stewart et al. have suggested that the first hit of NAFLD might start as early as *in utero* with excess lipid availability to the embryo leading to a lipotoxic environment and increased oxidative stress [11]. Furthermore, clinical cases of NAFLD in children suggest that the pathogenesis of NAFLD might indeed have an intrauterine origin [12].

## Human studies

Maternal obesity has been shown to alter gestation metabolism and promote placental abnormalities [13]. A positive correlation between maternal BMI and offspring adiposity has also been demonstrated [14] such that offspring exposed to maternal obesity have high lipid accumulation in arterial walls, insulin resistance and glucose dysmetabolism. Maternal weight reduction prior to offspring birth significantly reduced the risk factors for metabolic disease. This study focused on pre-pregnancy weight reduction in obese women with a previous child showed that after weight loss during the second pregnancy, weight-related parameters and metabolic risks of obesity in the second child were reduced compared to those in the first child [15]. Evidence from magnetic resonance imaging technique has moreover shown an association between maternal body mass index and hepatic lipid profile in infants [16]. Further evidence from a retrospective autopsy study in stillborn offspring from diabetic mothers drew a link between maternal programming and NAFLD [17]. Steatosis was found to be isolated to the liver, suggesting a preferential deposition in the liver at the embryonic stage.

## Animal models

### Rodent

Due to the ethical dilemma of interventional studies in humans during the perinatal periods, rodent models of perinatal programming has been the most used approach in this field. Furthermore, the short rodent lifetime allows the study of perinatal programming effects later in life and also becomes a useful tool for transgenerational studies.

A study from White et al. showed that offspring of obese mice had higher weight, hyperleptinaemia and insulin resistance [18]. A further study also showed that exposure to maternal obesity during the gestation period increased the risk of obesity in offspring [19]. As obesity and insulin resistance are closely associated with NAFLD, it is logical therefore to propose that maternal obesity might also predispose offspring to NAFLD.

A role for maternal obesity in offspring liver phenotype was first observed by Guo et al. They described that rats whose mother were subjected to a high-fat (HF) diet during gestation and lactation exhibited higher insulin/ glucose ratio, body fat mass and liver weight at weaning [20]. The subsequent study by Oben et al. explored the long-term effects of maternal obesity on offspring liver phenotype, the relative importance of the intra- and extrauterine periods and the mechanisms therein. This study demonstrated that the intrauterine period and the immediate post-partum periods influenced offspring behaviour into adulthood, and the liver phenotypes were further exacerbated by an obesogenic diet post-weaning [21]. These findings were confirmed in a similar experimental set up by Bouanane et al. [22]. A cross-fostering technique suggested that although the gestation period has a role in offspring metabolic profile, the lactation period might have a more important role in programming of the offspring [21]. A separate study by Bayol et al. also agrees that the lactation period might be predominant in programming the offspring [23]. Finally, the importance of maternal feeding during lactation has been highlighted in a recent study in which maternal obesogenic intake during this period accelerated early offspring weight gain and liver fat accumulation [24].

## Non-human primates

Non-human primate models of perinatal programming are the closest animal models for comparison with humans. A study in a Japanese rhesus macaque model demonstrated that the insulin profile of the mothers also has a role in offspring programming, independent of maternal obesity. Furthermore the altered lipogenic profile was irreversible despite the subjects being weaned onto a healthy diet, suggesting a long-lasting effect of programming [25].

## Cellular and subcellular mechanisms

Previous studies have observed that the breast milk of obese dams contains elevated amounts of leptin, which may act on the neonatal hypothalamic appetite centres to engender a leptin-resistant state in adulthood such that the offspring phenotype might be programmed via the leptin axis. This is consistent with the cross-fostering data that lactation appears to be a most critical period in developmental programming [21].

Developmental programming might also be mediated via mitochondrial-related mechanisms. It is known that mitochondrial inheritance is maternally transmitted [26]. Mitochondrial electron transport chain has been shown to be altered by maternal HF feeding in a rodent model, in which offspring showed NAFLD progression in parallel to an up-regulation of hepatic lipogenesis [27]. Similarly, altered mitochondrial function was observed in maternal over feeding-induced NAFLD offspring. In a study by Alfaradhi et al., subjecting rodents to maternal obesity led to increased activities in mitochondrial complex I and II, accompanied by reduced hepatic cytochrome c levels [28]. Additionally, maternal obesity altered the mitochondrial membrane potential, the levels of oxidative phosphorylation and the function of oocytes [29]. Offspring of obese rats also showed a reduction in mitochondrial protein content, electron transport chain effectors and hepatic sirtuins [30], with SIRT3 being localised in mitochondria and responsible for fatty acid oxidation.

## Nervous system

Maternal HF diet can also alter neural circuitry in the offspring, leading to hyperphagia and a preference for HF food [31]. An involvement of sympathetic nervous system (SNS) in liver regeneration by hepatic progenitor cells has been suggested by Oben et al. [32] and Soeda et al. [33]. The development of portal innervations occurs *in utero*, whereas the parenchymal innervation and maturity of liver occur after birth. In a non-human primate model, it has been shown that exposure to a maternal HF diet reduced SNS innervation to the liver and was accompanied by an increased hepatic apoptosis [34].

## Epigenetic mechanism

The term epigenetics refers to changes in the transcription of the genetic information contained in the DNA sequence without changes in the nucleotide sequence [35]. Epigenetic changes involve gene expression regulation predominantly through DNA methylation, histone amino acid tails modification and reactions mediated by microRNA. It has been proposed that epigenetic profile is established in early development and that maternal nutrition plays an important role in offspring epigenetic profile [36]. There is evidence that maternal HF diet can influence the modification of histone in the fetal liver [37]. In a rodent model where the offspring were subjected to a maternal HF diet during their gestation and lactation, NAFLD was associated with an up-regulation of genes related to lipogenesis, such as Fas, Instig, LXRα, Pgc1α or Pparα, accompanied by changes in hepatic

DNA methylation [38]. Similar findings were also demonstrated by Dudley et al. [39]. Other studies focusing on the lactating period and NAFLD development have described the importance of maternal diet composition in both macro- and micronutrients during the period of liver fat accumulation, plasma cardiovascular risk markers and DNA methylation programming in offspring [24] (Figure 26.1).

In a primate model of HF diet during pregnancy, the offspring at birth showed increased deposition of triglyceride in the liver associated with increased acetylation of histone H3 gene [42]. Chen et al. have further described how in rats restriction of methyl donors in maternal diets during gestation and lactation in offspring leads to modifications of DNA methylation in the promoter regions of 1 032 genes out of 14 981. These genes are mainly involved in glucose and lipid metabolism, ER stress, mitochondrial function and NAFLD [43]. According to other epigenetic marks, namely, microRNAs, seem also to play an important role in liver development and programming during the perinatal period. A maternal HF dietary consumption has been shown to affect offspring hepatic lipid metabolism and microRNA density cellular pattern [44, 45].

## Immune mechanism

The liver is a major organ in immunity, housing resident macrophages known as Kupffer cells (KC), which expresses Toll-like receptors (TLRs) on their surface. The pathogenesis of NAFLD that has been proposed might involve the activation of TLRs and as a result the production of cytokines and chemokines involved in liver inflammation and fibrosis [46]. Involvement of the innate immune system in the developmental programming of NAFLD phenotype was shown by Mouralidarane et al. who demonstrated in rodents that offspring subjected to maternal obesity had an increase in the number of KC, with increased production of ROS but paradoxically with impaired phagocytic ability [47]. Additionally, natural killer cells were reduced in offspring born to obese mothers [47].

## Gut microbiota

Obese individuals have been found to have a reduction in the relative proportion of Bacteroidetes by comparison with lean people, and the proportion increases with weight loss on two types of low-calorie diet [48]. There is also evidence that in neonates the microbiota community is

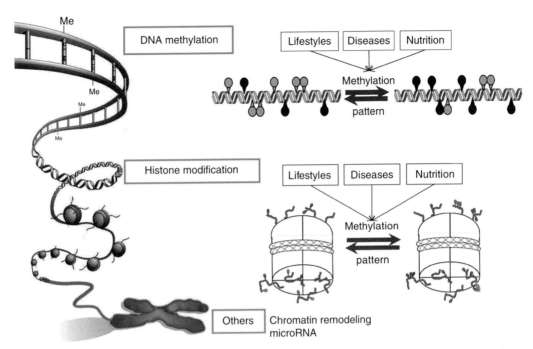

**FIG 26.1** The main epigenetic reactions are the methylation of CpG sites and the modifications on amino acidic tails of histones such as by methylation, acetylation or phosphorylation. These reactions could be influenced by factors such as lifestyles, diseases and diet, and the final conformation of DNA could facilitate joining of the transcription factors (*Source*: (left) Qiu [40], reproduced with permission of Nature Publishing Group and (right) Cordero et al. [41]). (*See insert for color representation of the figure.*)

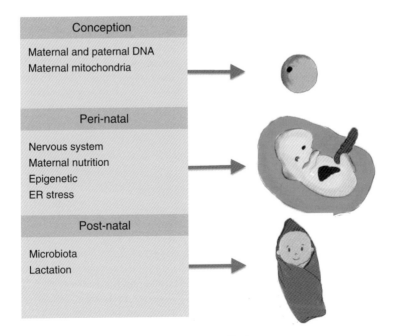

**FIG 26.2** Factors that might impact on the development of NAFLD in offspring.

different depending on the mode of delivery, with vaginal-delivered babies having microbiota resembling the microbiota of the mother's vagina and caesarean section-delivered babies resembling the microbiota of the mother's skin [49]. During childhood the microbiota change and gradually resemble the pattern observed in their mothers [50], suggesting maternal inheritance and programming. However, the role of maternal direction of offspring microbiota on the development of NAFLD is currently uncertain.

## Conclusions

In conclusion, there is emerging evidence of an interplay between the intrauterine environment, the postnatal diet and the development of NAFLD. However, the exact underlying mechanisms are unclear. There is also evidence that the innate immune system and the gut microbiota, perhaps through epigenetic mechanisms, may be implicated in the developmental programming of NAFLD. A summary of the factors that might contribute to the programming effect is depicted in Figure 26.2.

## References

1. Alfaradhi, M.Z. and S.E. Ozanne, Developmental programming in response to maternal overnutrition. Front Genet, 2011. 2: p. 27.
2. Barker, D.J. and C. Osmond, Infant mortality, childhood nutrition, and ischaemic heart disease in England and Wales. Lancet, 1986. 1(8489): p. 1077–81.
3. Hales, C.N., et al., Fetal and infant growth and impaired glucose tolerance at age 64. BMJ, 1991. 303(6809): p. 1019–22.
4. Armitage, J.A., et al., Developmental programming of the metabolic syndrome by maternal nutritional imbalance: how strong is the evidence from experimental models in mammals? J Physiol, 2004. 561(Pt 2): p. 355–77.
5. Wells, J.C., The thrifty phenotype: an adaptation in growth or metabolism? Am J Hum Biol, 2011. 23(1): p. 65–75.
6. Bugianesi, E., et al., Expanding the natural history of non-alcoholic steatohepatitis: from cryptogenic cirrhosis to hepatocellular carcinoma. Gastroenterology, 2002. 123(1): p. 134–40.
7. Day, C.P. and O.F. James, Steatohepatitis: a tale of two "hits"? Gastroenterology, 1998. 114(4): p. 842–5.
8. Lake, A.D., et al., The adaptive endoplasmic reticulum stress response to lipotoxicity in progressive human nonalcoholic fatty liver disease. Toxicol Sci, 2014. 137(1): p. 26–35.
9. Ma, K.L., et al., Inflammatory stress exacerbates lipid accumulation in hepatic cells and fatty livers of apolipoprotein E knockout mice. Hepatology, 2008. 48(3): p. 770–81.
10. Tilg, H. and Moschen A.R., Evolution of inflammation in nonalcoholic fatty liver disease: the multiple parallel hits hypothesis. Hepatology, 2010. 52(5): p. 1836–46.
11. Stewart, M.S., M.J. Heerwagen, and J.E. Friedman, Developmental programming of pediatric nonalcoholic fatty liver disease: redefining the "first hit". Clin Obstet Gynecol, 2013. 56(3): p. 577–90.
12. Alisi, A., et al., Non-alcoholic fatty liver disease and metabolic syndrome in adolescents: pathogenetic role of genetic background and intrauterine environment. Ann Med, 2012. 44(1): p. 29–40.
13. King, J.C., Maternal obesity, metabolism, and pregnancy outcomes. Annu Rev Nutr, 2006. 26: p. 271–91.
14. Reynolds, R.M., et al., Elevated fasting plasma cortisol is associated with ischemic heart disease and its risk factors in people with type 2 diabetes: the Edinburgh type 2 diabetes study. J Clin Endocrinol Metab, 2010. 95(4): p. 1602–8.
15. Smith, J., et al., Effects of maternal surgical weight loss in mothers on intergenerational transmission of obesity. J Clin Endocrinol Metab, 2009. 94(11): p. 4275–83.
16. Brumbaugh, D.E., et al., Intrahepatic fat is increased in the neonatal offspring of obese women with gestational diabetes. J Pediatr, 2013. 162(5): p. 930–6.e1.
17. Patel, K.R., F.V. White, and G.H. Deutsch, Hepatic steatosis is prevalent in stillborns delivered to women with diabetes. J Pediatr Gastroenterol Nutr, 2015;60:152–8.
18. White, C.L., M.N. Purpera, and C.D. Morrison, Maternal obesity is necessary for programming effect of high-fat diet on offspring. Am J Physiol Regul Integr Comp Physiol, 2009. 296(5): p. R1464–72.
19. Shankar, K., et al., Maternal obesity at conception programs obesity in the offspring. Am J Physiol Regul Integr Comp Physiol, 2008. 294(2): p. R528–38.
20. Guo, F. and K.L. Jen, High-fat feeding during pregnancy and lactation affects offspring metabolism in rats. Physiol Behav, 1995. 57(4): p. 681–6.
21. Oben, J.A., et al., Maternal obesity during pregnancy and lactation programs the development of offspring non-alcoholic fatty liver disease in mice. J Hepatol, 2010. 52(6): p. 913–20.
22. Bouanane, S., et al., Hepatic and very low-density lipoprotein fatty acids in obese offspring of overfed dams. Metabolism, 2010. 59(12): p. 1701–9.
23. Bayol, S.A., et al., A maternal "junk food" diet in pregnancy and lactation promotes nonalcoholic Fatty liver disease in rat offspring. Endocrinology, 2010. 151(4): p. 1451–61.
24. Cordero, P., et al., Maternal methyl donors supplementation during lactation prevents the hyperhomocysteinemia induced by a high-fat-sucrose intake by dams. Int J Mol Sci, 2013. 14(12): p. 24422–37.

25. Thorn, S.R., et al., Early life exposure to maternal insulin resistance has persistent effects on hepatic NAFLD in juvenile nonhuman primates. Diabetes, 2014. 63(8): p. 2702–13.

26. Camus, M.F., D.J. Clancy, and D.K. Dowling, Mitochondria, maternal inheritance, and male aging. Curr Biol, 2012. 22(18): p. 1717–21.

27. Bruce, K.D., et al., Maternal high-fat feeding primes steatohepatitis in adult mice offspring, involving mitochondrial dysfunction and altered lipogenesis gene expression. Hepatology, 2009. 50(6): p. 1796–808.

28. Alfaradhi, M.Z., et al., Oxidative stress and altered lipid homeostasis in the programming of offspring fatty liver by maternal obesity. Am J Physiol Regul Integr Comp Physiol, 2014. 307(1): p. R26–34.

29. Igosheva, N., et al., Maternal diet-induced obesity alters mitochondrial activity and redox status in mouse oocytes and zygotes. PLoS One, 2010. 5(4): p. e10074.

30. Borengasser, S.J., et al., Maternal obesity during gestation impairs fatty acid oxidation and mitochondrial SIRT3 expression in rat offspring at weaning. PLoS One, 2011. 6(8): p. e24068.

31. Sullivan, E.L., M.S. Smith, and K.L. Grove, Perinatal exposure to high-fat diet programs energy balance, metabolism and behavior in adulthood. Neuroendocrinology, 2011. 93(1): p. 1–8.

32. Oben, J.A., et al., Sympathetic nervous system inhibition increases hepatic progenitors and reduces liver injury. Hepatology, 2003. 38(3): p. 664–73.

33. Soeda, J., et al., The β-adrenoceptor agonist isoproterenol rescues acetaminophen-injured livers through increasing progenitor numbers by Wnt in mice. Hepatology, 2014. 60(3): p. 1023–34.

34. Grant, W.F., et al., Perinatal exposure to a high-fat diet is associated with reduced hepatic sympathetic innervation in one-year old male Japanese macaques. PLoS One, 2012. 7(10): p. e48119.

35. Bird, A., Perceptions of epigenetics. Nature, 2007. 447(7143): p. 396–8.

36. Waterland, R.A. and R.L. Jirtle, Early nutrition, epigenetic changes at transposons and imprinted genes, and enhanced susceptibility to adult chronic diseases. Nutrition, 2004. 20(1): p. 63–8.

37. Suter, M.A., et al., A maternal high-fat diet modulates fetal SIRT1 histone and protein deacetylase activity in nonhuman primates. FASEB J, 2012. 26(12): p. 5106–14.

38. Pruis, M.G., et al., Maternal western diet primes non-alcoholic fatty liver disease in adult mouse offspring. Acta Physiol (Oxf), 2014. 210(1): p. 215–27.

39. Dudley, K.J., et al., Offspring of mothers fed a high fat diet display hepatic cell cycle inhibition and associated changes in gene expression and DNA methylation. PLoS One, 2011. 6(7): p. e21662.

40. Qiu, J. Epigenetics: unfinished symphony. Nature, 2006. 441: p. 143–5.

41. Cordero, P., et al., [Nutritional epigenetics: a key piece in the obesity puzzle] (Spanish). Rev Esp Obes, 2010. 8(1): p. 10–20.

42. Aagaard-Tillery, K.M., et al., Developmental origins of disease and determinants of chromatin structure: maternal diet modifies the primate fetal epigenome. J Mol Endocrinol, 2008. 41(2): p. 91–102.

43. Chen, G., et al., Identification of master genes involved in liver key functions through transcriptomics and epigenomics of methyl donor deficiency in rat: relevance to non-alcoholic liver disease. Mol Nutr Food Res, 2015;59: p. 293–302.

44. Zhang, J., et al., Maternal high fat diet during pregnancy and lactation alters hepatic expression of insulin like growth factor-2 and key microRNAs in the adult offspring. BMC Genomics, 2009. 10: p. 478.

45. Benatti, R.O., et al., Maternal high-fat diet consumption modulates hepatic lipid metabolism and microRNA-122 (miR-122) and microRNA-370 (miR-370) expression in offspring. Br J Nutr, 2014. 111(12): p. 2112–22.

46. Farrell, G.C., et al., NASH is an inflammatory disorder: pathogenic, prognostic and therapeutic implications. Gut Liver, 2012. 6(2): p. 149–71.

47. Mouralidarane, A., et al., Maternal obesity programs offspring nonalcoholic fatty liver disease by innate immune dysfunction in mice. Hepatology, 2013. 58(1): p. 128–38.

48. Ley, R.E., et al., Microbial ecology: human gut microbes associated with obesity. Nature, 2006. 444(7122): p. 1022–3.

49. Dominguez-Bello, M.G., et al., Delivery mode shapes the acquisition and structure of the initial microbiota across multiple body habitats in newborns. Proc Natl Acad Sci U S A, 2010. 107(26): p. 11971–5.

50. Palmer, C., et al., Development of the human infant intestinal microbiota. PLoS Biol, 2007. 5(7): p. e177.

# Index

Page numbers in *italics* refer to illustrations; those in **bold** refer to tables